Know

Guide
tution
ves

t

Civetta Press
PO Box 1043
Portland, OR 97207-1043

Published by:

Civetta Press
PO Box 1043
Portland, Oregon 97207-1043
(503) 228-6649

Library of Congress Catalog Card Number:
2004113492

ISBN:0-9623318-3-X

Printed and bound in the United States of America

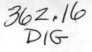

Dedication

To each one of us who will need care as we age.

Who will take care of us?

Acknowledgments

Special thanks to Dick and Mary Lutz of Dimi Press for their expertise in the production of this book. And, to Bruce DeRoos for his artistic talents in designing the book cover.

Contents

Why I Wrote This Book and Who It's For

*My Sixteen Years of Caregiving *My Mother's Brain
Cancer Recovery *My Mother's Head Injury and Coma
*Overview: Inadequate Hospital Care; The Feeding Tube;
Ignorance of Hospital Discharge Staff About Nursing
Homes and Alternatives; Inadequacies of Nursing
Homes; Who Really Needs Nursing Homes?; The Fallacy
of 24-Hour Nursing Care at Nursing Homes; How Com-
plaints are Handled by Nursing Home Staff; Avoidance
of Treating Patients at Nursing Homes; Right-to-Life
Issues; *Why This Book Is for Everyone

Selecting a Nursing Home

*How to Judge a Nursing Home: Beware of Government
Ratings/Beware of Referrals from Other Families *Rehab
vs. Long-Term Care Facilities *Corporate Nursing Homes
*Non-Profit Nursing Homes *Visiting a Nursing Home
*Skilled vs. Intermediate Units/Staff-to-Patient Ratios
*Nursing Home Management *Private vs. Shared Rooms
*Other Costs *Waiting Lists to Enter *Dumping Patients
*Checklist of Other Things to Consider

The Feeding Tube Fiasco

*To Feed Or Not To Feed By Mouth *Letter to The Doctor About Speech Therapy *Letter to The Doctor About Recreational Feeding Ban *The Double Standard For Feeding Patients By Mouth *Things to Consider About Swallowing *Feeding Tube Dangers *Other Feeding Tube Problems and Dangers *Recreational Feeding Suggestions *Postscript

Alternatives to Nursing Homes

*Beginning Your Search *Adult Day Care *Checklist For Adult Day Care *Assisted Living Facilities *Taking Your Elder Home & Hiring Private Caregivers *Checklists For Identifying Your Elder's Needs For Home Care *Hiring Home Help Through An Agency *Checklist of Typical Agency Tasks Performed *Checklists of Questions and Comments For Agency Management *Foster Home Care *Checklists of Questions to Ask Foster Home Owners *Residential Care Facilities *Hospice

You Can Care For The Bedridden

*Getting Started *Keeping Your Elder Clean: Sponge Baths *Incontinent Care and Repositioning Your Elder In Bed *Bowel Care *Respiratory Problems *Bandaging Sores and Tumors *Physical Maintenance: using the hoyer lift; Range of Motion Exercises; Massage; Physical Therapy; Splints *Nutrition *Medications *Miscellaneous

Care and Troubleshooting *Laundry and Linens *Sample Schedule of Care For The Bedridden *Supplies: regular and specialized health products; household products; clothing and linen; foods; appliances *Keeping Yourself In Good Health As a Caregiver

Stimulation For The Elderly Person

*Stimulating Your Elder's Communication *Sensory Stimulation

Long-Term Care Insurance

*To Have Or Not To Have *Types of Coverage *What To Do Without Long-Term Care Insurance

How Family Members Can Cope With Illness and Death

*Ways For Caregivers to Find Strength *Coping With The Negative Attitudes of Others *Dealing With Fears and Stress *Dealing With Death *Planning For Your Future After Your Elder's Death

Where Do We Go From Here?

*The Nursing Home Dilemma *The "Reinvention" of Nursing Homes *The Flawed Healthcare System In

General *How Society Regards Elders *Preparing For Our Care

Organizations Offering Information About Care Options For The Elderly and Help For Caregivers.

General Healthcare and Legal Terminology
Nursing Abbreviations

Warning-Disclaimer

This book contains information and opinions to aid in caring for loved ones and assisting in making healthcare, financial, and legal decisions on their behalf. The author isn't a healthcare, financial, or legal professional.

The author and Civetta Press shall have neither liability nor responsibility to any person or entity with respect to any loss or damage caused, or alleged to have been caused, directly or indirectly, by the information and opinions in this book. Every effort has been made to make the information as complete and accurate as possible. However, there may be errors. Readers should always consult their healthcare providers and seek professional financial and legal advice in making individual healthcare and related financial and legal decisions.

If you don't wish to be bound by the above, you may return this book to the publisher for a full refund.

Throughout this book, I haven't identified any nursing home facilities. I have also substituted fictitious names in the sample letters that I wrote to healthcare personnel.

In this book, many references are made to a hoyer lift. "Hoyer" is a trademark. Many references are also made to "Toothette." It is also a trademark.

Charlotte Digregorio

Introduction

Why I Wrote This Book and Who It's For

This book is one that I never thought I'd write. I'm a professional writer, and I always have titles in mind that I sooner or later get around to writing. However, I never thought I'd write this book, because I never thought I would ever put my mother in a nursing home, and certainly not for four years and five months. She was 76 years old at the time she entered her first nursing home and she stayed at three, before I took her home to care for her, for what turned out to be the final eight months of her life. I was no stranger to caregiving, however, as I had cared for her in the home for nearly ten and one-half years before she entered a nursing home.

This book is an exhaustive work, and an authoritative, eyewitness work on nursing homes, based on observation and interaction with all staff members, some of whom became friends over this lengthy period of time. Although I'd cared for my mother for more than a decade before she entered a nursing home, ironically, the caregiving I performed became more extensive once she reached the nursing home. I literally lived at three nursing homes with her, doing the majority of her care, fourteen hours a day, seven days a week during that four year and five month period. This is the irony of the situation. One pays thousands of dollars each month for care at a nursing home. One believes that it will provide specialized care that an adult child can't in her own home, when in fact, minimal care is performed, and it is in the form of custodial and not nursing care. In particular, family members who have bedridden parents at nursing homes end up picking up the slack or doing virtually all the care themselves.

Since there are growing care alternatives for the elderly these days, there is often no need for an elderly person to even go to a nursing home unless she/he is bedridden. However, nursing homes, due to extremely low staffing, are not set up to care for precisely the type of patients they were meant to care for — those that need nursing care. This book will drive home this point.

Let me give you some background on how my mother ended up at a nursing home. At the age of 33, I moved back home, after living two thousand miles away, to care for my mother. When she was in her 50s, she had breast cancer that was misdiagnosed for two or three years. Normally, a patient wouldn't have survived so long a period of misdiagnosis. However, since my mother had a slow-growing cancer, she survived. After a radical mastectomy on her right side, (lymph glands removed, too), she left the hospital and never returned until eight years and eight months later when it was discovered that her breast cancer had spread to the brain. (The brain cancer had been undetected for years. My mother had strange symptoms that none of her doctors understood, such as squinting/twitching eyes. After her brain cancer became evident due to a seizure and tests performed, in hindsight, an eye specialist at a medical school determined that her eye problems were most likely caused by the brain tumor. She was 65 at the time her brain cancer was discovered.)

With the brain cancer, she was not expected to live, as the disease is almost always fatal. Miraculously, she recovered. She had surgery, was temporarily paralyzed for six weeks on her right side, had five weeks of radiation, and returned home for nearly ten and one-half years. Though she wasn't expected to recover from the brain cancer, I was committed to taking care of her and did so for those many years. As one can imagine, you may be "cured" of the disease, but the radiation treatment takes its toll on your brain. It fries your brain. My mother's forgetfulness and dementia were particularly evident about seven years after her brain cancer surgery. They call it late effects of radiation and the brain rots prematurely. People who didn't know my mother, thought she had Alzheimer's. Despite her mental diminishments, her physical health was absolutely remarkable. She was very strong, and never even got colds or flu.

Feeling fortunate to have her alive and in good physical health, I tried to focus on the positive, despite the rigors of caregiving. My mother was still very intelligent and wise, despite memory problems. She was capable of very intellectual thought processes, despite not always being able to remember such easy tasks as how to dress herself, due to the brain damage.

Throughout this book, I will continue to give details about her illness, as each becomes appropriate, to illustrate caregiving techniques, for example.

However, focusing on the nursing home experience, and how she got there, I'll now explain. Late effects of radiation can involve mini-strokes years after brain surgery, or a return of seizures. My mother had not taken anti-seizure medication since two years after her brain surgery. She was not having seizures, and the doctors felt that she could most likely get along without the medication. After going for years without any spells and no anti-seizure medication, she began having infrequent "blackouts" while she sat in her chair. She would lose consciousness for a few minutes, not being able to wake up. At this time, though the doctor didn't know if she was having mini-strokes or seizures, he chose not to put her back on her anti-seizure medication. One day, during an episode of dementia, she became upset and in walking around the house confused, she fell and hit her head. I believe she had a seizure that caused her to fall.

At any rate, she was taken to the hospital and had surgery for the bleeding in the brain, due to the fall. She was expected to recover, and appeared to be on that course in the hospital, when two weeks later, she mysteriously lapsed into a coma, confounding the doctors. They said the coma was totally unexpected. Ironically, she had recovered from brain cancer, and tragically fell prey to a head injury. In retrospect, my brother and I wondered if perhaps there was a medication error. Most people have heard through the media that medication errors are prevalent in hospitals. Nurses have too many patients and they go too fast, giving medication to a patient that was intended for another patient in the next bed or the next room. Or, a wrong dose is given by an inexperienced nurse who doesn't know how to measure the correct dose.

If these errors occur in hospitals, you can imagine that at nursing homes, where the staffing problems are even greater, and where nurses are even more inexperienced, care is even worse. In fact, the hospital care that my mother received was just an introduction to the type of problems we were to encounter at nursing homes.

After my mother's surgery for her head injury, a cerebrovascular accident,(CVA), she had been speaking in complete sentences, eating, and feeding herself, and was even trying to lower the bedrails to get out of bed. The care in this major hospital was poor. One of the nurses in the acute neurology unit where my mother was in, asked me if I wanted to give her a sponge bath. Since her insurance was paying thousands of dollars a week for her care, I thought to myself, "Why does she think I should be doing her job for her?" Being confounded by her attitude, I took the towel, not wanting to get into any discussions about what her duties were. In this unit, the nurses did no personal care, such as brush teeth, and the nurses were pleased that the surgeon asked me to supervise my mother's meal time and assist her with eating. If I hadn't been there, and she needed help holding her fork, would they have fed her? One day, another nurse complained loudly in front of visitors that she had nine "total care" (totally dependent) patients who couldn't help themselves.

After my mother had improved and left the acute neurology unit, she was put into the skilled nursing unit at the hospital where she eventually lapsed into her coma. Medicare patients are put in the skilled unit of the hospital when they need regular nursing care that isn't classified as acute or specialized. In the skilled unit, there were eleven patients to a nurse, and one nurse there was shouting about having too many patients. My mother contracted a bladder infection in the skilled unit. I had noticed that sponge baths there involved no more than a nurse's aide wetting a terrycloth washcloth with no soap, and "cleaning" around the urinary area. Worse, the nurse's aides often wetted the washcloth by throwing it into the sink, rather than holding it under the faucet. Sinks, of course, are often not clean. Further, when she had a bowel movement, the aides would not bother to turn her on her side and wipe the feces in the direction away from her urinary area. In wiping the feces toward the urinary area, one can get a bladder infection. After her bladder infection, my mother's health kept deteriorating. She stopped swallowing well and coughing up food, but the doctor thought that this problem would clear up once the bladder infection was cured. He said even a bladder infection or any infection in a brain-damaged person could cause swallowing problems.

But did my mother get a bladder infection from the unclean practices of the aides, or due to the catheter she immediately got after surgery, that they soon took her off of? I later learned that oftentimes, catheters in institutions aren't sterilized properly after each patient use, so patients run the risk of bladder infections. I wondered why the doctor hadn't taken the precaution of putting her on an antibiotic after surgery because of the catheter insertion. Sometimes, even introducing a foreign object such as a catheter in the body of a weak person causes infection.

After the successful treatment of the bladder infection, she became lethargic, and a couple of times, I noticed a whiteness in my mother's eyeballs. When I reported this to the nurse, she said she didn't know what it was, and she didn't follow up with the doctor. This is often the case in all healthcare situations. Nurses often ignore problems and go on to the next patient. The whiteness in her eyes disappeared, and I had already called the doctor with other questions, so I didn't follow up with that one. In retrospect, could she have been allergic to some medication she was taking? Or, was she having a seizure? The neurologist had thought it was better not to put my mother on anti-seizure medication after her CVA surgery, because sedating her with medication might hamper her alertness and recovery.

Little by little, my mother stopped talking, began to lose her motor skills, and looked as if she wasn't alert. The care in the hospital's skilled nursing unit was poor. For example, when my mother was receiving medication through an IV for her bladder infection, the nurse didn't know how to run the IV. The medication wouldn't flow because she didn't unlock the IV. I had the call light on, but the nurse didn't come. I went out to the nurse's station only to find the nurse chatting with another nurse. They had the radio blasting. If I hadn't been there to help my mother, she wouldn't have been able to walk out of the room to get the nurse or even use the call light. It would have been at least another hour before she checked back in. I was told by the nurses that they check in every hour or so, but in reality, it was more like two hours with so many patients. Some nurses were visibly angry that they had too many patients, and they were just focused on their anger and weren't doing their job.

One nurse asked me if I was a registered nurse. He said, "Many patients have family members who come to help like you and stay all the time and sleep over." I knew I wasn't the only one. This was obviously a bad sign—that the patients were not getting adequate care.

As for the uncleanliness, we were to learn that the skilled nursing unit of a hospital is just a miniature nursing home. As with nursing homes, staff members come to work sick, coughing and sneezing. Worse, they don't bother to wear a surgical mask. Fortunately, my mother didn't catch a respiratory bug, but I did, and I wore a mask, not wanting to give the bug to my mother.

One day my mother was sitting in her wheelchair and she urinated, leaving a puddle of urine on the floor. When the registered nurse came in and saw it, he said nothing. I'd assumed he'd go get someone to clean up the mess. An hour later, when no one had come, I had to ask for it to be mopped up. What if someone had slipped and fallen?

When my mother was in bed, oftentimes I'd walk in, only to find her bed soaked in urine, clear up to her back. It was obvious her diaper hadn't been changed in hours. If a patient isn't ambulatory, a bed pan isn't an option in a hospital or a nursing home, even if the patient can ring for help. The staff usually isn't available when a patient needs to void her urine. Therefore, elderly patients who aren't ambulatory are given diapers.

I lived at the hospital 18 hours a day. The doctors kept saying my mother would recover, that her lethargy was a temporary condition. However, her condition worsened.

When my mother had trouble swallowing, she was evaluated by a speech therapist at the hospital. The gastro-enterologist — a physician who specializes in the physiology and pathology of the stomach, intestines, and related structures such as the pancreas and esophagus — said that based on the evaluation of the speech therapist, my mother should have a nasal gastric tube inserted, whereby nutritious formula could be lowered into her stomach so that she wouldn't have to swallow food. The tube was inserted up her nose, delivering food down the esophagus and into the stomach. Since she was having difficulty swallowing, they thought she would run the risk of developing pneumonia with liquids and food mistakenly traveling down the wind pipe to the lungs. Obviously, choking was also a concern. I have devoted a full chapter, (Chapter 4, "The Feeding Tube Fiasco"), to the feeding tube issue. It is one that is complex because of the problems and dangers that a patient encounters, not only by having a feeding tube in an institutional situation, but often by the opinions expressed by speech therapists that prohibit patients in institutions to eat by mouth. These opinions can prove to be wrong, and it is sometimes discovered that the patient can, in fact, swallow. Eventually, this turned out to be the case with my mother and some other patients we've known.

By the time my mother left the hospital, she had a permanent feeding tube, a G-Tube (stomach tube), surgically implanted. Oftentimes, patients who are semi-alert, keep pulling out nasal gastric tubes, as was the case with my mother. We had asked the nurses to strap her hands to a chair while the formula ran, but the nurses and aides kept forgetting to do so. Therefore, my mother kept removing the tube from her nose. For basically their own convenience, they felt she needed, through surgery, a permanent tube, so they wouldn't have to deal with her removing her nasal gastric tube and reinserting it. We were leery of having our mother, in her weakened condition, go through another surgery, but the staff didn't want to be responsible for re-membering to strap her hands so she wouldn't pull out the nasal gastric tube. We didn't even know if her swallowing problem was a permanent condition at that time. However, we felt we had no choice but to put her through surgery, based on the doctor's recommendation.

It should be mentioned, too, that my mother became weaker and weaker due to a series of delays and goof-ups whereby she didn't get her stomach tube surgery for three days. The hospital staff forgot about taking her down for her surgery at the scheduled time. Despite our efforts to keep them on schedule, she was forgotten about. We've since heard that this isn't a rare occurrence with surgical procedures. Since she was prohibited from eating by mouth, and no longer had a nasal gastric tube, she wasn't getting nutrition. The doctor wasn't concerned. However, we felt she wasn't making progress in physical therapy because she didn't have the strength and physical endurance to stand with her lack of nutrition. And, she was getting more feeble, not following commands, we felt, due to a lack of nutrition.

The hospital kitchen, one evening, delivered a food tray to my mother's room, by mistake, even though she couldn't eat by mouth. I was tempted to test her and see if she could eat. However, if you don't follow hospital rules, you fear repercussions. In retrospect, it would have been a good idea to test her swallowing again.

After she got her G-Tube, I came into my mother's room on various occasions to find her in bed, so soaked in urine, that even her G-Tube was covered with urine. This is so unsanitary, since urine can seep in through the cap of the tube and go into the stomach. My mother even had an impacted bowel, because the staff wasn't keeping track of her bowel movements. The doctor told me I needed to keep track of her bowel movements. What we were to learn from this hospital experience was that staff at hospitals and nursing homes don't like to be monitored, and yet they don't do their jobs. I was a teacher for some years, and if the parents of my students had to monitor my teaching, I would have felt ashamed. However, I didn't see any signs of shame on the faces of the hospital's skilled nursing unit's staff.

My mother became weaker after her G-Tube surgery. She was no longer squeezing the doctor's hand on command. After 16 days of hospital care, I noticed she began having seizures. During the first seizure, she was having trouble breathing. I ran out of the room to get the nurse, and she couldn't even identify it as a seizure. She called a resident on duty at the hospital to assist, until my mother's doctor could come. The resident looked frantic and didn't know how to respond at first. He gave her an injection, and she quietly drifted off and wouldn't wake up. When her doctor arrived, he asked me that in the event that she were to stop breathing, if I wanted her to be on a respirator. I said that I didn't even know about respirators, but if it meant death without one, that we'd try a respirator. As it turned out, she didn't need one, but she lapsed into a coma nevertheless. I told the doctor that I was totally unprepared for the issue of death because I'd been told by the neurologist and neurosurgeon that they saw no reason why my mother wouldn't recover.

Of course, when staff members see a hospital patient every few hours, if a patient is having seizures, no one notices, unless the family is there to notify them. If my mother had continued to have seizures, she would have died, and no one would have known the cause of her death.

They moved her back to the acute neurology unit of the hospital so that she could be monitored in her room by camera from the nurse's station. However, the anti-seizure medication that they gave her wasn't working. She continued to have seizures, that only I noticed, because the nurses often weren't at the nurse's station to watch the camera in my mother's room. If they were at the nurse's station, they were often busy doing other things. If the seizure didn't last long, they didn't notice it.

After a couple of days of my not noticing seizures, the neurologist wanted to transfer my mother out of the acute neurology unit back to the skilled nursing unit. I told him I didn't think this was a good idea, because I didn't know if my mother's seizures were under control. As it turned out, I was right. Her seizures continued, and the doctor at least admitted that my concerns were well-founded. Here again, we were to learn what we learned throughout this healthcare ordeal. That is, doctors and nurses don't always know best. The family needs to trust its instincts. Although my brother and I have no medical background, we tried to use our common sense. Doctors and nurses often don't use common sense.

Although my mother was still having seizures, they were getting mild. She was just twitching her face or her hand would twitch. However, the nurses in the acute neurology unit didn't want to transfer her by a lifting machine (the hoyer lift) into a wheelchair, because they said that if she had seizures she could fall out of her chair. The doctors said she needed to get into a wheelchair, because if she stayed in bed, she wouldn't be upright enough to exercise her lungs and she may get pneumonia and die. The nurses refused to follow doctors' orders because they said it was against nursing policy. I said I would watch my mother while she was in her wheelchair and that they could even get her a seat belt to strap her in. They still wouldn't agree. This was yet another lesson we were to learn. At hospitals and nursing homes, nurses sometimes dispute or even ignore doctor's orders. They sometimes don't care what's in the best interests of the patient. They do what's easiest or best for them. How could my mother fall out of a wheelchair if she was just twitching her face?

When the doctor substituted a second anti-seizure medication, I didn't witness any seizures, though I didn't know if she was having any during the night when I was sleeping. To make a long story short, Medicare and her private insurance no longer would pay for the acute neurology unit, so my mother was transferred back to the skilled nursing unit.

However, a letter that my brother and I wrote to her doctor got my mother prematurely thrown out of the skilled nursing unit, that is, out of the hospital altogether. She was scheduled to stay about an extra week in the hospital, but she got thrown out when we sent a copy of the letter to the nurse manager of the skilled nursing unit.

While the following letter seems harmless, nurse managers often get defensive about care issues. We had wondered if our mother had lapsed into a coma because of a medication error made in the skilled nursing unit. Although we didn't mention this in the following letter, the doctor knew we were scared about transferring her back to a unit where she'd had problems with care issues and cleanliness. Further, it was here where they wouldn't strap her hand to a wheelchair, perhaps causing her to have a permanent feeding tube sutured into her body unnecessarily. The latter I had been very vocal about in my complaints. We could have disputed the premature "dumping" of our mother, but when we talked to the hospital ombudsman, who had an office at the hospital, she didn't go to bat for us. We thought she was probably chummy with the staff. She said both my brother and I had been upset with staff about care, and it was best my mother get into another situation, that is, a nursing home, which the staff had originally suggested for when she was to be discharged. This nursing home had been suggested even before we began complaining about care issues at the hospital. Our mother was in bad shape, still in a coma, and at this point, not knowing if she would live or die, we had no time to dispute anything. We didn't even know if her seizures were totally under control. The doctor said "she might die any day." We realized medicine was just guesswork, as we'd learned after our mother's brain cancer recovery.

However, you should know that dumping a patient out of the hospital prematurely, can be disputed, and I will discuss this in Chapter 10, "Where Do We Go From Here?"

Following is the "infamous" letter that got my mother dumped out of the hospital. As with all the letters in this book, fictitious names have been substituted, and dates have been omitted.

TO: John Smith, M.D.

Dear Doctor:

Following up on your conversation with us, we don't want to interfere with your decision to transfer our mother back to the skilled nursing unit as soon as possible. While we have been very satisfied with the level of nursing care she has received in the acute neurology unit, we share your hope that she may soon be able to benefit from the therapy available in the skilled nursing unit.

As we have discussed many times, our greatest concern is avoiding the possibility of further infections. Accordingly, we would appreciate any effort you can make in reiterating the emphasis on several basic care matters to the skilled nursing unit staff.

1) Continued elevation of the patient's upper body at all times for lung health.
2) All hygiene issues that involve possible skin breakdown and infections (i.e. frequent diaper changes, dry bed pads, etc.)
3) Averting patient contact with nurses and aides with colds or contagious diseases.

We know that you remain sensitive to our mother's guarded condition. We also have been impressed with the skills and experience exhibited by hospital staff members. However, we also have been discouraged by witnessing the demands placed on nurses and the time constraints under which they work. As always, we deeply thank you for your persistent help and cooperation.

Sincerely...........................

As I've said, when my mother left the hospital, the nursing home care was no better, despite what nursing home administrators told us about their care being "better than hospitals." As we were to learn in healthcare, everyone points the finger about poor care to another institution. Or, they point the finger about poor attitudes to others in their profession. People in healthcare always tell you that they and their institutions are giving "excellent care."

The doctor had told us that he didn't recommend nursing homes, but he didn't have a solution on what to do as far as needing a nurse to monitor our mother 'round the clock. He said privately hired nurses were hard to find, unless you knew someone, and agency help with an R.N. was too expensive for 'round the clock care, (today about $70 an hour or more). What he didn't tell us, nor did the hospital discharge staff know, was that my mother was entitled to up to 27 hours a week of free R.N. care through an agency in her home, just by virtue of the fact that she had a feeding tube. The reason for this is that feeding tubes are considered to be life support. This care would have been sustained beyond the usual 100 days of skilled home care benefits. If we'd known this, with that generous benefit of nearly four hours a day of free R.N. care, we'd have taken our mother home. The hospital discharge staff whom we'd talked to in the very beginning of her hospital stay —when it looked as if she'd only need to spend a week in the hospital, instead of nearly a month — said that she wasn't entitled to any substantial free registered nurse care at home. Even the nurse who coordinated my mother's private insurance care out of the doctor's office, knew of no substantial R.N. benefits. With nearly four hours a day of a free nurse and my care, plus some supplemental nurse's aide care that we would have paid for, we could have managed financially. In fact, we could have spent less money than we would have spent at a nursing home and have gotten private care. My mother was also entitled to some free home care equipment, such as a hospital bed, wheelchair, and hoyer lift. Further, in not being ignored by nursing home staff, she would have had a chance at meaningful recovery.

In addition, her doctor never mentioned the extraordinary benefits of hospice, which are perhaps the best benefits of care available to any patient. Upon leaving the hospital, the doctor said our mother "could die any day." If he believed that, he could have authorized hospice care that would have been at least a temporary solution. If she didn't die, and made progress toward recovery, she would have been dropped by the hospice program, but her home care benefits with her feeding tube situation would have picked up where hospice left off. You will read about hospice benefits in Chapter 5, "Alternatives to Nursing Homes."

Surprisingly, none of the hospital discharge staff, including social workers, seemed to have a clue about viable alternatives to nursing homes. (We didn't find out about the missed opportunity for free R.N. care at home, until four years later. At that point, we first began seriously talking to hospice about taking our mother home, and we asked if free care was available besides hospice.) The hospital staff had said 'round the clock care at a nursing home was the best way to go. Ironically, 'round the clock care is non-existent at a nursing home, as you'll find in reading this book.

It also should be noted that there are other tragedies to this story, beyond my inexperience at knowing the full alternatives to nursing homes, including substantial home health benefits. My mother had been cancer-free after her brain cancer for eleven and one-half years. She had decided not to take anti-cancer drugs two years after her brain cancer surgery, and she still recovered. However, because of her weakened condition in a coma — although she never got brain cancer again — her breast cancer came back in her other breast a year after she lapsed into a coma. The oncologists and her internist said that she would never have gotten cancer again had she not gone into a coma and also become dependent on feeding tube formula to sustain her. They said if she'd made a full recovery after her cerebrovascular accident, her cancer cells would have stayed dormant for ten or more years. That means she could have lived until the age of 86 or longer.

Even though she got cancer again, she didn't die of cancer. She died five years after her CVA. The cause of her death, the doctor said, was due to her long-standing problems resulting from her head injury—that is her bedridden state and resultant weakness. What's more, is that her oncologists and internist had actually recommended surgery for her breast cancer, something my brother and I declined because we knew she'd never survive the surgery. The doctors' rationale was that the tumor on the surface of her breast would ulcerate and that she'd die a painful death of infections. This never happened, largely because I took her out of the nursing home, and took care of her at home, using precautions. As her tumor got larger, I dressed the "wound" myself. At institutions, aides are careless with patients. If a tumor is on the surface, they will carelessly touch and rupture it. With a surface tumor, care must be taken in giving sponge baths, and moving a patient in bed to change her diaper and clean her up. Often doctors offer highly impractical options. Why cut our mother up one last time, we thought? Someone who is bedridden has no business going through cancer surgery. Again, exercise your common sense at all times in dealing with healthcare personnel and institutions. That's one of the points I'd like to hammer home in this book.

As one can see, if your elder is hospitalized before entering a nursing home, as is often the case, you have had perhaps a primer in the healthcare system and some of the attitudes of healthcare personnel. However, all in all, the system does get worse at nursing homes.

You'll often consider a nursing home, "long-term care facility," as we did, if you feel you can't care for your loved one and she is bedridden, particularly if she is too heavy to lift. For example, if you're single and have no one else in the home to assist you, then you gravitate toward putting someone in a nursing home. There is no one else at home to share in the duties, and you can't always get out of the house for an important errand.

As I've said, despite my ten and one-half years of caregiving at home when my mother was ambulatory, in institutionalizing her, my caregiving duties increased. I found the care to be so pitifully minimal at the three nursing homes my mother was at in her four years plus, that I needed to do the majority of care. These three nursing homes were praised and rated as being the best in the area, two of which were religious-affiliated facilities. I merely relied on staff to do the lifting or help me with it.

Nursing homes now cost on the average about $7,000 a month ($84,000 a year) for a private room. This is according to the Health Care Financing Administration, Office of the Actuary, National Health Statistics Group. Costs are typically higher in U.S. metropolitan areas. In the year 2011, it is estimated that nursing home costs will average $118,000 a year, and that in the year 2031, nursing home costs will average $224,000 a year, according to the Financing Administration and American Council of Life Insurers. When it comes down to it, for the average patient, it amounts to warehousing someone, a nurse distributing medication, meals, dressing a patient, and some activities for those who can participate. And, you often pay for the first month in advance of receiving the care.

In my opinion, nursing homes are not for people who are ambulatory and somewhat confused. There are alternatives for these people as I will discuss in Chapter 5, "Alternatives to Nursing Homes." Nursing homes should only be considered for a bedridden patient who is too heavy to lift. And, as this book will repeatedly give examples of, nursing homes can't adequately provide for these bedridden people that they were meant to serve. They don't offer 'round the clock attention, unless a family member is there to access care, and even then, patients are sometimes ignored.

Another reason you may decide on a nursing home is if your home is inadequate for caring for your elder. Though, considering the high cost of nursing homes, one can invest some money in adapting one's home for the handicapped. I will also discuss this matter in Chapter 5. I was leery of taking my mother home because her house was not insulated, and was very damp during the winter. We often had power outages. And, during the winter with some snow and ice, I thought it would be hard to get relief help to drive up to our hilly part of town when streets weren't plowed. However, when I took my mother out of the nursing home, despite these obstacles, we did manage.

This book is not intended to be a diatribe against nursing homes, though criticism that is due, needs to be fully addressed. It will be addressed in order for readers to completely understand care issues at nursing homes, so that they can decide whether their family members, or even their patients, clients, or they themselves should ever end up there. This book is really for everyone, not just families and adult children. It is for older adults, nurses, social workers, family counselors, hospital discharge personnel, doctors, physical, speech, and occupational therapists, elder law attorneys, gerontologists, gerontology professors, geriatricians, nursing school professors, nursing students, ministers, long-term care ombudsmen, and state inspectors of long-term care facilities. It is also for family members who already have loved ones at nursing homes, so that they can find solutions to problems with care and work with staff to resolve them.

While our mother was institutionalized, many nurses, doctors, and other healthcare people confided in me that they didn't fully comprehend how inadequate nursing homes were until they realized what my brother and I had been through with our mother. Some nurses I knew had never worked in such situations, and some had never had relatives in nursing homes. Even those who worked at nursing homes didn't realize what families go through when they politely complain about care to management, or lack thereof.

Although my mother came out of her coma to some extent, she was unable to speak for the most part, saying a few things in her five years of lethargy. She was unable to move for the most part, except she would sometimes lift her limbs when I told her to. I believe that had she been given the physical therapy and speech therapy my brother and I had advocated for, she would have come out of her coma to a greater extent. We had extreme difficulty convincing the nursing homes and her doctor that she was alert enough to swallow food, and for the first year and seven months, she wasn't allowed to eat anything by mouth. She had to rely on her feeding tube that had been surgically implanted at the hospital before she lapsed into a coma.

I will address issues of right-to-life and quality of life, and right-to-die issues. Quality of life should be a key issue at nursing homes, yet the patient is often considered not to have quality of life because of his condition. When in fact, the nursing home often hinders his quality of life by its policies and practices.

Though I have tried to address alternatives to nursing homes, in the event a family or guardian sees no alternative in the patient's individual case, I will show how to obtain some level of care at a nursing home, no matter how minimal. I will also discuss at length how to care for bedridden patients.

In our case, I chose to go it virtually alone with the help of hospice and some relief sitters the last eight months of my mother's life. Her condition had deteriorated, and the nursing home was not even providing the most minimal

of care, but also causing illness to my mother by doing nothing to remedy filthy practices by aides and nurses alike.
Nursing homes — even non-profit religious-affiliated ones
— are short-staffed. Aides are usually paid slightly above
minimum wage to start. The breakdown in care is often
due to an attitude of "I don't care," regardless of how they
say the care is "excellent" and how "loving" the staff says
they are toward patients. Oftentimes, the nurses don't want
to listen to specific instances of substandard care. Worse,
the social workers at these institutions and resident care
managers often tell you when you politely complain that
"If you don't like it, you can go someplace else."

While I did meet some outstanding nurse's aides, (nursing assistants as they are now called), and some outstanding nurses, they were few and far between. Those who were
truly good people often moved on, choosing not to stay
and defend the practices of the facility. Those who stayed,
believed that critical co-workers and family members, such
as I, who were polite and professional in their complaints,
were nothing but troublemakers. One good nurse, who was
nearing retirement and would soon leave, told me that
when she went to bat for patients who weren't receiving
good nurse's aide care, she was labeled a troublemaker by
other nurses.

Tragically, some staff members at nursing homes look
upon patients as being a nuisance, and they believe that
patients, such as my mother, shouldn't be alive. Amazingly,
some nurses, even at religious-affiliated facilities, will tell
family members to their face, "Why are you keeping your
mother alive?" I remember one nurse at a religious-affiliated facility asked me, "Did your mother ever tell you what
she would like done, if she should ever become like this?"
Why ask? The answer was obviously "no." The majority
of people in our parents' generation, now in their 80s, didn't
consider "advance directives." That is, they didn't consider
whether or not they wanted to be on a respirator, or receive tube feedings if they are unable to swallow.

At a non-religious-affiliated facility, one nurse, when I remarked that my mother looked sad, said, "Is she sad because she's being kept alive against her will?" I was already feeling so scared and anxious about my mother's condition, and this was like a dagger to my heart. At this same nursing home, a Catholic nurse, trained at a four-year Catholic nursing school, asked my brother and I, in front of my 12-year-old niece, "Why do you want to treat your mother for pneumonia, she's comatose?" The nurse looked so annoyed and offended. It's amazing how these people take it as a personal offense.

The sad part is that nursing homes often cause a patient's health to decline. The patient often gets pneumonia when doctor's orders are not followed to get the patient out of bed and into a wheelchair, and to do range of motion exercises, or merely to move their body in bed. Not doing this causes lung problems. What nurses often fail to realize, too, is that they see a patient a few minutes during their eight-hour shift when they pass out medication. My mother was not totally comatose. She was in a "vegetative state", and had periods of alertness. For a nurse who doesn't see her periods of alertness, perhaps the patient's life is worthless.

The gross unprofessionalism aside — if you can block it out of your mind — leaves one wondering about something else. What kind of human beings would be so cruel as to think, and worse, say things like these to a family member? My mother was alert at the time these nurses said these things, and I'm sure she processed the statements. It must be a combination of extreme insensitivity, unintelligence, and unprofessionalism. One wonders if the nurses pick up this attitude from working around others with poor attitudes. A resident care manager, (a nurse in charge of the paperwork in my mother's unit), had a poor attitude. She was gossiping behind my mother's back about what a foolish person I was, in thinking that my mother had a chance to recover. In fact, when one nursing student

— from a local community college who was doing her internship at the nursing home — remarked that my mother was alert, she told me this resident care manager laughed at her, flipping her hand at her. The next day, when I tried to awaken my mother, the resident care manager looked at me in a shocked way with her mouth open. This was the same resident care manager who ignored doctor's orders to get my mother out of bed, leading to her worsening condition. The doctor had ordered that my mother was to receive movement, transferring her from her bed into a wheelchair. This wouldn't only give her comfort, but keep her lungs healthy, allowing her to breathe more deeply in an upright position. Just the motion of transferring someone out of bed into a chair, changes his body position and exercises his lungs. Also, it's good for circulation in the legs, to have the legs dangling from a wheelchair with no leg rests, as opposed to laying in bed. This resident care manager told us that the doctor wasn't right in his assessment that bedridden people need to be transferred out of bed. She ignored his orders for a month, and my mother's lungs deteriorated. First she got pneumonia. Then the following week, she was rushed to the hospital late one night after suffering lung embolisms (clots). These were blood clots in her legs that shot up to her lungs. Her hands were turning blue when a nurse found her. She lost oxygen to the brain. After my mother returned from the hospital to the nursing home, she got pneumonia again, and started having seizures. With this major setback, she suffered further brain damage. It's a wonder that in the following months, she awakened from her coma. Had she not had this setback, and received proper care, it's possible that she would have come out of her coma sooner, and to a greater extent.

As I mentioned when I talked about my mother's hospital stay, nurses sometimes ignore doctor's orders when they feel it's too much trouble to do the work. At nursing homes, they sometimes get into power struggles with the doctor over the phone, challenging his/her judgment, and refusing to carry out orders. The doctor can't fire them, and doesn't have the time to report them to the nursing home administrator. The nursing home where my mother developed lung embolisms, that was rated as one of the best nursing homes, didn't even own a hoyer lift, standard equipment. If it had, this would have made the process of getting my mother out of bed easy, taking only a few minutes.

One could make the case that my mother could have gotten these lung clots anyway. The doctor hadn't ordered constrictive hose which sometimes prevents blood clots in the legs. And, of course, no one at the nursing home suggested these tight-fitting stockings. So, you can't sue a nursing home. Nursing home staff members know that they can never get in trouble for poor care, because the patient is in such bad shape anyway that you can't prove that her deterioration resulted from poor care.

Further, nursing home staff often deny care problems that you've witnessed. If you witness that your elder was the victim of an error made by a nurse or nurse's aide, and your elder becomes sick, they find an explanation that would point to some other cause. They blame the patient for becoming ill due to old age. For example, if a nurse's aide opens the patient's window on a cold day to air out odors of a bowel movement, and then forgets to close the window, if the patient develops pneumonia, they'll say that the patient would have gotten pneumonia anyway. Blatant denials often border on the absurd.

Why not report problems to the ombudsman? Particularly if doctor's orders aren't being followed? Because the resident care manager of a unit knows by the nature of the complaint, who complained, and rather than improve care, she often ignores the patient more.

Why can't you complain to the nursing home administrator? Because the administrator won't fire anyone because he has trouble finding help. Therefore, the employee stays on, bad-mouths you to other employees, and then nearly everyone shuns your elder.

A director of nursing once told me that if you fire one person, you end up replacing her with one who is just as bad. Then, why, you wonder, would any self-respecting director of nursing not realize that it diminishes her to work in such a situation?

As for the nurses who felt my mother was unjustly being kept alive by her children, one also wonders if healthcare personnel see some adult children as being evil for choosing life for a family member. If your elders don't want to discuss death, and in my mother's Italian culture of her generation it was taboo to do so, then family members must decide for their elders about what to do if they become totally disabled. Normally, one errs on the side of human life, particularly if one has had an accident that caused her condition. You want to give your elder a chance to recover. It's an agonizing decision to have to make, but it hurts even more deeply when a healthcare employee questions you in a reprimanding way for your decision. Would they have more respect for someone who said he wanted his parent to die quicker to receive an inheritance?

Even after my mother died, I asked a close family friend in her 70s, if she had made it known to her son about her wishes, should she become totally disabled. She replied that she hadn't, and that it would be up to him to decide. You see, this woman had visited my mother three times a week during the last five years of her life, and knew exactly the kind of condition my mother was in. This didn't motivate her to make out an "advance directive," stating under what conditions she would want her life prolonged. In her generation, one didn't make these kind of advance plans.

Some nurses who became my friends told me in confidence that they wouldn't want to be patients at a nursing home. They also said that if they had their parents at nursing homes, they would be spending just as much time as I did there monitoring care and doing it myself. These nurses did eventually move on to jobs elsewhere.

When you complain about care, the nursing home staff doesn't address the problem and often merely flips you off telling you they have an excellent facility and you can go someplace else. These people haven't taken a good look at themselves. They haven't admitted to themselves that they don't want to care for sick people. If they seek employment at another facility, they carry the same attitude with them, not wanting to care for the patients there, either. They are simply in the wrong field. We, as healthcare consumers are customers. We pay their salaries, and if a facility loses business because the staff flips off family members and takes their elders elsewhere, administrators will further reduce their staffing. These individuals may find themselves out of work. With their attitudes, the best they can hope for is to find work at another shabby nursing home.

We need to do better as a society, because before long, we may end up in nursing homes ourselves. We can't afford to let the care get shabbier and shabbier without reform. This book will address daily nursing home problems and offer solutions to coping reasonably with the situation, working with the staff to attempt to resolve problems. This book will serve as a means of effecting change. As our aging population increases, no one can afford shabby warehousing for thousands of dollars each month. Actual care and accountability for care is needed. In comparing notes with friends who've had parents in nursing homes, a common response to complaints from family members is not only "We give excellent care," but "You're the only one who complains." The pat answers that staff gives to avoid resolving the problems become all too predicable. Hostility and belligerence from staff isn't uncommon.

The healthcare profession has always done a bad job of monitoring itself for the care it's supposed to provide. We used to think that doctors weren't accountable, but in my 16 years of caregiving, I've realized that a poor "customer service" attitude has filtered down through all rungs of the healthcare field. It's as if no one cares, and even worse, standards become lower and lower, and the less that is done for patients in nursing homes, the more staffers believe they are doing "excellent work."

Why is healthcare so non-customer-service oriented? If a schoolteacher flipped off parents, people would be astonished at how unprofessional he was. What if he told the parents that the student was a lost cause, wasn't fit to learn, and didn't deserve an education? I believe something would be done about it. If the teacher couldn't be fired, he would be demoted, or at least reprimanded by a superior and shunned by colleagues. We care more about children than we do about elders. Perhaps that's why no one demands better healthcare for seniors.

One social worker at a religious-affiliated facility said, "Our staff doesn't want to work with you. We don't work with the family member. We work with the patient." I replied, "The reason I'm trying to work with the staff is because my mother can't speak and can't advocate for herself. If she could speak about the care, she wouldn't be as polite as I've been with you." The staff member was merely saying in a rude way that she didn't want to hear complaints.

If one can excuse poor care due to a lack of adequate staffing, one cannot forgive the belligerence and poor attitudes of staff. It's not unusual at all for nurses to chew out family members and even shout at them, after a polite complaint is made. Worse, the supervisory staff which is meager — often just a director of nursing and an assistant director of nursing — pretends not to hear.

In healthcare, any attitude seems acceptable. As I said, at the hospital where my mother was a patient, I routinely heard nurses loudly complain about working conditions.

When I was a teacher I had a total of 250 students in all my classes. If I had complained about the workload or shouted at parents, I wouldn't have been able to hold on to my job.

What I observed during my mother's years at nursing homes, is that the bad nurses and other poor personnel often choose to work there, not because they "love older people," but because they can't do any better. If they aren't fresh out of nursing school and inexperienced, sometimes they've failed at hospital jobs that they previously held. It's not necessarily that the bad nurses lacked nursing knowledge. It's that they had trouble functioning in larger situations with many co-workers, patients, supervisors, and doctors. They lacked the skills in getting along with people. At nursing homes, they work alone — the only nurse out on the floor in a unit. They have no one to answer to. Yes, they often work in a stinking nursing home that isn't pleasant, but nobody bothers them.

The good nurses who work at nursing homes do want to provide good care. Often, their morale becomes low, knowing that all they have time to do is to pass out medications. They can't use the nursing skills they have because they have time to just pass out medications. That's why patients don't often get nursing care. According to current statistics, practically anywhere, nurses can get a job at hospitals for $25 an hour or more. They are never laid off, have great benefits, and they can work overtime to make more money. Therefore, good nurses subject themselves to conditions at nursing homes only if they really love the patients.

As for aides I knew, the bad ones who left for higher paying jobs at hospitals, came back to the nursing home within a couple of months. They complained, for example, that their hospital supervisors were too critical of them.

One wonders if in their nursing education, nurses are taught how to communicate with patients and family members. Are they taught about responsibility, ethics, and attitude?

Or, do bad nurses slip through the cracks? When I ask my nurse-friends about bad nurses, they say, "It just happens."

At nursing homes, I routinely saw nurses walk away from patients with bad colds and coughs who normally didn't have respiratory problems. When my mother started coughing and was developing a cold, the nurses would always adopt a wait-and-see attitude. Despite my initial concerns, they wouldn't do anything. They would wait a day or two or even more, until it was really bad. They'd finally call the doctor when it was full-blown pneumonia. My mother couldn't blow her nose, so her drainage would go down her throat, and straight to her lungs. Merely getting a doctor's order for a cold remedy would have worked. (I gave her a cold remedy when I took her home to care for her in her final months. She didn't get pneumonia, despite her very weakened state, as she did each winter at the nursing home.)

At nursing homes, when the cold escalates to pneumonia, the nurses don't want to treat it. I remember the first winter at a religious-affiliated nursing home, my mother was struggling to breathe for days. The nurses didn't want to call the doctor until seven days after her respiratory problems began. When it was obvious that she had pneumonia, the nurses didn't want to treat her. They wanted to send her out in 25-degree weather to the hospital to be treated. I remember one nurse raising her voice on the phone to the doctor who said she must treat my mother. She even told the director of nursing she had too much work and didn't want to deal with my mother. My brother and I protested that our mother would die if she were transported to the hospital. Then, the nurse looked mad at us for insisting that our mother be treated. She reluctantly did her job.

In many cases, the patients get pneumonia because the nurses and nurse's aides come to work with bad colds. They do not even bother to wear masks, coughing and sneezing in the patient's face.

Patients die of pneumonia, too, because the nurses don't want to bother to suction phlegm out of their throats. The patients aren't strong enough to cough up the phlegm. The nurses feel they don't have the time to do it.

It always amazed me how the postponement of delivering vital care or even medication to treat the ill patient didn't bother the nurses. Either they didn't care if the patient lived or died, or purposely were trying to "put them out of their misery" once and for all. One nurse who routinely ignored patients' respiratory problems told me she didn't like to see patients suffer. Then, why didn't she treat the illness before it became worse?

Besides the instance of the nurse wanting to send my mother out in 25-degree weather to be treated at the hospital, there were two other atrocious instances. I remember another winter when my mother got pneumonia. There was a nurse who, after my mother's medication arrived to treat her pneumonia, found excuses not to give it to her. My mother was no longer in a coma, and was responding quite well and eating by mouth to some extent. The nurse said she wouldn't give my mother the medication because it was the wrong medication. I had the doctor call her twice to tell her that it was the right medication and that she should administer it. She still didn't give the medication. Later, she kept saying, when I asked, "Yes, dear, I'll give the medication, when I can." My mother didn't get her medication until nine hours later from another nurse on the next shift. I reported the problem to the social worker and to the director of nursing. They not only never did anything about it, but a few months later, this substitute nurse was hired as a full-time nurse on another unit. On this other unit, one nurse's aide told me that this nurse was acting the same way with other patients who needed medication. The aide said one patient died from the nurse not giving medication to her, and that she reported what the nurse had done to her daughter. Who knows if a lawsuit was ever filed? I doubt it, because it would have been hard to prove that the patient was a victim of neglect unless the aide testified. This nurse, when she did allow patients to have their medication, often asked aides to deliver the pills. This was against the law. The nurse's aides were not even certified as medication aides.

Yet another instance of a nurse not wanting to treat pneumonia was at the nursing home my mother was in when she got the lung embolisms. This nurse was the resident care manager, a nurse who not only does paperwork on a particular unit, but who gives instructions to the nurse on the floor. (Oftentimes, this nurse who does paperwork is less experienced than the nurse on the floor who treats patients, according to what many nurses say.) When she and the nursing home administrator met with my brother and I to discuss lingering care problems, she actually said in front of the administrator that if my mother were to get pneumonia again, she would "have trouble" seeing her treated. She said my mother couldn't talk and therefore "give permission" to be treated. She asked, "How do we know she doesn't want to die?" It's not only astonishing that she asked this, but it's astonishing that she made such statements in front of the administrator. More astonishingly, the administrator didn't say anything to her about how despicable her attitude was. He said absolutely nothing. We plainly and firmly stated, "We expect you to treat her." A few weeks later, we moved my mother out of that nursing home, as soon as space was available at the next one.

When patients die, oftentimes, the patient's relatives don't know they died because of neglect and refusal to care for the patient. Many relatives who've had elders at nursing homes, even over a period of a few years, don't know what kind of care their family members are receiving. I remember an elderly woman who could make it to the nursing home twice a week to visit her husband, when she got a ride there. When he died, she thanked the nurses and the aides by letter and sent flowers to them. She thanked them for the care they gave him. She said she wished he could have lived longer. The fact is, he could have lived longer. He was coughing very badly for a few days, and each staff nurse ignored him until his daughter showed up. She didn't know that he'd been coughing for a few days, but she reported to the nurse that he was having trouble breathing, and that she wanted him treated. The nurse reluctantly called the doctor to have x-rays done. It was discovered that he had pneumonia. The next day, he died. The daughter probably thought his illness came on suddenly.

Before I put my mother in a nursing home, I assumed nurses were bound by some ethical standard or oath to care for patients. If they are bound, some nurses defy the principles of their vocation. I saw it over and over again at each nursing home. Nurses would ignore ill patients, and only reluctantly call the doctor for x-rays or medication if the family members visited and notified them they wanted the patient treated. It remains unfathomable to me how some nurses can be so derelict in their duties, and worse, make judgment calls as to whether your loved one should live or die.

Again, you often don't report these things to the ombudsman, because you try to work within the nursing home channels. If problems persist, you move your loved one someplace else. You try to get the care needed without reporting them or "tattling" on their practices. You use your best judgment without trying to alienate the staff, as you are often accused of doing with your complaints. Despite my efforts to deal with each problem as it came up, and not report problems to governmental regulating agencies, often social workers and nurses accused me of "alienating" their staff by complaining. One response I used was, "If you really love your patients as you say you do, and you give excellent care, then you'll be happy to know about problems so you can correct them." The family member is always accused of alienating staff despite her most careful efforts not to blame or be impolite. In fact, when you complain of persistent problems that haven't been resolved, the staff begins complaining about you. I remember at the first nursing home, if my mother was given a sponge bath at all each morning, it was performed so poorly that she stunk afterwards. When I gave up on repeating my complaints and decided to do the sponge baths myself, the resident care manager told me I was using too many towels! If I were a nurse, I would first feel ashamed that a family member would have to resort to providing personal care for her elder, care that they are being paid for, and can't even execute.

A patient smells after a sponge bath, usually because the aide uses two washcloths to clean the entire body and a hand towel to dry. If he uses two washcloths, this means that if one is used to soap the patient with, and the other one is used to rinse, then the one with soap is used for the face, neck, armpits, arms, stomach, urinary area, bowel area, and the legs and feet. Especially with a bedridden, incontinent patient, using one soapy washcloth means the aide is just spreading germs and stink around various parts of the body. Therefore, a patient comes through the sponge bath smelling worse than before. What is especially unsanitary is, that because they don't use enough towels, they are continuously dipping dirty towels into the sponge bath tub after cleaning up sweat, urine, and feces, to get more soapy water. Worse, the sponge bath tub is never cleaned before the next usage. The tub itself is often a cesspool. The next time, the sponge bath is given, the face is washed with the washcloth, dipped in the contaminated tub, etc. The aides are instructed to start a sponge bath by washing the face first and working their way down the body. However, I've even seen aides start with the urinary and bowel area, and finish off with the face.

Often, the aides don't even wear latex gloves in cleaning the patient. In fact, one nurse from a third world country erroneously told me that aides didn't have to wear gloves when cleaning a patient. Some aides go from room to room giving personal care, patient to patient, without gloves or even washing their hands. If this doesn't spread infection and disease, what does? When my mother entered a nursing home, I realized that unclean practices were just as bad there, as in the poor countries of the world. This uncleanliness at nursing homes is among the worst of the problems. Until it is resolved to monitor the aides' care for cleanliness and fire personnel who don't follow procedure, nothing will change, and patients will fall prey to unnecessary infections, get weak, and die. When I witnessed aides not wearing latex gloves in cleaning my mother's body and I asked them to wear gloves, I was sometimes later condemned by nurses for "supervising" their employees. The aides would report me, and the nurses would forget about the poor care issues and scold me.

Among the reasons why nursing homes don't improve their care, is that some staff, don't realize that patients deserve care. That's what they pay money for. As you will find in this book, amazingly nonsensical and bureaucratic responses are given to family members by staff when questions about care issues are raised. The routine in institutional settings involves bureaucratic thinking and practices. This thinking is not in the best interests of patients. Rather, it damages the patient's well-being and health. As one nurse I was fond of told me, "Standards of caring for the elderly are lower than those standards of caring for others. It shouldn't be this way."

Sometimes complaints lead to solutions, but these solutions are often temporary ones. After about two weeks of improvement in aide care, for example, it's business as usual and basic care falls apart again.

It's interesting to me that some nurses and nurse's aides suggested that I write this book. They thought that improvements in care could result if families became aware of practices in nursing homes and advocated for better care for their elders. We must hold management accountable.

While I've known some home health care agencies to send out surveys to families regarding their level of satisfaction with employees, you'll rarely, if ever, get a satisfaction survey from a nursing home. While many families don't really show up enough to visit their elders at nursing homes, and therefore, can't judge the quality of care, wouldn't it be helpful for nursing home staff to know at least something about how well they're doing? I believe that many nursing homes don't care how the family feels. They feel they are doing excellent work and don't want to hear otherwise.

Some nurses, though, told me in confidence, that they don't believe their facilities offer excellent care, and that if they told the truth to a family member about care, they'd get in trouble for it.

We often read of overt nursing home abuse in the way of aides pushing, shoving, bruising patients, and yelling at them. But, we don't hear of bedridden patients being abused and neglected behind closed doors, or of family members being verbally abused and intimidated by professional staff. You will hear of all common occurrences of abuse in nursing homes throughout this book.

Nursing home personnel need to take a good look at themselves. While working conditions may not be ideal at nursing homes, improvements can begin with supervisory personnel who set the tone for the attitude of everyone working there. Supervisors must improve their communication skills with family members. If not, their subordinates follow suit and express hostility to family members, and ultimately to the patient. Common statements made by professional staff such as "This patient will never talk or walk," or "Only a miracle will help this patient," often are not only inaccurate, but they are unprofessional. If they don't believe that some patients can have some quality of life, why are they there? My mother's quality of life was not only scoffed at by professional staff, but in doing so, they neglected her, so her quality of life diminished. My mother, when she improved and came out of her coma after five months, was alert and wakeful in her lethargic state. It didn't seem like she wanted to die. In one instance, she said she was happy, and she asked "Will I make it?" She said this in Italian, so she still knew two languages. Other times, she smiled and even laughed. In her periods of alertness, she seemed to recognize me, my brother and his children. (I am single and have no children.)

The most pathetic aspect of her condition was perhaps not the condition itself, which a family member somehow learns to reconcile herself to, but the attitude of the nurses toward her. I had to whisper to my mother that she would get well, otherwise the nurses would scowl at me, and say otherwise in front of my mother, and talk behind my back. When I told my mother, who was semi-alert one morning, that she had to get better so I could take her home, one nurse said in front of her, "Oh, don't tease her." It's commonly known that doctors lack bedside manners, but what about some nurses?

Back in 1991, there was a study that showed that out of 84 patients diagnosed as being in a "permanent vegetative state," 58 percent recovered consciousness within the first three years. However, studies show that if a patient is to improve, most of her improvement takes place in the first year. Therefore, if they regain consciousness as my mother did, are not neglected, not exposed to illness and infection, receive adequate stimulation by movement and physical therapy, and are allowed to eat by mouth, their chances of meaningful recovery are greatly improved. In a nursing home situation, as we found, a patient in my mother's condition isn't given a chance.

There are about 17,000 nursing homes in the U.S. They are depressing places, just by virtue of the fact that they house frail and mentally-impaired adults. One of the saddest things I saw, was a husband and his second wife coming to help his elderly and demented ex-wife who screamed all day long. She had no one else to advocate for her.

At another nursing home, there was a pleasantly confused woman who spoke gibberish most of the time. However, in one instance, she was truly lucid. I knew her to be a Medicaid patient, because her daughter told me she was. She wheeled herself up to me and said, "This is homelessness." Even being poor, she felt a nursing home was inadequate.

The reality of the situation is that no matter how scrupulous you are in planning for your old age, often no one will take care of you. Often, they will accept your money, and give you little, if any care.

Whether or not nursing home care improves, if you can, either take care of your loved one at home or follow the options in this book. I've attempted to write this book in plain, simple English, trying to avoid medical jargon. It is my sincere hope that it will help everyone who reads it.

CHAPTER 1

Selecting a Nursing Home

Just after my mother had surgery, hospital discharge personnel came to talk to us about what our plans were when she left the hospital. They thought she would be out in a week. As I've discussed in the Introduction of this book, her doctor, the nurse liaison in his office who dealt with my mother's HMO, and the hospital discharge personnel apparently didn't know that my mother had rather extensive home health care benefits including some free R.N. care. Because of her feeding tube, she was a life support patient, and she was entitled to benefits that most patients aren't. These professionals insisted that she didn't have benefits that would make it possible for her to go home, and that my brother and I should check out nursing homes where she would be given 100 days of free skilled care with her Medicare and private insurance. (This is still available today through her insurance.)We were to learn that skilled care is a nebulous term. Basically, it's no different care than intermediate care at a nursing home, except that the patient foots the bill for the latter. Also, in intermediate care, the nursing unit has more patients. I will later discuss nurse to patient ratios and nurse's aide to patient ratios.

Had we known that my mother was entitled to extensive home health care benefits, we either never would have put her in a nursing home or certainly not have kept her there beyond the expiration of her skilled nursing benefits.

This is a lesson for you. Before putting an elder in a nursing home, specifically determine what home health care benefits are available in the way of R.N. visits, equipment, and supplies by speaking in person to a supervisor at your elder's insurance company. If possible, also speak to someone at your local social security office about Medicare, and at a local Welfare office about Medicaid. You need to talk specifics about your loved one's medical condition. If good home health benefits are available, your loved one could do much better at home. Remember that in a nursing home, although a nurse is on duty 24 hours a day, in an emergency or in the case of illness, it may be hours before anyone responds. Therefore, if your motivation for putting someone in a nursing home is that a nurse is already on duty, and one doesn't have to be called in from the outside as you would have to at home, a nursing home doesn't necessarily mean you'll get faster care. Staff only checks in on a patient every few hours at best, and the nurses often drag their feet in placing a call to the doctor unless the patient is dying right then and there. (When my mother had lung embolisms at the nursing home, she was probably losing oxygen for a while before the nurse found her. My mother's room was right across from the nurse's station. Otherwise, she probably wouldn't have been found at all for hours. Then, the nurse dragged her feet. It took over an hour to get a call back from the doctor. If my mother had been at home, instead of delaying, I would have dialed 9-1-1. Apparently, the nurse was debating what to do, instead of reacting in an emergency situation. Besides giving oxygen, she should have rushed her off to the hospital.)

You should also consider what I experienced when I took my mother home in her final months of life. She didn't get pneumonia and other infections from being in an institution, so she didn't even need a nurse most of the time. The hospice nurse visited once a week, and even skipped one week when I didn't have any concerns or questions. And, in my mother's final days, the hospice nurse came more frequently as needed.

How To Judge a Nursing Home

If you have determined that you need to place your loved one at a nursing home, you must realize that doctors and hospital discharge personnel such as social workers, will often speak with confidence or authority on facilities. Bear in mind, their recommendations are often not good. These social workers may tell you they've visited certain facilities, but often one visit doesn't tell you anything. Further, facilities go through a lot of changes in staff or management in just a matter of a few months. In reality, the healthcare professionals go by the rumor mill, and rarely have they themselves ever had a parent at a particular facility in the recent past. What was once considered one of the best facilities, may have turned into a bad one. We were told by hospital discharge personnel and my mother's doctors that the nursing home she ended up going to was "top of the line." In reality, it hadn't been top of the line for about 20 years. Even the state inspectors still rated it as among the best. However, it was a hellhole with nurses and resident care managers laughing about patients and their families behind their backs, and telling family members outright that they should let their elders die.

The state rates facilities based on its annual inspection of them. You can find out the ratings through your state's Long-Term Care Office. However, when the state comes to inspect, you'll find that the inspector often doesn't even walk down the halls. He sits at the nurse's station reviewing charts on patients. The charts tell part of the story, such as a patient's infections, but not necessarily the whole truth. The first nursing home we put our mother in had a high rating from the state. We knew that a lot of patients were being treated for bedsores, including my mother, who was being left for as much as eight hours soaked in urine in her bed. You know if this is happening to your mother, it is happening to others. (One day, I wasn't at the nursing home "on duty" as I normally was. Having left for eight hours, I came back, finding her in the same position in bed as I'd left her. Her whole bed was soaked and she was laying in her feces.)

This nursing home was great in maintaining all kinds of paperwork about care given to each patient—care that in many cases wasn't done. Of course, this is fraudulent to chart care not given to the patient, but who's to know? Unless a family member is there all the time, he can't say with certainty that certain care wasn't given. The nursing home patients themselves are usually not in good enough shape mentally to complain about care. Incidentally, it's a good idea to ask to read a patient's chart, from time to time. It's very revealing, as nurses even include their complaints about family members. In my mother's chart, I read that I was "unrealistic" about her chance for recovery.

In the records inspectors read, the staff also doesn't include letters family members have written to the director of nursing or to the resident care manager about problems with care.

If the state inspector walked into the patient's room to observe how an aide delivers care, she would most likely note all kinds of unclean practices. It should be noted, too, that even for the three, four, or even five-day inspection, the nursing home staff is on its best behavior. The nursing home staff makes sure the place looks clean. They call in extra employees for those days. The resident care manager who usually doesn't leave the nurse's station, is walking up and down the halls, making sure there are no problems.

And, believe it or not, the state inspection isn't impromptu. The staff seems to know when the inspector is due to visit because she comes back around the same time every year, or she's just visited another facility in the area.

Making use of what information is available to you, a way of finding out what a nursing home is like may be to contact the state's Long-Term Care Office to find out who the ombudsman is for a particular facility. It will give you the name and phone number of the ombudsman who is a volunteer. This volunteer may be able to shed more light than what the state inspection reveals. This may be true if the ombudsman has been visiting the particular facility for a long time and is diligent about talking to family members. We called the ombudsman at one facility before we transferred our mother there from another nursing home. She was a retired nurse. We asked her what kinds of complaints she was getting from family members at the facility. Because she had been an ombudsman at another facility before, and because of her nursing background, we felt she was as good a source as we were going to get. She told us she hadn't gotten many complaints, and not serious ones. She said occasionally a family member complained that his elder wasn't being kept clean, but that she didn't get as many of these complaints as one would normally hear of at nursing homes. She said she thought this facility was the best we were ever going to find. Interestingly enough, we were to learn that this ombudsman apparently had not heard of a major complaint against the facility that had occurred six months prior. At the present facility my mother was at, coincidentally, we talked to another family member we met a few days after we talked to this ombudsman. She said her mother had a terrible time at the facility we were thinking of transferring my mother to. (I should mention that we often met family members at facilities who had previously had their parents in other facilities. They are sometimes a good source of information.) This family member said she filed a suit against this nursing home we were looking into. Apparently, she claimed the facility had caused her mother to have a head injury. Her mother had been recovering from a stroke and was mobile. However, due to this head injury she claimed her mother had sustained, she was now paralyzed from the waste down. She claimed the nurse's aides there had been turning her mother and pulling her body up in the bed when they hit her mother's head on the bedboard. Worse, the brain hemorrhage wasn't discovered until three days later. The staff apparently noticed no change in her level of alertness, etc. When she told us this, it didn't make us feel too confident anymore about this other facility. We wondered why the ombudsman hadn't heard of it. We must admit, however, that this didn't surprise us, because at the present facility we had our mother at, I witnessed one nurse's aide hitting my mother's head on the bedboard when pulling her up in bed. You need to put a pillow flat against the bedboard when pulling someone up. In my mother's case, fortunately this hadn't caused her injury, though it's obviously not a good thing for a head injury patient to sustain. We did end up transferring our mother to the facility anyway, because we'd felt we'd had enough of the poor attitudes at the present facility, where some of the professional staff believed people in my mother's condition were vegetables who didn't deserve to live. We didn't expect to find the same attitude at the facility that we transferred our mother to—the one that the woman suffered the head injury and paralysis at—because it was a Catholic facility. Disappointingly, we did find that attitude even there among three staff members—though not as many as we'd run across in the previous facility.

Yet another method of finding out about nursing homes in your area is to dial 1-800-Medicare. The federal government does rate nursing homes in your area. Their website is www.medicare.gov. The Medicare website is courtesy of The U.S. Department of Health and Human Services. Nursing home data it keeps may help you select a nursing home in your area. Over three million people live in nursing homes in the U.S. An estimated one-half of women and one-third of men will spend some time there during their lifetime. Federal data includes that of certified Medicaid facilities, besides that of Medicare facilities. It compares nursing homes for care of short-term stay patients (rehab) and long-term patients, and rates quality. For short-term patients, for example, data shows the percentage of patients whose walking has improved. This data may or may not reveal that the patients are receiving good physical therapy or are being walked a lot by aides, rather than being left in wheelchairs. For long-term patients, for example, the data shows percentages of patients who have certain types of infections, such as bladder infections, and there is data on patients who have bedsores. Bladder infections can often be prevented by keeping a patient well-hydrated. A bed-ridden patient can often avoid bladder infections by being turned in bed to facilitate urination, and by being kept clean after urinating and having bowel movements. Bedsores usually come about from not being kept clean, nor turned from side to side in bed.

Federal ratings also involve the number of complaints filed. This information is often deceiving, since a lot of facilities don't get as many complaints as they should. If family members get fed up, they move their elders out and try some other place. You'll find that nursing homes that were for years highly rated, often slack off in care, to where they are now bad ones. However, their ratings haven't slid.

Ultimately, it's not what the government—federal or state long-term care office— says about a nursing home. It's what your individual elder ends up getting in a particular facility.

Even if a family member swears that his loved one got excellent care at a certain facility, that doesn't mean she did. Yes, go ahead and ask a family member you have located who had an elder at a certain facility. He may not have known what goes on there, though. After my mother's roommate at a facility died, I saw her daughter show up for the very first time in two months. She told me what wonderful care her mother had gotten. It's funny, I thought, that in my fourteen hours a day there in those two months,

I never saw the daughter. Perhaps she thought that just because her mother lived to be in her 90s, she must have been getting good care. That's not necessarily so, because some people survive anything. Even a family member's daily visit for an hour can reveal little. Unless a family member spends a few hours a day there, spread out over different shifts—morning, swing, and graveyard—he can come away with wrong assumptions. If you inquire of a family member who has had a loved one at a certain facility, be sure to ask how long his loved one was there, how long ago she was a patient there, and the frequency of the family member's visits. If, for example, his elder was at nursing home for just a few months, you can't always get a good indication of what the "long-term care" was like. One doesn't know if they often had a high turnover of staff, for example, thereby causing patients inconsistency in the level of care they were receiving.

Rehab vs. Long-Term Care Facilities

Consider, also, that at certain nursing homes, they may deal better with certain types of patients. For example, care for bedridden patients may not be as good at a rehab facility as it is for rehab patients. Ultimately, you never know until you find out firsthand when your family member gets there. When we first put our mother into a nursing home that was reputed to be top of the line in rehab and long-term care, we went there hoping that she would recover enough to make use of the rehab therapy. Being bedridden, she was ignored, and her condition plummeted whereby she wasn't able to be rehabilitated. Not being at a facility that specialized in long-term care, it had little equipment for bedridden patients, such as wheelchairs and no lifts to get the bedridden out of bed. Their nurses and nurse's aides didn't like caring for bedridden patients. If patients weren't well enough to benefit from rehab, they were considered vegetables, and treated that way. Nursing homes that are primarily rehab facilities try to make money off of providing speech, physical, and occupational therapy. If you've got a bedridden elder or one in the advanced stages of Alzheimer's, they are seen as not being able to benefit from these services. The patient is not seen as being profitable enough, and is ignored.

A long-term care facility doesn't have the rapid turn-over in patients that a rehab facility does. A rehab facility takes hospital discharges and patients come and go once they are rehabilitated. Consequently, your loved one might get better care at a long-term care facility if she is bedridden, because here the aides get used to the routine of caring for the same patients. It's possible that nurses and nurse's aides just might develop an attachment to their patients, and give better care to patients they've gotten used to.

A rehab facility usually appears more chaotic, with patients being admitted and discharged more often. Ambulances are often parked outside. Nurse's aides at a rehab facility see new patients coming in on a regular basis and have difficulty learning their individual needs. They are not well-oriented to each patient.

If your loved one has Alzheimer's or a related memory illness, perhaps he'd be better served in an assisted living facility or foster home. (Read Chapter 5, "Alternatives to Nursing Homes.") However, if you don't feel these would be acceptable, consider whether a nursing home would be equipped to handle him. Does it have an Alzheimer's Unit? Are the patients there given any freedom? Is everything done for them? Sometimes an Alzheimer's patient deteriorates more rapidly in a nursing home because the staff doesn't have the time to assist him in certain tasks like dressing, and they quickly do it for him. Or, if an Alzheimer's patient becomes incontinent, they don't have time to get him to the bathroom on a regular basis. They prematurely put him in diapers, so he doesn't have an "accident."

Further, if your loved one has Alzheimer's, are there enough activities for him at a nursing home? Are the other Alzheimer's patients drugged heavily, sitting in wheelchairs? Does the nursing home have door monitors? That is, if your loved one tries to escape, will the door not open because he is wearing a metal bracelet that prevents the door from opening for him? (If the facility doesn't have a separate Alzheimer's Unit that is kept locked, a patient can easily slip out of the doors of a facility, if a visitor enters and opens the door while he is trying to exit. I've seen this happen. Even if the patient is wearing a metal bracelet, if the door is opened by someone else, an alarm won't sound.)

Believe it or not, some nursing homes accept Alzheimer's patients but they say they don't want their patients to wear I.D. bracelets. They say it's a privacy issue. This is ridiculous, because who would go up to the patients and read their bracelets, except for the staff who need to know who they are. Without I.D. bracelets, medication errors can occur when agency or substitute nurses care for them who don't know who they are. Often the patients can't tell them their names. Often, policies at nursing homes make no sense.

Some nursing homes have Alzheimer's units with different levels of dementia. Ask them about these different levels, and what kind of independence patients are given at each level. Are they allowing them to walk or be confined to wheelchairs at certain levels? Ask them what their policies are about medicating patients. I would ask the latter to the director of nursing.

Corporate Nursing Homes

Nursing homes can be owned by corporations with stock traded on the New York Stock Exchange. These public companies make up about 20 percent of the nursing home industry. The chief executives of the big corporations are very well compensated. One nurse that I met at a non-profit nursing home told me she once worked at a nursing home owned by a very large corporation and that the patients got excellent care. Some believe, however, that profit is more of a priority with them than at other facilities. These corporate-owned nursing homes pay high salaries to administrators, and some believe patients often come away with less than they would normally get. In the early 1990s, as cash-strapped hospitals began sending their sicker patients to nursing homes, operators of some of these public companies turned to a Medicare loophole favoring nursing homes. There were no reimbursement caps on treatments such as respiratory, physical, and occupational therapies. Later, to cut soaring costs, Medicare instituted a new policy consisting of a daily price cap that in one fell swoop wiped out rehab margins by at least 50 percent. The blow to these public nursing home companies was catastrophic by the late 90s—those that had counted heavily on rehab services. However, the impact on privately-owned nursing homes, that is 80 percent of the industry, wasn't as bad, because they didn't count on the rehab business.

Today, some public companies are instituting big cost cuts, and some are facing debt. Some experts claim some public companies profited from Medicare, and are now paying the price.

Non-Profit Nursing Homes

So what about non-profit nursing homes—those that are religious-affiliated? Catholic? Jewish, etc.? The good thing is that they often get outside contributions, that they say they need to meet their costs. And, in contrast, profit-making institutions are often heavily taxed. Non-profit administrators don't have the large salaries that their profit-making counterparts do. Consequently, non-profits are commonly less expensive than for-profit nursing homes, but not by that much. The non-profits generally tend to be more generous with equipment, linens, towels, and blankets. This is what I noted. At one religious-affiliated nursing home my mother was at, each patient was assigned his own wheelchair. However, as far as care, non-profits often have the same problems other nursing homes do.

If they tell you they "love their patients," and give "superior" care at a religious-affiliated facility, don't necessarily believe them. You're inclined to think that this is their philosophy, however, the reality may be different. If you check out the care when your elder is there, you may realize that you're facing the same problems you faced at others, and that staff has a harder time admitting they can't deliver on their philosophy of care. Catholic and Jewish nursing homes often give priority to elders of that faith, but they accept everyone.

Visiting a Nursing Home

In selecting any nursing home, there may be something you can check out. If you read the Classified Want Ads under "Healthcare" in the newspaper you may discover something important. I noticed that there was a particular nursing home in town that was constantly advertising for nurses and nurse's aides. This signaled to me that it had a bad problem with staffing. High turnover of employees means your loved one will constantly have new nurses and nurse's aides working with her who don't know what her needs are. By the time they learn her needs, they quit and go someplace else.

I also noticed that the worst nursing home my mother was in was doing radio ads to lure patients. Because hospitals do so much dumping of patients, nursing homes usually have enough patients, so they don't need to advertise.

Before you place your loved one at any nursing home, you obviously must visit it. Try to visit three facilities to compare. In fact, make a few visits on different shifts. Day shift is 7 a.m. to 3 p.m., and evening shift is 3 to 11 p.m. On your first visit, try to make an appointment to see the administrator, and also while you're there, see if you can ask a few questions to the director of nursing. If she isn't available, call her later on the phone with questions.

In visiting nursing homes, you will often find an administrator dressed in a suit. If it's a Catholic nursing home, the administrator will most likely be a nun. You will see pleasant faces among the nurses and the nurse's aides. They are dressed professionally in white, of course. They may smile, be polite, and even shake your hand. But the question is, what is the care like? What goes on or doesn't go on behind closed doors with the patient?

Don't judge a nursing home by its manicured lawns and fancy lobby with antiques, or its wallpapered patients' rooms with tall plants in brass vases. Some do have these, despite being among the worst as far as care and attitudes of staff. Yes, some nursing homes look less institutional than others, and if so, are more pleasant to visit, but again, the primary concern is care, unless the distance is really far from you, such as an hour away from your home.

People do really extraordinary things to find what they feel is the best facility for their loved ones. At one nursing home my mother was in, she had an 86-year-old roommate, before she got a private room. We were to learn that her roommate's 86-year-old husband had taken his wife out of the same facility that our mother had transferred out of. This previous facility was only three blocks from his home. But for what he felt was better care at the new facility, he drove twelve miles round-trip in heavy traffic, twice a day, to feed his wife. He had bad eyesight and hearing, but he made it there!

When you visit a nursing home, if you called ahead of your visit, you probably won't notice any smells in the hall. Believe me, nursing homes smell most of the time, though administrators deny it. If you drop in unexpectedly and the place is a mess and smells, the receptionist will tell you that there is no one to show you around, or they'll make you wait until they can spruce up and spray air freshener along the hall they'll take you down. The air fresheners aren't really that. They are usually sprays with an ineffable institutional smell. I remember the smell was routinely bad at one facility my mother was at, so much so that I complained to the nurse. You couldn't walk down the hall without gagging. When I complained about the smell, she laughed and called me a wuss. However, I didn't see her venture down the hall. The state can fine nursing homes for excessive odors, but they don't. One hospital nurse who lives in my neighborhood, told me there's no excuse for the smells, and I know she's right. What nursing homes do is they clean up bedridden patients and place soiled diapers in barrels in the hall. (At one facility, they didn't even have barrels. They had a garbage bag with a lid over it that they hooked up to a wheeled device. Most unsanitary! I'm sure it was in violation of state rules.) Nursing homes that have the garbage barrels don't cart away the barrels for hours. Even in the winter, the aides just open all the windows in the patients' rooms, leaving some patients in their rooms directly in the cold, to air out the facility. The aides must think they are airing out the halls, too, when in fact, the barrels filled with waste are the source of the stench and they haven't been removed from the halls. All this accomplishes is that heat is wasted. The janitorial manager at one nursing home told me they waste thousands of dollars a year in heating which drives up nursing home costs. Of course, it leads to patients dying from pneumonia when the windows are left open. The professional staff walks down those frightfully cold halls and doesn't bother to close the windows or ask the aides to cart away the barrels. They seem oblivious to everything. It defies common sense. (The foul smells put off family members enough so that many don't want to visit and consequently, they don't see even greater problems there.) One woman who was dying in her room had the blowing cold from the open windows next to her bed. No nurse was attending her, as is often the case when patients are dying because nursing homes don't bother to put an extra nurse on duty to help. (This was also true of a Catholic facility my mother was at, incidentally.) Further, especially around meal time, for those who eat in their rooms, in a television room on their unit, or in the dining hall, it's certainly not very appetizing to eat close to halls that smell of stench.

When we took a tour of a nursing home with one administrator, we thought it might be a good facility since nurses and nurse's aides were bustling around, looking very busy. We thought they must be working hard. What we later found when we moved our mother in, was that the place was in total chaos. Too many patients, not enough staff. On the other hand, if you visit a facility that's very quiet, with staff standing around, that's bad, too. There shouldn't be staff standing around, since all nursing homes are short-staffed. There should be plenty of work to do.

Skilled vs. Intermediate Units

If a patient is discharged from the hospital, he first goes into skilled care at a nursing home, completely paid for by Medicaid, or Medicare and private insurance. In a skilled unit, there may be as many as 17 patients to one nurse at a private facility during day shift and evening shift. Some of these patients are at death's door. Seventeen patients for a nurse to handle is humanly impossible, yet this is what private facility skilled care is like. Skilled care for my mother lasted 100 days, and today she could still get this from her private insurance, if she were still alive. Once a patient's skilled benefits are used up, she pays for intermediate care. It's mind boggling, but intermediate care at a private facility with a private room often runs $225 a day or more. (Read the statistics in this book's Introduction.) In intermediate care, there is anywhere from 25 to 40 patients to one nurse on day and evening shifts. Usually about all a nurse can do is to pass out multiple medications to each patient and bandage bedsores that the patient has gotten from poor nurse's aide care. My brother and I often thought that since there was little care at the nursing home, we should check our mother into a nice hotel for the deluxe prices she was paying.

State laws often stipulate that a patient in a nursing home must be checked in on every two hours. That means, for example, that a nurse's aide should change the diaper of a bedridden patient and turn his body to the other side to avoid bedsores. However, even at the better facilities, one is lucky to be checked in on every three or four hours. Often, if a family member doesn't show up, a patient could go for eight hours without being attended to. The nurse, with her patient load, has no time to supervise or even check up on a nurse's aide. Often, nurse's aides are irresponsible and don't do their job.

Shockingly, at a Medicaid facility, there can be one nurse to 80 patients on day shift.

When you meet with the administrator of a nursing home, ask what the nurse to patient ratio is, and what the nurse's aide to patient ratio is. Beware that nursing home administrators will often tell you there are two nurses to 25 patients or two nurses to 40 patients on day shift, when in fact, the second nurse is the resident care manager who does just paperwork. I've seen the state's ratings for private nursing homes in my area. One year, the highest rating went to a private facility that had one nurse to 40 patients on day shift, when there were private facilities with much better nurse to patient ratios, such as one nurse to 25 patients. It's hard to judge the ratings.

On graveyard shift, at a private facility, a nurse usually has anywhere from 40 to 80 patients. The graveyard shift nurse at the last facility my mother was in had 80 patients, and she told me that one-third of them needed her care with medications and feeding tube nutrition during the night.

As for the nurse's aide to patient ratio at a private facility, on day shift, when most of the care needs to be done, you'll find anywhere from seven to eight patients to a nurse's aide. The aide on this shift is supposed to give a sponge bath to each patient, get the patient dressed, help him into a wheelchair, and feed him at noon. On swing shift, (evening shift), at a private facility, each aide may have as many as fourteen patients. The aide must deal with incontinent care, feed each patient dinner, and get him ready for bed. On graveyard shift at a private facility, each aide can have as many as 20 patients to which she gives incontinent care, changing diapers and turning bedridden patients from side to side.

As you can see, day shift has the best ratio for care, and graveyard shift has the worst ratio for care.

When you first visit a nursing home, try to visit in the morning when most of the care that a patient will get should be given. At 7:30 a.m. or 8 a.m., the patients are fed and at 9 a.m., they are given sponge baths. So, by 10 a.m., you should see patients dressed with their hair combed and men shaven, sitting in wheelchairs around the facility. If you see a lot of patients sitting in bed at 10 a.m. or even 11 a.m., this is a bad sign. Don't let the staff tell you that the person is bedridden and doesn't get out of bed. Bedridden people, in particular, should be moved and gotten into a wheelchair at least for a few hours each day to exercise their lungs. If bedridden and ambulatory patients aren't gotten out of bed, the nursing home is a real warehouse, and you're better off caring for them at home or putting them in a foster home for less money.

Is the nursing home noisy? At one nursing home my mother was at, they had an intercom system just like a hospital with staff being paged every minute from 8 a.m. to 5 p.m. This was very annoying. In contrast, at the next nursing home my mother was at, the professional staff carried around pocket phones, so the receptionist could dial them up individually. After business hours, here, you could dial up your loved one's unit to speak to a nurse. And in an emergency with a patient, the nurse could dial 9-1-1 or talk to a doctor without running back and forth to the nurse's station to use the phone or wait for the doctor's call, leaving the patient unattended. (If a nurse doesn't carry a pocket phone, then after 5 p.m., if you want to reach a nurse, you have to catch her when she happens to be at the nurse's station.)

Nursing Home Management

What you will find in talking to an administrator of a nursing home is that he / she seems to have a different view of what really goes on there than what the staff has. You'll hear about "loving care," and "The patients are our extended family." You'll hear this in particular at a religious-affiliated nursing home. While we found individual staff members who were truly genuine people and did care about their patients, there were others who worked there because they couldn't find jobs doing anything else. For example, some nurse's aides didn't speak or understand English very well. This can, and often does, endanger a patient who needs care such as that of a feeding tube. Patients with feeding tubes need to have certain precautions taken in working with them. (This will be covered in Chapter 4, "The Feeding Tube Fiasco.")

Since turnover of staff is high—especially with nurse's aides who are paid minimum wage or not much higher—ask the administrator what kind of continuity of care there is. If the patient is at the nursing home for six months or more, can she expect many new staff members to come in?

Ask him how long, on average, do their nurses, aides, and director of nursing stay? At one facility I visited, there had been a new director of nursing each year for the past three years. Something was obviously wrong. You should also ask the administrator if they often call upon agencies for staffing. If so, this signals lack of staff, or staff often being absent.

A nursing home administrator will often dance around the question of staff turnover. He will tell you they have several staff who've been there for years. While it may be true that some have worked there long-term, most nurse's aides stay six months. And, most nurses stay a year.

Two hospice nurses I met, after my mother left the last nursing home, told me that they noted there was very little difference between "good" and "bad" nursing homes. This is true because all fail to give the basic care they promise. One of these hospice nurses started her career at a nursing home and left a few months later. She said, "You start out at a nursing home upbeat and excited about doing a good job, just like the nurse's aides. Then, after a few months, you get discouraged because you realize you have so many patients that you can't do your very best."

At the first private nursing home my mother was at, believe it or not, many of the family members hired private aides for their elders, on top of paying thousands of dollars each month to the nursing home. In fact, a few aides at the nursing home were telling family members that they had too much work and that their loved ones were too much of a burden to them. Of course, the administrator and resident care managers knew their staff was saying this, and they obviously knew about the hiring of private aides. They felt no shame. Worse, the administrator said he would "provide" private aides for a price. Aides on their days off could work privately and the nursing home would get a cut of what they were paid. Then, you wonder, what, if anything, the nursing home is doing to earn the thousands of dollars a month you pay. Is it just for a nurse to pass medications and a roof over your loved one's head? It seems illegal to double dip, doesn't it? At least if you're hiring private aides, why should the nursing home that isn't doing its job take even more from you?

The hiring of private aides goes on with family members at many nursing homes. A family friend who had his mother at another private nursing home had to do the same for her. (When he tried home care for her, it was hard to find adequate aides to staff his mother's home 'round the clock, even with the help of a home health service. He would alternate. He would take her out of one nursing home, bring her home, put her in another nursing home, bring her home, etc. Nothing worked, neither home care nor nursing home care. I will discuss this more in Chapter 5, "Alternatives to Nursing Homes," because it can work under certain circumstances.)

When my mother was in skilled care, getting free benefits, we hired private aides to sit with her when I wasn't there. The private aides I hired on my own were there to monitor the nursing home's aide care, remind the nurse's aides to care for my mother, and brief them on what needed to be done for her. Again, the professional staff at nursing homes doesn't have the time to monitor their aides. We even hired a registered nurse, a family friend, to stop in one hour a day (that's all she had time for) to check my mother's condition and do range of motion exercises with her, on top of the range of motion exercises I was doing with my mother.

When I told an elder law attorney I knew about the hiring of private aides to supplement care at nursing homes, he said it didn't surprise him. He knew it went on at nursing homes. He said he didn't recommend any nursing homes in the area to clients.

As far as staffing, nursing home administrators won't admit they are short-staffed, when you first go to visit them.

Later, when your elder is there, and you complain of care problems, they will blame it on staffing problems. (I knew an aide who worked at a hospital and later came to work for me through an agency, when I took my mother out of the nursing home for good. She said her nurse supervisor at the hospital would tell nurse's aides they weren't even allowed to say they were short-staffed. Her supervisor said they were "optimally staffed.")

Beware of nursing homes that are long on administrative staffs and short on "care" staff. At the first nursing home my mother entered, the rehab facility, the administrator and assistant administrator wore nice suits and there were a lot of social workers who didn't work with families to resolve care issues, but who worked with hospitals on discharging patients and sending them to their facility. There were enough bookkeepers, too.

In considering a nursing home, ask the administrator what kind of care they pride themselves for. If he says "rehab," then maybe their long-term care for patients, whom they feel can't be rehabilitated, isn't good. When we told the administrator at the first nursing home, that we were taking our mother out of there, we reiterated to him that care issues had never been resolved for my mother in her bedridden condition. He then told us what he hadn't admitted before. That is, that he felt they were a good rehab facility, and that "You can't be everything to everybody." When you first go talk to any administrator, he will lead you to believe otherwise, just to get your business. (It should be noted that many nursing homes don't provide care for patients on respirators because they require too much monitoring.)

In meeting with the administrator, discuss what particular care your loved one requires and ask for an honest answer if that kind of care can be delivered. In asking this question, it's helpful if the director of nursing (DNS) is present, too, or the assistant director of nursing. If the administrator is not a nurse, she may not know the details of care involved. Often, administrators say their facility can handle any patient, just to fill up their beds. The DNS may be a little more truthful. If your loved one is presently at another nursing home, tell them what problems you've encountered there, and ask if they have those problems, too. Or, ask how they are able to prevent those problems.

Realize that when a nursing home administrator or DNS says they provide excellent care or superior care, this is an impossibility at any institution. The patients who are nursing home candidates are the type who need anywhere from extensive to private attention. This type of care isn't possible to offer at a nursing home that delivers a few minutes of care every three or four hours at best.

The DNSes I've known are often less than truthful about their facilities. I knew a DNS at a religious-affiliated facility that told me their nurse's aide care was always rated as excellent by the state. In reality, two months prior to that, the state classified their aide care as "substandard," and the facility lost its privileges to train nurse's aides for certification. It had been highly-rated before. When you consider that the state already has minimal standards for care, rating a facility substandard, reveals just how substandard it is.

Although when you visit a nursing home, the management will be on its best behavior, it's better than not speaking to them at all. If you can, ask to speak with the resident care manager of the unit they will most likely put your elder on. She does the paperwork and often gives instructions to the nurse on the floor. She's supposed to draw up a written care plan for each patient. You want to determine what her attitudes are like towards patients in your loved one's condition.

If your loved one is bedridden, when you visit a nursing home, you should ask the DNS, in particular, if they have problems with bedsores. I remember at the first nursing home my mother entered, the resident care manager bragged that none of the patients had bedsores. She was either a smiling liar or a delusional psychotic. After we moved our mother in there, we overheard nurses talking about some of the patients with bedsores "down to the bone." A special dermatology nurse would make visits. We also learned from a nurse there that state inspectors usually don't shut down a facility unless there is something severe like murder, repeated overt abuse, conditions that have caused injuries to patients, or conditions that threaten life. For example, with the latter, if patients slip and fall on wet floors and break their bones, then maybe a facility will be shut down for a few months. They could even lose their Medicare or Medicaid funding. However, federal regulators hardly ever crack down on nursing homes. If a nursing home does lose Medicare or Medicaid funding, it can later regain it if it corrects its violations. Inspectors don't like to shut down facilities because there is often no place to transfer all the patients to. One of the honest nurses we knew told us that even with bedsores down to the bone, inspectors don't shut down nursing homes. At worst, they'll be fined. Or, they will monitor the nursing home and tell staff that if they don't remedy the problems, they will lose their privilege to accept new patients. Bedsores occur with bedridden patients who are not kept clean and their bodies aren't turned in bed. This nurse told me that antibiotics for bedsores often weaken patients. They can then come down with some affliction and die.

Don't accept the explanation from management that bedsores are always caused by poor circulation. They often try to blame the patient for their shabby care.

In chatting with management, they should acknowledge that they go through good and bad periods of care. This may last a few months at a time, when they hire new aides who may not have learned the ropes, may not be performing well, and not be cleaning up patients. This obviously

won't sit too well with family members who, in the meantime, are paying tens of thousands of dollars for either care
that isn't being delivered on time or is being done so poorly
as to infect the patient. However, if management admits to
having periods of rough times with care, at least it's an
admission.

Another question for management is whether they have
certified nurse's aides who also are certified medication
aides who are allowed to dispense medications. I would
definitely not place a loved one at a facility that allows this.
Statistics show that it's not uncommon for nurses to make
mistakes with medication. Can you imagine someone who
often has no more than a high school education and isn't
even good at giving personal care, handling medications?

Beware, also, that at some nursing homes, they sometimes hire nurse's aides who are untrained and not yet certified to do nurse's aide work. If they have nurse's aides
who are not certified, ask management if they work with
bedridden patients, (if your loved one is bedridden), and
how long it will be before the aides become certified. Even
certified nurse's aides (CNAs) have difficulty providing
adequate and clean care for the bedridden.

Often when you visit management prior to placing your
loved one at the nursing home, they will tell you your loved
one's specific needs are "no problem" for their staff to carry
out. After your loved one has been admitted, however, excuses are found by another professional staff member not
to carry out these specific needs. For example, before we
placed our mother at the first nursing home, the administrator told us that it would be no problem for our mother
to be lifted into a wheelchair two times a day as the doctor
would order. The administrator assured us that doctor's
orders would be followed. However, the resident care manager on the unit they placed our mother in, obviously felt it
was too much trouble to do so. She said that it really wasn't
any more beneficial to lift our mother into a wheelchair to

exercise her lungs that to just elevate the back of her bed. When we complained to our mother's doctor and asked him to call and reiterate that the nursing home do this, despite his efforts, the resident care manager didn't comply. My mother fell prey to pneumonia, then to lung embolisms, and almost died. Perhaps if we'd gotten the ombudsman involved, we could have gotten the resident care manager to change her tune. However, at the time, we were trying to get other care issues resolved, and we felt we couldn't harp on every issue with them. We felt we had to trust the resident care manager's judgment and that she wouldn't harm a patient. As it turned out, she was both an ignorant nurse and she didn't care about our mother. We later found out, that she was always talking behind our backs about how our mother shouldn't be alive.

Perhaps after you visit a nursing home, and before placing your loved one there, write a letter to the administrator going over the care points he agreed on, and copy the DNS and the resident care manager. This way, if they later decide they don't want to carry out the care they promised, you can show the ombudsman your letter, besides having the doctor's order in place. They not only didn't follow doctor's orders, but they deceived a family member by initially promising care that they didn't want to provide.

After my mother had the lung embolisms, they did start getting her up in her chair. While a doctor can't say with certainty that my mother with her brain injury, wouldn't have gotten lung embolisms anyway, not moving her body out of bed certainly wasn't good for her. This shows that nursing homes can hardly ever be liable for lack of care. This facility, incidentally, had only one lifting machine. It was not the type of lift my mother needed. She needed a hoyer lift. When they finally agreed to getting my mother out of bed and into a wheelchair, since they didn't have a hoyer lift, they unsafely lifted her out of bed by rolling her on to a bedsheet and rounding up four aides to grab hold of each corner of the sheet. She was then transferred to a stretcher that folded up into wheelchair position. If one aide had dropped his corner of the sheet, my mother would have been injured. Even more ridiculous and unsafe, one day two aides, right in front of me, told me they could lift her on their own. They rolled her onto the bedsheet, flipped her body off the sheet about six inches into the air, and caught her before transferring her into the wheelchair. What if the bedsheet had torn when it caught her? I told them never to do it again. Incidentally, this was the most expensive nursing home in town, and it had the least equipment.

Besides care issues, ask management about equipment your loved one needs. If your elder is bedridden, make certain they have enough wheelchairs and hoyer lifts so they can't use the excuse that your loved one can't get out of bed because the equipment is already being used by other patients.

At another facility my mother was at, each patient was given her own wheelchair. This works well so that germs aren't transferred from one incontinent patient to another. Recognize that aides and housekeeping staff are not religious about disinfecting equipment before another patient uses it.

The facility should have shower chairs so patients aren't given showers sitting in a wheelchair, as a substitute. (They did this to my mother once when she was hospitalized.)

Surprisingly, most nursing homes don't have air conditioning. When you ask about whether they have it, they'll often respond, "We'll get it this summer." What we found was that this was equivalent to "The check's in the mail." Usually, during the summer months, they'll keep the doors propped open, so the flies and bees come in. And, if it turns drafty in the early evening hours, they don't close the doors for the patients' sake. The staff is overheated from moving around and working with patients, so they don't realize that it may be drafty for the patient.

One nurse who worked at a nursing home told me that before she went to work there, she thought all nursing homes had air conditioning, since elders can die from heat and dehydration. Why isn't it a law? Air conditioning should at least be available in the halls to aid staff. Some patients don't like it in their rooms, so it should be able to be regulated to the "off" position in each room. Further, nursing home room windows should open easily and should have screens.

A lot of nursing homes are lacking in the basics. Their linen and towel supply is minimal. They really run into problems when a washing machine breaks down, as sometimes happens. The chemical-smelling stained towels were so bad at one nursing home, the most expensive one, that I brought towels from home. When they use face washcloths to wipe all areas of the body including rear ends and urinary areas, of course these get stained, and they need to heap on the bleach.

In addition to these basics, you should also consider if food is available in between meals, should a patient become hungry. At one nursing home my mother was at, they had a kitchenette in each unit with a refrigerator. It had some sandwiches, juice, cookies, pudding, and ice cream for snacks or just in case a patient wasn't hungry at lunch or dinner and later got hungry.

Private Rooms vs. Shared Rooms

As for accommodations at a nursing home, should you place your loved one in a private room, double room, four-bed room?

After my mother was discharged from the hospital, she entered the skilled care unit at the nursing home. Her stay was covered for 100 days by Medicare and her private insurance for a shared room with one other patient. We tried to get her into a private room as soon as possible. It took about two weeks. In the meantime, we arranged with the nursing home to be billed for the difference in price between a shared room and a private room. Often, private rooms are not available, so the patient spends a few weeks or even a few months in a shared room. If you're persistent and pay your bills on time, they'll accomodate you. The pluses of a private room are that one doesn't catch the germs of a roommate, and one doesn't smell the odors of incontinence of another patient. Also, if a patient shares a room, nurse's aides have been known to confuse the patient's personal possessions with the other patient's. This happens even if the possessions are clearly marked. A really gross error occurred in my mother's case when she first shared a room. The aide used my mother's roommate's toothbrush on her! (Actually, the aide didn't even know my mother wasn't supposed to be using a toothbrush, just tooth sponges, because of her swallowing difficulties. Tooth sponges are just used to swab a patient's mouth.) After the mistake, we cleaned my mother's mouth with peroxide. Again, frail and elderly patients in facilities often get sick and die due to the errors of staff. When it happens, no one discovers the real cause. It's just due, they say, to "old age."

A friend of mine told me his father had a roommate in a nursing home. Both he and his roommate were helped out of bed at the same time. When each was returned to bed, the aide got them confused and put each back into his roommate's bed. His father's roommate had defecated in his bed and the sheets weren't even removed. Consequently, his father ended up in the contaminated bed of his roommate. Beyond this grossness, if a substitute nurse had been on duty that day, she would have confused the patients who often don't wear wristbands, and given each the wrong medication.

As in hospitals, nursing home patients who have roommates who acquire communicable diseases like pneumonia usually end up catching their germs. The staff won't remove the healthy patient from the room. My mother caught a roommate's lung infection years before when she was in the hospital trying to recover from her brain cancer surgery. I took her home at that time with the added burden of trying to cure her lung infection. I had asked the hospital nurses to move her into one of the many vacant rooms they had, but they didn't. At nursing homes, if they have vacant rooms, they won't do this, either. Therefore, if your loved one will share a room, ask if the roommate has a history of colds and pneumonia. If so, ask for another roommate.

As far as a private room vs. shared room, a friend of mine had a different take in institutionalizing his father. He felt patients in private rooms are forgotten about, and that it is less easy for staff to forget two patients in the same room. I told him I didn't see his logic, because I thought most patients were neglected anyway. In a double room, perhaps there is less chance of abuse, if one has a roommate who is somewhat alert. However, most patients are drugged up and not very aware. It should be noted that husbands and wives are often not permitted to share the same room. A private room with private full bath can run $225 or more a day. A private room with a private toilet and sink can run $220 or more a day; and a private room with a shared toilet and sink with the adjoining room can run about $215 a day or more. A double room can run about $210 a day or more. A four-bed room can run $205 a day or more.

Consider, too, that it's helpful to have a room close to the nurse's station where the nurse frequently walks past the room, in the event that your loved one is in distress.

Other Costs

Residents are classified by the level of care they need. For example, there are additional charges of about $150 a month for catheter care. About $250 a month is charged for feeding tube care. While your elder's insurance will cover feeding tube formula and related supplies, the patient foots the nursing home bill for the nurse to administer the tube feedings which basically involves hooking the patient up to the formula and flushing his tube with water after-wards—simple tasks. If, for example, a patient is "severely disoriented," and needs such services as catheter care and "more supervision," he is charged $200 a month extra. "More supervision" means the nurse spends more time on medication issues, such as evaluating the patient and con-ferring on the phone with the doctor to subdue the patient with medication. Sometimes, nursing homes have flat fees based on classifying a patient as being at level 1, 2, or 3, meaning from being fairly self-sufficient to totally depen-dent and bedriddden.

Some nursing homes charge extra for doing personal laundry. Some charge extra for having an aide feed a pa-tient. The latter is ridiculous, since many nursing home patients are there simply because they need assistance with feeding themselves.

It's becoming more and more so that the room fee cov-ers room and food, and much of the care is becoming an extra charge. It's interesting that a patient who is on a feed-ing tube and gets free formula and feeding tube supplies through her insurance, doesn't get some adjustment on her bill, considering the fact she isn't eating nursing home food.

There is also an initial charge of about $250 for the nurse to do an assessment when the patient enters the nursing home. This involves looking over the patient's body and charting her general condition. They note skin problems and other health problems, for example.

The room rates also don't include inhalation therapy (oxygen), medication, or supplies such as diapers and la-tex gloves for the aides to use in working with the patient. These are billed extra each month. It's not unusual for the aides to make mistakes in recording usage of supplies. At most facilities, you have the option of bringing in personal care products such as diapers, soap, toothpaste, shampoo, etc. This is cheaper than having the nursing home bill you, particularly if you buy in bulk from discount stores.

At non-profit, private facilities, after about three years of being a paying customer, if a patient runs out of money and has no assets, they may let her stay as a charity case on Medicaid. Often 20 percent of their patients are Medicaid patients. (Consequently, one doesn't have to transfer to a Medicaid facility that is even more short-staffed.) However, I'm sure that if family members complained about their loved one's care, the administrator wouldn't want to give the patient a free ride.

At nursing homes, patients often run out of money or get behind on paying. In figuring out rent, I'm sure management factors in this loss. Therefore the "rich" patients end up paying more and sometimes get care that most people don't even want for free.

Waiting Lists to Enter

All things considered, if you want to get your loved one into a nursing home, and there is a waiting list, oftentimes placing phone calls each week to the social worker there will keep them focused on your need, so they won't forget about you.

If your loved one is discharged from the hospital, and her insurance covers skilled nursing care for a limited time at a facility you don't like, if you can afford it, place your relative in another facility and pay for it. There's no sense in letting your loved one go downhill in a facility that is unsuitable.

When you place your loved one in a nursing home, it might not be a bad idea to keep checking out other nursing homes. Perhaps it's a good idea to put him on a waiting list at another one in case the present one doesn't work out. If he's not ready to go in when you're called, tell them to drop your loved one down a little further on the list.

At the last nursing home we put our mother into, we actually bribed her way into it. The previous nursing home would have probably killed our mother from neglect, so we were desperate to find another. This last nursing home was a non-profit religious-affiliated facility that had a long reputation as being the best rated. For three months, we hounded the administrator and were told that there were no openings because there were no deaths out of 126 patients. I really doubt this was true. She also said there was a waiting list. I then took action. I sent a $250 contribution to the administrator telling her that we had always supported religious institutions. A few days later, the waiting list mysteriously evaporated, and they called with an opening for our mother. Connect the dots! Bribery does work at non-profit institutions. They like contributions. This facility wasn't too much better that the others at the time she entered it. And, at the time we took her out, it was terrible. Again, reputations and ratings mean little in the nursing home business. It is a business, not healthcare. Recognize, too, that it means little to you if most of the patients are receiving good care. All that matters is what kind of care your loved one is receiving. As time went on, and our complaints became more frequent, the social worker told us what we'd heard at other facilities: "If you don't like the care here, go someplace else." During the time my mother was there, if my mother was receiving good care, we'd often make a contribution of $100 at holiday time. We'd enclose a note to the administrator with our thanks for the staff's efforts. Later as care dwindled and became downright wretched, we began complaining to the social worker. That's when she said we could place our mother elsewhere. Needless to say, our contributions stopped, and we eventually took our mother home.

This brings me to another point. Sometimes people feel, even if they are not religious themselves, that it's helpful to place their loved one in a religious-affiliated institution run by the clergy. They feel that they and their loved ones can get some emotional and spiritual support from having the clergy greet them. Frankly, in the religious-affiliated facilities my mother was at, we found the clergy to be pretty aloof. I felt, however, that the other family members we got to know were helpful to talk to and get some support from.

Incidentally, if your loved one is already at a nursing home and you want to put her at another one, if you've gotten to know some good aides and nurses at the present nursing home, you can ask them questions about some other nursing homes they've worked at. Nursing home staff tends to move around from one to another. Ask them what was good and bad about the other nursing homes.

Dumping Patients

It should also be noted that although nursing homes like to fill their rooms, they may dump patients, particularly those whose families harp on them for care they promised that isn't being delivered. They may say the family member is mistreating staff or disrupting their routine. They would have to give 30 days notice and give a legitimate reason. For example, if you had a loved one with Alzheimer's, and you didn't want them to heavily drug him, but he was trying to escape, they'd say they couldn't keep him. This could be a valid reason. Or, at some point, if your loved one stopped swallowing and the facility didn't offer feeding tube care, but you wanted your loved one to get a feeding tube, that would be a valid reason to dump him. Usually they try to keep patients for as long as they can do the absolute minimum for them, as long as the patients can be controlled through medication, and as long as the family members don't complain much.

Remember that at nursing homes the rule of relativity applies. They really are rated not by how good they are, but if they aren't as bad as the others. This is how the government judges them when it comes right down to it. Further, if you complain to staff and they get off of their "We're an excellent facility" jag, they sometimes finally admit their shortcomings and say, "We might have some problems, but we're not as bad as the others." They don't really realize what they are saying. It's as if I, as a teacher said, "I've taught at schools with bad teachers, but our school doesn't have as many bad teachers as the others, so we're a good school."

Checklist of Other Things to Consider

Finally, here is a checklist of other basic things to consider in selecting a nursing home:
- Is the facility certified for Medicare or for Medicaid?
- Is the nursing home licensed, regulated, and inspected by the state for the particular level of care your loved one needs?
- Does the nursing home allow visitors 24-hour access? (Many do, if the patient is in a private room, and there won't be a disturbance to other patients.)
- Does the staff communicate with patients by name?
- Are patients lined up in the halls or sitting in their rooms being ignored by staff?
- Are there private areas for family members to visit with physicians who come, so that they are not discussing sensitive issues in front of the patient?
- Does the nursing home have a policy on restricting the use of physical restraints?
- Can the physical therapy services benefit your loved one?
- Can the speech therapy services benefit your loved one?
- Can the occupational therapy services benefit your loved one? (Services involving daily skills such as dressing oneself).
- How often does a registered dietician visit? Does

the facility prepare physician-ordered therapeutic diets?

- Are meals served in an appealing way? Do they serve a lot of foods that don't have much nutritional value—hot dogs, fries, baloney sandwiches? (You'll see these at some.)
- Are handrails in the hall and grab bars in the bathroom secure?
- Do call lights actually light up?
- Are there sturdy and comfortable chairs in rooms?
- Do they offer a lot of activities, and are all patients transported to them? (Ask to see a calendar of activities, and attend one. If they have a full-time activities director, then you know that all activities listed will take place. At one nursing home my mother was at, there was a variety of enjoyable activities, such as musical programs that every patient liked.)

On a final note, the topsy-turvy world of institutional care is often mind-boggling. We knew the DNS at one nursing home our mother was at, who ran one of the "best" facilities, according to state ratings. In reality, many patients were plagued with horrible bedsores there, because the aide care was so bad and patients were lying in urine-soaked beds for entire eight-hour shifts. This DNS left the facility, and a year later, became an independent consultant to nursing homes. The state recommended her as a consultant to nursing homes that it had deemed "substandard" in care.

Chapter 2

Understanding The Routine at Nursing Homes and Solving Problems

Nurse's Aide Care

When you place a loved one in a nursing home, you know he won't get private care, but you will probably assume that the care from a nurse will be the most important part of the care. This is not necessarily true. Nursing homes operate on the premise that the nurse's aides will be doing most of the care that one receives. The care is intended to be custodial care, not so much professional care. As stated before, when one nurse has anywhere from 25 to 40 patients (or even 80 patients in a Medicaid facility), what kind of professional care can one expect to get?

Further, as discussed before, many of the problems requiring attention from a nurse arise due to the uncleanliness of the staff, resulting in infections.

If you ask a doctor what the worst problems are in a nursing home, she will tell you that skin breakdown is high on the list. We know the state often dictates that nurse's aides need to check on patients every two hours to change diapers, for example, and yet with the aides not being supervised or monitored by staff, a patient will often go for four hours or more without attention. Most patients who are in nursing homes have problems with incontinence. Frequent urination is worse with a bedridden patient who receives just tube feeding formula to sustain life. She is always urinating.

If an incontinent person isn't kept clean every two hours, skin breakdown can result. What is especially disheartening is to find that often nurse's aides go on the assumption that if they slather a patient's skin with skin barrier creams or cover the inside of a patient's diaper with powder, that this can help prevent skin breakdown. Barrier creams are supposed to be used sparingly, perhaps a couple times a day. Nurses in hospitals and nursing homes often get a doctor's order for these creams so that when patients urinate in their diaper, the cream acts as a shield for the skin. Use of barrier creams is really an admission that the patient isn't being kept clean. Further, if one is kept clean, barrier creams don't need to be used at all. Frequent use of creams is bad for the skin, wearing the skin down. Barrier creams, when used a lot by the aides, cost the patient about $75 a month or more. As for loading layers of baby powder on a diaper, this does nothing to prevent skin irritation when a patient urinates without being changed for hours.

What is particularly hard for family members is the all too common problem of finding a loved one lying in a bed soaked with urine, or finding his ambulatory elder sitting in a chair with his clothes soaked with urine. One assumes he hasn't been checked on for hours. However, when you complain to a nurse, a common response is that he urinated just after his diaper was last changed two hours ago.Therefore, he unfortunately sat in urine for two hours. You can accept this argument if you want. Realistically, if you repeatedly find your loved one soaked in urine, you know this argument "doesn't wash." (No pun intended!) As for a bedridden patient, part of changing his diaper also involves the routine of repositioning his body from side to side so he doesn't get bedsores. For example, if the patient is lying on his right side, the next time he is changed, he should be positioned on his left side. If you want to do a test of whether your loved one is being regularly changed, then arrive every three hours (give the aides a grace period of an hour), and see if your loved one has been changed and turned in three hours.

At the first nursing home my mother was at, we had to complain repeatedly that we were finding her soaked in urine, and that she was developing rashes and sores on her skin. After listening to the resident care manager's usual excuse, that my mother must be urinating just after the aide left the room, we asked the resident care manager to post a sign-in schedule in my mother's room and have each aide sign in to show that she had been regularly changed. Of course, you say, the aide could "doctor up" the schedule so if he missed a few hours, on his next visit, he could sign in and fill in the missing time slot. However, as we found, in checking on our mother, there were missing slots on the schedule when aides completely forgot to come in. Therefore, we proved our point to the resident care manager.

While nursing homes that charge "deluxe" prices claim individualized care, nothing could be farther from the truth. For example, if you find that an aide has changed your elder's diaper and cleaned her up, but ten minutes later, your loved one urinates, you can't expect the aide to come back in and change the patient again. Your elder must wait at least another hour and fifty minutes. Being short-staffed, the aide needs to go on to the other patients. Therefore, the family member ends up changing the patient if he is around.

The majority of care that a bedridden patient should get in a nursing home involves being wiped clean before a new diaper is changed, and being turned in bed at regular intervals. The question is, will the nursing home do it? The answer is often no, unless you, as a family member, are there to constantly monitor staff. As a bedridden patient who can't speak, your loved one could conceivably get no care on any given shift, outside of the nurse delivering medication or giving feeding tube formula, if he has a feeding tube.

The methods that aides use to clean up a patient often do more harm than good. What we first saw when my mother was in the hospital, and later saw at nursing homes, is that aides often dirty the washcloths before cleaning up a patient, if they use washcloths at all. In between a daily or twice daily sponging of the patient's urinary and bowel area (morning and evening), diaper wipes are used to clean up incontinence. Beware that alcohol-based wipes often cause irritation to a patient's skin. Aloe-based wipes are better, but really wipes of any kind are often harsh on bedridden patients, especially "tube feeders" who take in only feeding tube formula and urinate frequently. Ideally, an aide, in between sponge baths, should use a terrycloth washcloth when changing a diaper, one with soap and another one to rinse the urinary and bowel areas. Then, he should dry those areas with hand towels.

When aides use washcloths, they often throw them into the sink to get them wet. I have witnessed aides do this even in front of nurses who said nothing to them about this uncleanly habit. To wet a washcloth, it is so simple just to hold it under the faucet. Or, it is easy to drop it into a plastic sponge bath tub to be filled with water. Oftentimes, nurses and nursing supervisors don't want to correct aides at the expense of patients catching infections.

Too often, aides don't wash their hands in going from patient to patient, or they merely splash water on their hands. Then, they often don't wear latex gloves in cleaning up a patient's body including his private parts.

I was shocked to observe the uncleanly routine at nursing homes that were touted for decades by the state and the community as being the best. They'd "clean up" my mother just by merely wiping her off after urinating and defecating. If they did wear latex gloves, they didn't immediately remove them after cleaning her. With dirty gloves, they would touch bedrails, doorknobs, the wheel-chair, and the handles of the hoyer lift to prepare to get her out of bed. The transferring of filth from her body to things in her room was obviously not a common sense thing to do. Often the aides would put on gloves before cleaning the patient, but then go out of the room and get a wheel-chair and a hoyer lift with their clean gloves, wheel those in, thereby dirtying their gloves before even working on the patient. Hoyer lift handles and wheelchair handles were not disinfected. I did see bedrails being cleaned about once every six months. When I reported this uncleanliness to nurses, they would be angry with me.

Despite my constant washing of my hands at the nurs-ing home, and wearing latex gloves, I got 40 warts on my two hands, which I had to be treated for by a dermatolo-gist. The place was filthy. If a healthy person such as I, could get warts, colds and flu, that I never got before my mother was institutionalized, how is an older, frail person going to fare?

Further, while nursing homes often blame bedsores on the frail patient who is unable to even wiggle around in bed, if the bedridden patient is turned from one side to another every two hours, and is cleaned up so that she doesn't sit in urine or in feces, bedsores can usually be avoided. Perhaps, the patient who has bad skin or bad cir-culation is the exception.

Bedsores can eat deep into someone's flesh. Bedsores can be horrifying to look at. Besides bedsores in nursing homes, I was told by a good nurse who became my friend there, that yeast infections were also common at nursing homes. She said yeast infections were so common there, that many nurses would ignore them. My mother devel-oped a variety of yeast infections.

Many nurses will also blame yeast infections on the immobility of a bedridden patient. More often, yeast infec-tions occur due to the uncleanliness of staff. I believe you can't teach cleanliness to an adult if she didn't grow up practicing cleanliness. My mother didn't have yeast infections before she entered the hospital and nursing homes. In being institutionalized, she would get yeast infections in between her thighs, for example, not being cleaned up regularly after urinating. At my request, the nurse would call the doctor to get prescription creams to treat them. The nurses wouldn't do anything about them, otherwise. (Of course, these creams would lead to further expense for us, in addition to skin barrier creams.) It should be noted that nurses often felt they were too busy to apply the prescription creams to treat a yeast infection. They would ask the nurse's aides to do it, which technically they shouldn't be doing because it was a prescription treatment. The aides didn't understand that the creams needed to be used sparingly, nor were they shown where to apply them.

One nurse's aide who told me she wanted to become a surgical nurse would spread creams around my mother's urinary areas with her bare hands. At least if the nurses didn't want to take the time to apply the creams, they could have instructed the aides on how to do it. At one other nursing home, the nurse actually asked me to apply the prescription creams.

It wasn't uncommon to see nurse's aides wipe up floors using terrycloth washcloths intended for patient use. They could have easily used paper towels. What particularly shocked me is that after one aide wiped up the floor with a washcloth, she proceeded to give a sponge bath to my mother using that same terrycloth towel. I objected, and I went out of the room to get a clean towel.

If nurse's aides spot bedsores or yeast infections on the skin, they sometimes don't bother to report the problems to nurses. I knew only one nurse in my mother's years at nursing homes who took the time to pull the sheets back in bed and check a patient's body for skin problems each day. She ended up leaving the facility after less than a year to work at a hospital. Most nurses at nursing homes enter a patient's room to give medications and then walk out. I knew a doctor from my mother's doctor's office who made visits every six months to his patient at the nursing home where my mother was at. One day he came in and stood outside my mother's room to wait for the nurse to come out. He told the nurse plainly and firmly that his patient had a bedsore. He waited for her to respond. She said nothing. Apparently, the nurse didn't even know. He then proceeded to give her instructions on what to do. I noticed that nurses often stare blankly at a family member or someone else who reports a care problem.

If you read the Introduction of this book, you already know how poorly sponge baths are usually executed at nursing homes, compared to the proper way aides are trained to do the job. Nurse's aides keep dunking dirty washcloths into a sponge bath tub to keep "cleaning the body." Some cloths are soaked with urine and feces. To add insult to infection, they never disinfect the sponge bath tub or even wash it with soap and hot water. The sponge bath tub is filled with germs.

Some nurse's aides have learning disabilities and are not detail-oriented. They can't do the step-by-step-care of a sponge bath, for example, without forgetting a step. If they wash the patient with soap, they may forget to rinse her. Or, if they rinse her, they sometimes forget to dry the patient.

There are usually no state laws that say that a family member can't be in the room when a sponge bath is performed, or when a diaper is changed by an aide. However, the nursing home staff tells families to leave the room, so the aide isn't intimidated by the family member's presence. I usually stayed in the room and told the aide that I would help her turn my mother's body. The good aides were grateful for my help.

Some aides just rush from room to room, not greeting the patient nor communicating with her. They draw the curtains to give a sponge bath or to change the diaper of the patient. The room is dark and they start working on the patient, taking off her hospital gown, without telling her what they are going to do. I'm sure it is very scary for a patient not knowing who the aide is and what is going to happen to her. The aides sometimes turn the patient's body over in bed in a very rough way. Some aides look unkempt and bizarre. Some male aides aren't well shaven. Management who hire such people should ask themselves if they would like someone such as that taking care of them. Aides like these were also hired at religious-affiliated facilities.

Maybe the patient feels she will be assaulted by these aides. Aides need to be trained to communicate with the patient, by first greeting her and asking her how she feels, even if they know the patient doesn't speak.

At one nursing home, I remember there was such a callous disregard for patients, not only on the part of nurse's aides, but on the part of the nurses, too. The nurse's aides were allowed to dress up in witch's costumes on Halloween with faces painted. Can you imagine an aide walking into an elder's room, drawing the curtains to clean his body, and then leaning over him to give him care? An elder, either with Alzheimer's or a stroke victim might have a heart attack out of fear, not being able to process what's going on. Management allowed this. At nursing homes, sometimes the utter lack of common sense and lack of caring are unfathomable.

However, I can think of some wonderful aides. I knew one, for example, who would come in and talk to my mother, ask her questions, and then answer the questions for her, as if a dialogue was going on. Of course, she knew my mother couldn't respond.

For the comfort and safety of the patient, and for the comfort of aides who run the risk of straining their backs, nurse's aides should work in pairs with bedridden patients when they give sponge baths and change diapers. Turning a bedridden patient in bed and lifting her, is easier on the patient if two aides are sharing the task. Usually, however, aides work alone.

Besides bedsores and yeast infections in between the legs and inside the body, if sponge baths aren't done well, sores and infections can result under the armpits, and in between the toes and fingers. In these places, nurse's aides don't often bother to clean. When a patient, over a period of time doesn't get cleaned in these spots, you will see little slits in the skin appear. You may also see the skin turning brown in between toes and fingers. Of course, the armpits will smell of perspiration, too, if one doesn't clean them.

Lack of Supervision of Nurse's Aides

At nursing homes, there is a dire need for an additional nurse on each unit to work as a supervisor to the nurse's aides. This supervisor could ensure that the aides are giving each patient the care that they are supposed to deliver, including giving the patient adequate sponge baths and changing his diaper. With those aides who are having trouble performing, she could work along with them on tasks until they improved.

An additional nurse could also routinely assist with showers and baths in a bathtub.

On some occasions, at one nursing home, the nurse would assist the aide with a bathtub bath, if another aide wasn't available, though this is rarely done at nursing homes. It should be done for bedridden patients who must be lowered by hoyer lift into the bathtub, and be left suspended in the lift halfway into the tub.

At some nursing homes, patients are only given showers or baths in a tub once a week. Sometimes aides do not know how to give a proper shower or bath. I found, for example, two long-time nurse's aides giving my mother a bath in the bathtub with the window open on a windy day.

If a patient misses his shower or bathtub day due to an illness, you will have to negotiate with the nursing home to get it made up. They don't volunteer to reschedule a patient. They forget about him until the next week. Worse, if a patient misses a shower or bath, due to an aide being absent, she must wait until the next week. And, after they wash a patient's hair in the shower or bathtub, they don't blow it dry. They just wrap it in a towel. At one of the "best" facilities, they had a tub to give baths, but sometimes in between patients, they would forget to disinfect it, or if they did, they wouldn't rinse out all the disinfectant.

I decided to check the bathtub myself, before my mother entered it, and offered to disinfect it. It often had hair from the previous patient. Do you think I was making the staff feel bad? If so, I'm sorry, but the alternative was a germ-filled bathtub. They didn't seem to be offended at my doing this. In fact, I knew a family member of a patient and she was a registered nurse at a hospital nearby. On her mother's shower day, she came in and demonstrated to the aides, how to give a good shower. You would think that a family member wouldn't have to do this. Incidentally, I have read that prisoners in jail get two showers per week (and two times a week of exercise). That is often more than nursing home patients get, and the latter pay through the nose for care.

At nursing homes, they often do care backwards. After a shower or bath, for example, they bring a bedridden patient back to her room to lay her down on her bed and dry her with towels. However, the patient is obviously wet, but they changed the bed linens prior to the shower. Her body then wets the pillow cases and sheets. I remember finding my mother lying in a bed with soaked sheets. I ended up changing the sheets myself. Surprisingly, this time the nurse had actually helped the aide dry my mother. The nurse told me it wasn't necessary to change the wet sheets again since they would dry. Often, their responses are so nonsensical, that you don't bother to try to respond. It leaves you thinking that what little care is done for a patient, is executed so poorly and without thought as to cause discomfort and even illness. Again, "comfort care" that nursing homes claim to give to bedridden patients doesn't exist.

An extra nurse needs to patrol the halls, doing spot checks, and discovering problems with care before a family member walks in on the problem. She can assist with difficult tasks where safety is an issue, such as transferring a bedridden patient to a wheelchair by hoyer lift. One nurse in each unit on the floor is not enough. She can't adequately give multiple medications to as many as 40 patients; record care in patients' charts; make phone calls to doctors; order medications as prescribed by the doctor; take care of skin problems; care for ill patients; and monitor nurse's aides.

Nursing homes might also be able to solve some of their problems if an experienced aide trained a new aide, working along with her. When a new nurse's aide arrives at a nursing home from another facility, he is simply put out on the floor, and it is not known if he knows how to do certain tasks. The aide may have worked with mobile Alzheimer's patients at the former facility and not know how to adequately care for a bedridden patient. Even if he already has a CNA's license (certified nurse's aide's license), he may have forgotten or never fully learned how to care for a bedridden patient.

A nurse who trained nurse's aides for certification once told me how she instructed nurse's aides. She said, for example, that she could get nurse's aides to wear gloves by telling them that if they did, they wouldn't bring germs home to their children.

As for changing diapers, nurse's aides often change diapers without first cleaning the patient's urine-soaked skin. Some are not careful in positioning diapers so the patient often urinates all over the bed pads or sheets. Sometimes it is a case of a new aide not having learned how to position a diaper.

A trick that nurse's aides use when they don't want to change a patient every two hours as required, is that they use two diapers at once. That is, they put two diapers, one on top of the other, so the patient doesn't soak the bed. Of course, the patient's skin breaks down by not being changed often enough. Often graveyard shift is the most lax in not changing a patient because there are even fewer aides on duty.

You can prove to the staff that your loved one isn't being changed on a regular basis by counting the diapers in her room each morning and recording how many have been used until the following morning. If a patient urinates frequently and is supposed to be changed every two hours, then she should go through about 12 diapers. If the staff says that perhaps she was dry when they came to change her a few times, that may be true. However, is her skin breaking down? Are you finding her bed soaked? You know if your loved one urinates frequently or not. With my mother taking vast amounts of liquid feedings, she was urinating every two hours.

When care was more lax than usual, I started taking extensive notes on what condition I found my mother in, on each shift.

Infections

Incontinent care is one of the major reasons people put their bedridden family members in nursing homes. The majority of these family members don't like catheters. Particularly in institutions, where catheters aren't sterilized well and staff doesn't use appropriate cleanliness practices, catheters often result in bladder infections. Therefore, family members usually don't want a catheter for a loved one, but do expect their loved one to be cleaned up properly after urinating and having bowel movements. For example, the Centers for Disease Control (CDC) urge doctors to remove catheters from patients in hospitals as soon after surgery as possible. In nursing homes, if a patient has a catheter, this means that the nurse's aides will do even less for a patient than they normally would, in not having to change diapers. The patient is at the nursing home largely because he needs incontinent care and diaper changes. Otherwise, you might be able to keep him at home with a catheter. Why give the nursing home even less to do, and place the patient in more danger of ill-health with a catheter?

The uncleanliness at nursing homes is often revolting. I was told by a nursing home nurse that in the 1980s at nursing homes, cleanliness standards were even worse than now. She said that nurses and aides were not required to use latex gloves when sticking their fingers up a patient's rear end to induce a bowel movement, as they sometimes try to do.

When my mother left the last nursing home she was at, to be taken care of by me at home, she left with a bladder infection—a strep infection, to be precise. Strep is a germ that is passed along from patient to patient. Her urine contained strep in it. The patient across the hall from my mother had a chronic bladder infection, as her son told me. I had constantly reported to the nursing home nurses and management that aides were not washing their hands, or even wearing gloves. I had also reported that if they did put on a fresh pair of gloves, they often would get sidetracked and do other things, not removing the gloves when they touched hoyer lifts and other equipment, before cleaning up my mother. The nurses were often angry at me when I reported this. One simply said, "I back these aides 100 percent." She didn't address herself to the problem, and other nurses would stare blankly at me when I complained.

Strep infections are hard to get rid of, even when a person is of robust health. My mother had the strep infection for the last six weeks of her nursing home stay, along with a horrid skin infection in between her thighs that couldn't be cured with even prescription creams. Her inner thighs were the color "burnt red" as if she had been burned in a fire. We were to later learn that since her urine had strep, urinating on her skin had most likely caused the skin infection. I was changing her diaper as much as every 15 minutes. To add insult to injury, the nurses even ignored the infection, saying they didn't know why she was urinating so frequently. Of course, the staff wasn't going to change her diaper every 15 minutes. That's private care which they don't do. So, I was her private aide and I did it. In my mother's final months, after eight months of care at home, my mother died of a recurring bladder infection. According to a Harvard University study in the journal "Nature," up to 40 percent of a strep family may be resistant to penicillin and thromycin. Did my mother die due to the strep infection which kept recurring? Or, did she die because a permanent catheter infected her when I brought her home? She needed a permanent catheter because her skin breakdown in between her thighs was chronic, and her urine couldn't touch her sensitive skin. Permanent catheters in weak patients can cause recurring bladder infections. Since her last weeks at the nursing home, her skin breakdown would recur if creams were discontinued. Her strep bladder infection and skin breakdown were caused by the nursing home, and she was never able to recover from them in her weakened state.

At the nursing home, nurses will tell you that if a patient's urine is smelly, and either brown or orange, this is a bladder infection. At any rate, bladder infections can be easily caused when an incontinent patient is not being kept clean.

Perhaps one of the most ridiculous statements made by the nursing home staff was when the nurse told me—the day before I took my mother out of the nursing home—that my mother's recurring yeast infections and strep infection happened because "she was kept too clean" due to my constant changing her and cleaning her. This was just plain ignorant, and made absolutely no sense.

The Centers for Disease Control says one in every 20 patients gets hospital infections. However, the statistics for nursing homes are hard to figure out, since nursing homes often don't treat infections and often don't even recognize that patients have them. Therefore, there isn't even a record of a lot of infections, unless the family member suspects a problem and asks that tests be conducted. The staff can usually ignore infections because the patient is often too feeble to complain or can't articulate.

The Centers for Disease Control says that the hospital patient should ask doctors, nurses, and aides if they have washed their hands, since that's where infections usually originate. However, whether in a hospital or in a nursing home, I soon learned that staff doesn't like to be monitored by family members, and that they even protest that you are telling them what to do, no matter how non-confrontational you are.

Discomfort of Patients

As I have said, the daily routine at nursing homes doesn't allow personalized care, which the management even goes so far as to falsely promise. For example, if a patient is in pain, sitting up in her wheelchair for too long a time, when it is time for all patients to be put back to bed for sleep time, they won't make an exception and put that patient back to bed first. She must wait her turn. When my mother had the painful strep infection and her inner thighs were burnt red, sitting up in a wheelchair for long periods of time with her legs close together was even more painful. When I asked for my mother to have priority in getting back to bed, the nurse and the aide on duty told me my mother wasn't in pain. How would they have known? They hadn't seen her. They always deny a problem so as not to have to react. My mother was piercing her lips and they were turning blue. My mother was in great pain from a condition that the nursing home caused. Further, because family members aren't allowed to use the nursing home's equipment and transfer a patient back to bed using their hoyer lift, my mother had to wait until they decided to help her. Just as a nurse is the only one authorized to give the prescribed medication, (a family member can't give the medication if the nurse is busy), so it is with the use of their equipment.

Using the hoyer lift properly to get a patient up and into her wheelchair, or back to bed, is often a problem for nurse's aides. At nursing homes, nurses will tell aides to work in pairs to operate a hoyer lift, due to liability issues. It is usually the nursing home's policy. They don't want a patient landing on the floor instead of into a wheelchair, or on the floor, instead of back into bed. (At home, hoyer lifts are operated successfully by one vigilant family member.) Often, however, an aide in a nursing home can't find another aide to help in operating the hoyer lift since they are short-staffed and other aides are busy. If they can't even locate the nurse, they often struggle in getting a patient hooked up securely to a hoyer lift. (If there was a second nurse on the floor, she could assist with this.) When being transferred to a wheelchair, the patient's body is attached to a hammock which in turn, is suspended by chains from the hoyer lift. If the aides aren't careful, the patient's head is smashed against the metal slabs of the hammock or the chains of the lift itself. This could cause head injury. One simple solution is to buffer the patient's head with a pillow, but many aides don't care, if they even notice the head is being smashed. My mother was brain-injured to begin with, and this was a particular added danger. They never buffered her head.

Another problem that aides have in using the hoyer lift is that they often use a hammock that is too small or too large for the patient's body. If it is too small, when the patient is transferred, the metal clamps of the hammock dig into the patient's legs. When the patient lands in the wheelchair, the aides don't bother to release the metal clamps of the hammock, and this cuts off the circulation in the legs of the patient. The patient may feel extreme discomfort for hours. No one notices because they often put a laprobe over the patient. My mother's legs were bruised. It's a question of the aides not paying attention to what they are doing. If the hammock they use is too large, the patient's body shifts and slides back and forth when being transferred, and she can hit her head on the chains of the lift.

I remember one time before two aides transferred my mother into her wheelchair, they put a wooden board on the wheelchair's seat so that they could then put a pillow on top of the board which wouldn't slide off the chair. My mother would be able to sit comfortably in her chair and she wouldn't get sores from the seat of the wheelchair itself, as sometimes happens. They had the right idea, however, they forgot one thing—the pillow. So my mother was sitting on top of a wooden board which is obviously harder than the seat of the wheelchair. Often, aides don't pay attention to what they are doing at all.

An aide in a nursing home told me that her grandmother had been a nursing home patient elsewhere. Her grandmother fell from the hoyer lift and landed on the floor, breaking her hip. Only one nurse's aide was operating the lift at the time. There was no malfunction of the lift. The aide simply didn't have the patient's hammock clamped securely. If one person is responsible and competent, he can see that the patient lands securely positioned in the wheelchair, while simultaneously operating the lift mechanism itself. It takes some practice, however.

Even with two aides operating the lift, they don't often position the patient securely once she lands in the wheelchair, and they leave the patient sliding halfway off the wheelchair. This often happened to my mother. They would actually leave the room, seeing that she was sliding out of her chair. I would have to call the nurse to get the aides to come back in and reposition her. It is a common sight, too, to see patients in wheelchairs in nursing homes with bare feet. If the patient is bedridden, she'll often wear a hospital gown and robe, but the aides will forget to put her slippers on.

Sometimes, our mother didn't even have a laprobe covering her when she was in a wheelchair. Her hospital gown and robe covered her only to her knees, so her lower legs were bare. A paralyzed patient feels especially cold with bare body parts.

It should be noted that nursing homes and hospitals alike are quick to put a paralyzed patient in a soft, vinyl lounging chair, instead of a regular wheelchair. They think it is more safe for liability purposes to keep someone in a chair where their legs are stretched out and supported, rather than in a wheelchair where they feel a patient can slide out of the chair. However, in putting the patient in a lounging chair, she can lose back muscle endurance. At one nursing home, it took us a year to convince the physical therapist that our mother would do fine in a regular wheelchair, even without leg rests, letting her legs dangle for circulation purposes. If the staff is leery of a wheelchair, ask them to first try a wheelchair with a seat belt. The physical therapist may argue with you and naysay the idea. As with many on a nursing home staff, egos and the idea they know better than you often keep them from listening to you.

If a nursing home does get a bedridden patient into a wheelchair, oftentimes they don't get her back to bed on a timely basis. Therefore, a patient can go for hours without her diaper being changed. She is uncomfortable in a chair, urinating and getting rashes. Further, if a bedridden patient is urinating while in her wheelchair, being seated on the hoyer lift's hammock beneath her, the urine can leak out of her diaper, onto the hammock. The aides never wash the hammock which is often made of material that can't go through a washing machine. The aides just hang up the hammock to dry. It not only stinks and smells, but often, it isn't dry before the patient uses the hoyer lift again. Consequently, the next time the patient gets up in her wheelchair, she is sitting on a wet hammock.

With patients who can stand and pivot into a wheelchair, many aides don't want to try to assist them with pivoting. They either use a hoyer lift, which diminishes their mobility, or they don't get them out of bed at all. Consequently, their lungs suffer because they aren't exerting themselves with any movement.

The routine at nursing homes is such that being short of staff, they adopt a warehouse attitude toward the patient. They don't have time to walk ambulatory patients so they keep them seated in chairs. They don't even have time to walk them to a toilet, so they let them become incontinent, urinating in diapers, and then they don't even change the diapers regularly.

More On the Myth of Comfort Care

When an ambulatory patient is too drugged, he falls down when he tries to get up from his wheelchair. He sometimes gashes his head, or he breaks his hip and never recovers from it, confined to his bed. Then his lungs go bad, he gets pneumonia and dies. Often ambulatory patients are drugged because they try to escape. A family member should question medication given to his loved one. Further, when nursing homes give tranquilizers, I have read that some of these drugs can interfere with memory. A patient gets more confused.

Nurses, with all their patients, don't always notice changes in an individual patient. They ask the doctor for medication and then the doctor sometimes prescribes too high a dose. A family member should write a letter to the resident care manager asking her to note on the chart that family members should be notified of changes in medication so they can themselves observe their loved one.

What is a pity, too, is that patients are not only left sitting in their wheelchairs in the hall, but often in their rooms. You never see aides wheel them outside in good weather. Often, the only time they are wheeled around is when family members visit and do it.

Bedridden patients have the worst time in nursing homes, particularly those who are completely paralyzed. They are often not kept well-elevated in bed by nurse's aides, and their bodies are positioned very uncomfortably. Often their bodies are not pulled up in bed, so they slide down the mattress, if the bed is elevated to some extent. Their legs are often twisted in bed. I guess aides don't bother to look at the patient and see if the patient looks uncomfortable and is grimacing. They often don't treat the patient the way they'd like to be treated.

Before you elevate the back of a hospital bed, the patient's body must be pulled up in bed. Otherwise, elevating the back of the bed, without pulling the patient's body up, results in just the neck being bent over. Many times I came into my mother's room, and found her this way. Sometimes the nurse uses the excuse that the patient must have slid down by herself. The reason aides don't take the time to pull a patient up in bed is that it is strenuous. However, it is especially necessary to keep a patient elevated in bed who is a "tube feeder," that is, one who has a feeding tube, otherwise he can choke while receiving feeding tube formula. Or, if he has trouble swallowing, and he is laying flat, he could aspirate even with just his saliva. (This will be covered in Chapter 4, "The Feeding Tube Fiasco.") Even if someone isn't a tube feeder, if she is paralyzed, keeping the patient's back elevated in bed helps her breathe better, and is often more comfortable, particularly if she starts coughing.

It isn't uncommon for even nurses to walk into a patient's room and see him in an uncomfortable position or pose, and not reposition the patient. They, too, often ignore patients' obvious discomfort, all the while telling family members their loved ones receive comfort care. I often saw aides who did elevate my mother's back. However, they positioned her so that she was too elevated to the point of being bent over at the waist with her neck against her chest. Sometimes she was curled over into a ball as they left the room. The family member is left to reposition her loved one. There is sometimes no compassion for the patient or pride in work done.

If patients with brain injuries are not positioned well in bed, their contractures become even worse. Brain-injured patients, over time, do get twisted arms, legs, and wrists, but this can be delayed by not only adequate range of motion exercise (restorative aid) but by proper positioning in bed.

The worst case of abuse that was inflicted on my mother was right before I decided to take her home from the last nursing home. The graveyard shift aide must have been mentally ill, as some of the employees of nursing homes are. The aide had positioned my mother's body in bed so that her 165-pound body was supported by her left wrist that was already badly bent inward by a restorative aide who had previously abused her. In other words, the aide had tilted my mother's body slightly toward the right and used her left wrist like a kickstand on a bicycle. The aide did this in front of me once and I asked her if she really meant to position my mother that way. She looked at my mother who was gritting her teeth with her lips spread wide from cheek to cheek. The aide didn't respond, and just looked at my mother. I told her this was obviously excruciatingly painful. She said nothing and did nothing. I repositioned my mother's body. I thought this would be the end of the abuse. However, a couple of weeks later, I came in one morning at 8 a.m. only to find my mother in this same horrible pose, moaning. I wondered if she had been positioned like that all during graveyard shift, and how many graveyard shifts my mother had been in an excruciating position like that. Even a few seconds of that position would have tortured me. I called to the day shift nurse down the hall to witness the horror on my mother's face. I doubt this nurse did any reporting of this in her chart. She merely admitted that many aides don't care about patients. The graveyard shift nurse had already left that morning, but in the evening I waited to talk to her at 11:30 p.m. when she was on duty. When I reported this to the graveyard shift nurse, she said, "That's not torture." She also told me that by reporting this aide to her, I had alienated the aide and she no longer wanted to work with my mother. Instead of the graveyard shift nurse reporting this to the director of nursing to have the aide fired, she started blaming me for reporting the problem. She defended the aide for flagrant abuse. When I spoke to the director of nursing about this, she looked at me very puzzled, and merely said what a good aide this aide was. I told the director of nursing that I planned to take my mother out of the facility in two months, and that if I ever witnessed that again, I would call the state to investigate. (This was a religious-affiliated facility.) I did end up reporting the facility to the state when my mother left for this and other abuses that I will cover in this book. Through the long-term care state office, facilities are penalized with fines and sometimes monitored. However, the penalty fine, I'm sure, is passed along to the nursing home residents. Each year, you get a notice from the nursing home that fees are being increased to raise staff salaries. The staff members usually told me they hadn't been notified of a raise. Or, if they did get a raise, the nurse's aides, for example, got a ten-cent raise per hour. At some nursing homes, aides get a 25-cent raise per hour each year. It becomes obvious, therefore, why they don't fire staff. Who will replace them, given the management's "generosity"? The administrator likely got a raise, and the rest of the residents' increase probably went to cover not only penalty fines but even legal fees for malpractice suits. It isn't uncommon for nursing homes to have on their boards of directors a medical malpractice attorney. There often needs to be a pattern of malpractice occurrences with patients in order for a family to be successful in litigation with an elderly patient. Even if a patient dies, since the patient is elderly, frail, and ill, it is hard to prove that she was a victim of abuse or neglect. Her death can be blamed on old age. That is why the staff is sometimes so bravado in either not responding to complaints, nor following up to investigate, and even making up excuses. They know it is almost impossible to point the finger at them.

As for the proper positioning of a patient in bed, I often posted signs above my mother's bed hoping that the aides who were good and conscientious would be reminded of what to do. Because nurse's aides have so many patients, they often don't remember each patient's condition or needs associated with that condition. One nurse who didn't like me, took down my reminder signs. Another one childishly made little tears on the signs on the edges of the paper. Some nurses feel that they are in charge and what a family member wants is irrelevant. I decided that it was time to get the director of nursing involved. I asked her to put up official signs. She took color paper, and made computer-printed signs in big, bold letters. Then, she laminated the signs.

For example, one sign read, "Attention: Please be sure the head of the bed is elevated at all times at 45 degrees." (I'm not sure it helps, however, to mention degrees, because some people don't know what the 45-degree angle is.)

At one point, I posted another sign: "Attention R.N.s/ CNAs: My goal is to get my mother standing. This won't be possible if her legs, knees, ankles, and feet are bent and twisted unnecessarily. Could you please have two people position her in bed by pulling her up?"

Most often, if you tape signs above the patient's bed, they aren't even noticed. Nurse's aides' work becomes for some aides like assembly-line work. They have so many patients that they just run from one room to another, not thinking about what they are doing. They feel they are so rushed that they don't have time to read signs. You can even remind an aide verbally that a patient should be elevated when he leaves the room. Two minutes later, he leaves and forgets to elevate the patient.

One other attempt at trying to get aides to read signs is to get a "physician's order," for example, to keep the patient elevated, and specifically post the sign as "physician's order."

An aide needs to reposition a patient in bed after changing her diaper, for example. Even with a patient who has swallowing difficulties, he can lay her flat for a limited time while he changes her diaper. He can elevate the back of the bed if the patient begins coughing or is in discomfort. Unless the patient has major swallowing difficulties, laying her flat for a limited time shouldn't hurt her. After changing a diaper, that's the time aides forget to reposition the body and elevate the back of the bed. I have not only seen aides leave a patient flat, who should have been elevated, but they even leave the room forgetting to cover the patient with sheets and blankets. Or, sometimes they will cover the patient with only a sheet. I once posted a sign that said: "Please be sure to always cover the patient with a blanket. She has a tendency to always feel cold, when the rest of us may feel hot." If aides are perspiring from working hard, they will think the room is hot, and cover the patient with only a sheet.

One thing that often defines a nursing home as far as care is aides giving enemas. Nurses need a doctor's order for everything, from Preparation H for hemorrhoids, to suppositories and enemas. Nursing homes like to give enemas instead of suppositories because they work faster than the latter. Nursing homes are often fined if patients get bowel impactments three times. With a bowel impactment, a patient can vomit.

Enemas are a routine at nursing homes. However, often they are given when they aren't needed, because of mistakes made by aides. For example, on many occasions at nursing homes, my mother would be given an enema because the aides forgot to chart the bowel movements she had. I can remember an instance where each day my mother had large bowel movements for three days. On the third day, she was given an enema. Apparently, three aides forgot to chart her bowel movements, or confused her with other patients, and "credited" them for her bowel movements. Often, the nursing home's policy is that if one doesn't have a bowel movement in three days, an enema is given.

When a patient enters a nursing home, the staff gets a doctor's order to give enemas when needed. When I began noting mistakes made by aides in charting enemas, I called my mother's doctor to cancel his authorization for enemas, but to allow suppositories. For my mother, I felt if mistakes were going to be made, at least she wouldn't have enemas, but suppositories that were milder.

Further, although nursing home nurses never told me this, I learned from an agency nurse who was substituting at the nursing home that even a feeding tube patient can be given juices, including prune juice, through her tube. Prune juice obviously stimulates a bowel movement. As with anything else at a nursing home, a doctor's order is needed for prune juice to go through a feeding tube. I then phoned the doctor for an order, and I gave my mother prune juice through her tube myself. Yes, the nurses often did allow me to operate the feeding tube since it saved them time. (However, they didn't want the administrator to find out about it, since family members pay extra for the operation of the feeding tube.)

What I was disturbed about was that the nurses never told me that juice or even broth can be run through a feeding tube. Obviously, these are more nutritious than feeding tube formula. If I had known this, I would have gotten a doctor's order in the beginning. If the nursing home wouldn't allow her to eat by mouth for such a long time, they didn't have to deprive her of better nutrition through the feeding tube.

The only drawback to prune juice in the feeding tube is that if you give it frequently, such as every day for a period of a month, it usually clogs the feeding tube and the tube needs to be replaced. This is due to its consistency and thickness. Cranberry juice, which is acidic, doesn't usually clog a feeding tube. Even if you flush the tube with a glass of water after giving the prune juice, the juice still ends up clogging the tube. (I was to find this out when I took my mother home and the feeding tube clogged up during her late night feeding. I couldn't finish the feeding tube formula. I had to wait until the morning when the nurse could come to replace the tube.)

In your own home, you don't need a doctor's order for suppositories, juice through a tube, or anything except prescription medications. For a nursing home, it is simpler to give a patient an enema, once there is a doctor's order. If the nurse has to give a glass of prune juice to a "tube feeder" it takes her extra time to get the juice, run the juice through the tube, and afterwards flush the tube with water. It is just another task added on to the load of having 40 patients who need multiple medications.

As for other bowel matters, diarrhea isn't rare at nursing homes. It is easy to spot the uncleanliness at nursing homes. When one patient gets diarrhea, often many patients get it on the same unit. Why? The aides don't properly wash their hands nor wear latex gloves. Therefore, diarrhea spreads just like infections.

Personal Care

Personal care, such as shaving a man's face, or removing face hair from women, is something that should be routine at a nursing home, but hardly ever is. (It isn't even done at hospitals.) Friends of mine who have had parents in nursing homes have also complained that it wasn't done. You see women patients, with hair above the mouth like mustaches on men, that detract from their appearance. If they had family members who visited, they would do it. If the nursing home management should feel that they can't entrust this care to an aide, then a nurse should do it.

It is rare for a nursing home, or even a hospital, to brush a patient's teeth regularly or even swab a patient's mouth with a "toothette," (a small disposable sponge attached to a stick). When my mother was hospitalized for her head injury, it was not considered part of the care.

If hospitals don't do it, of course nursing homes often won't. At one nursing home my mother was at, however, they had a special aide, hired to do just oral care for a few hours each evening. What I saw repulsed me, so I decided to do my mother's oral care myself. The "tooth fairy," as she was ironically called, would go from one patient to another, up and down the halls, without changing her latex gloves. She'd even touch the patients' toothbrushes by the brush's end with her gloves when rinsing the toothbrush. She would also clean dentures wearing dirty gloves.When she was absent, one aide who had better cleanliness skills, would dunk my mother's toothette heavily in water, instead of dipping it in. This water-logged toothette would make my mother gag because she hadn't swallowed liquids in a long time.

Some nursing homes have a particular dentist visit every two months or so. He bills the patient's family directly. You are under no obligation to schedule a visit for your elder. Or, you can have a dentist of your choice visit, if he's willing to make private calls. For a patient with swallow-ing problems, dentists don't usually recommend that you have her teeth cleaned by them. A patient could easily choke during the process. They say that even using "throat packs" to keep a patient from swallowing plaque is dangerous for a patient with swallowing problems. They usually recom-mend that if there is plaque and receding gums they shouldn't be treated for a patient in this condition. Even if there is abscess or decay, usually a dentist won't treat it.

As for other personal care, two of the nursing homes my mother was in, had hairdressers on premise, working three to five days a week. Of course, the patient's family is billed extra for these services, if they are requested.

Nutrition

A basic service at nursing homes is feeding the patient. You've probably read investigative reports in magazines about nursing home residents and dehydration, leading to death. What appalled me at the three nursing homes my mother was at, is that there weren't enough aides to feed the patients. It was disheartening that routinely at these private nursing homes family members showed up at lunch and dinner to feed their elders, something they paid the nursing homes to do. My friend told me that for the eight months her mother was in another private nursing home due to Alzheimer's, she, her father, and her sister would take shifts, each showing up for breakfast, lunch, and din-ner to feed her mother.

At nursing homes, you witness as I did, one aide lining up as many as fourteen patients at dinnertime, taking one spoonful, assembly-line fashion, to give to each patient one after the other. Afterwards, she'd start again at the front of the line. I even witnessed a patient falling asleep before getting her next spoonful. This assembly-line feeding sys-tem is hardly conducive to getting the patient to eat well.

One family member I knew hired a private aide to show up at each dinnertime to feed her father. When you're paying thousands of dollars each month for care, can't a nursing home keep a patient clean and feed him? These are the basics. A family member doesn't ask for extraordinary service. However, when you complain, management often treats you like you're asking for too much for your money. Why should family members pitch in to do any work?

At one nursing home, I witnessed that if a patient wasn't hungry for breakfast or lunch, they would set aside her tray for later on, but wouldn't bother to reheat the food. Therefore, for all intents and purposes, the patient would have to wait until the next meal to get hot food. At only one of these three nursing homes were snacks like yogurt, pudding, cookies, ice cream, juice, and sandwiches available in between meals in the unit's own refrigerator. Snacks such as fresh fruit would have been nutritious, no doubt, but I never saw them.

Further, at nursing homes, second helpings of food aren't available. I watched as a patient asked an aide for more hot food at lunch. He was told he would have to wait for dinner. The portions of food aren't generous, either.

I remember at the last nursing home my mother was at, a patient was in her room eating a bar of soap. None of the staff noticed this. They were notified of this by a family member of another patient. I overheard two nurses talking about how demented this patient was. I thought to myself that the patient was probably demented, but also hungry. I was shocked that the nurses didn't bother to ask themselves if the patient was hungry. I thought, why is the patient always blamed for things that go wrong?

I remember that if a nurse's aide from an agency was substituting for an absent aide, it was common for a food tray to be delivered by mistake to my mother's room. One agency aide even tried to feed her. I stopped him. The nursing home staff didn't want her to be fed by the facility or even by her family. One would think that nursing homes would be organized enough to label each tray with a patient's name, particularly because some patients eat only soft foods or semi-soft foods, and may get the wrong tray. If a patient is even assisted by a staff aide who isn't familiar with his diet, he could choke on food that wasn't appropriate for him.

After a few incidents where an agency aide mistakenly delivered a food tray to my mother, the director of nursing posted a sign above her bed, "NPO," which means "Nothing by Mouth." (Some aides didn't know what this abbreviation even meant.) Just like stroke victims, Alzheimer's victims, in the late stages of their disease, can lose their ability to swallow. Nursing homes have a speech therapist to evaluate the patient's swallowing ability. Family members are notified as to what the speech therapist's evaluation reveals. It is up to the family to decide if the patient should continue being fed despite the risks, or whether they wish the patient to have a feeding tube. If a patient, such as my mother, already arrives at the nursing home with a feeding tube, it's extremely difficult to convince a speech therapist to allow her to eat by mouth. I will discuss this double standard of allowing some patients with swallowing difficulties to be fed by mouth and not others, in Chapter 4, "The Feeding Tube Fiasco."

Other Basic Care

As for other care that one would classify as basic and that deals with comfort is the issue of clipping fingernails and toenails. At only one of the three facilities my mother was at, did they clip fingernails and toenails. Unless someone is diabetic, there is usually no problem with clipping toenails. However, at most facilities, nurses won't even file nails. Nurses say they are afraid of causing someone infection. It does need to be done. A stroke victim, such as my mother, can get contracted whereby her fingers dig into the palm of the hand. If one has long fingernails, this can cause infection. At this one facility where they did clip nails, the aides and nurses alike did a good, careful job. However, often they needed to be reminded to clip nails.

Nursing homes, as a rule, don't check a patient's ears for wax, unless asked to do so. After my mother's bath and shampoo, I saw an aide try to dry the inside of her ear by poking her little finger inside of it with a towel. This accomplished nothing except to push the wax further into her ear, having my mother run the risk of infection. Before my mother entered a nursing home, every six months the nurse at her doctor's office would remove a lot of wax by first shooting warm water through a syringe in the ear. At nursing homes, the nurses often don't want to take the time to do this. Instead, they'll insert wax remover (with a doctor's order), and let it do its work for a few days. Afterwards, the wax is easily removed. However, I found a pattern to this procedure with my mother. On two different occasions, when it was done, my mother got pneumonia afterwards. The second time it was done in the summer, not winter when pneumonia is common. I maintain that, at least in my mother's case, the coldness of the wax remover caused a congestion in my mother's nasal passages and it was if she was catching a cold. Not able to blow the mucous out of her nose, it traveled down her throat into the lungs, and it turned into pneumonia. Only one nurse agreed with me that this was possible.

As for yet other basic care, range of motion exercises should be done every day. However, at nursing homes, one is lucky if they are done two times a week, ten minutes each time, as promised. At the last nursing home my mother was in, we negotiated having a restorative aide give a half hour of range of motion five days a week and paid the nursing home extra in the way of a contribution. This was a non-profit nursing home. This was on top of one hour to an hour and one-half of the range of motion exercise I gave my mother. The nursing home calls range of motion "restorative aid." If one is bedridden and paralyzed, it feels good to have this done at different intervals during the day.

After a period of time, the restorative aide at the nursing home started torturing my mother. My mother was crying in pain and gritting her teeth as the aide vigorously tried to unbend my mother's badly contracted arm and straighten it out. It was amazing to watch this aide who acted as if she was in a different world, oblivious to my mother's cries. I reported the aide, and told the nursing home I'd do the exercises all by myself. As is often the case, what little care is done, is done so poorly that it's better not to have it done at all. After this aide tortured her, my mother's arm was permanently straightened out like an upside down walking cane with her left wrist hooked inward. My mother's arm looked deformed and atrocious. The aide was most likely mentally ill. Not surprisingly, I knew another family member at the nursing home who reported to me of an oddly similar occurrence for which the staff had no explanation for, as usual. His sister, who was paralyzed from multiple sclerosis, had developed a badly twisted ankle all of a sudden. She was moaning one day when he went to visit. She was receiving restorative aid from this restorative aide. We wondered if this aide had abused her, too. When you complain, the staff often doesn't investigate and you are left to complain to the state. The staff hopes the problem will go away automatically.

By the end of my mother's nursing home experience, it became painfully clear, that as care is performed less and less competently, you can't complain about everything. You end up doing each task yourself so as not to cause injury or infection to your loved one, as the aides do.

It always disappointed me, too, how if a staff member who performed a certain task, such as restorative aid, was absent or on vacation, the task was completely skipped without a substitute intervening. Similarly, if an aide was absent and an agency aide wasn't available, some patients wouldn't be bathed, dressed and gotten out of bed. I was always there to advocate for my mother so that if anyone was slighted in the case of an absent aide, it wasn't going to be my mother. I remember, at the beginning of my mother's nursing home stay, a restorative aide who was quite good became ill for a week. I asked if the physical therapist's assistant could do the restorative aid. They accomodated me even though they dragged their feet at first.

Lack of Continuity of Care

Lack of continuity of care is such a big issue at nursing homes, particuarly with aide care. With nurse's aides rotating on each unit that has as many as 40 patients, they can't memorize each patient's needs. They forget which patients need to be kept elevated in bed to keep their lungs healthy. However, sometimes aides just don't know that bedridden patients are prone to pneumonia because they can't get up and move around to give their lungs a workout. After my mother's lung embolisms, we had a lung filter implanted to block further clots. Perhaps this weakened her and made her even more prone to pneumonia.

It should be noted, too, that there is no continuity in care when a nurse's aide (or nurse) is absent, and agency help replaces her. Agency help, of course, has no familiarity with the patient. Agency aides often feel they have no incentive to do a good job, since the next night they'll be working at a different facility. At one facility that my mother was in, they tried very hard to avoid having agency help. They asked staff aides to work on their days off, if they were willing, in order to cover for absent aides. Here, I asked that agency aides not be allowed to work with my mother, and that if an agency aide was assigned to my mother's hall, a staff aide from another wing work with her. They did oblige me, since previously, an agency aide had been careless in operating a hoyer lift to move my mother from her bed to her wheelchair. My mother's thumb got trapped on the side of the wheelchair and was badly cut. This agency aide didn't even notice it. Since my mother couldn't speak, she couldn't complain. Didn't the aide notice an expression of pain on her face? Some aides are merely automatons, not looking at their patients or even listening to their moaning. It's often as if the patients are just objects to them. There are excellent aides, however, who don't fit into this category. The latter treat patients the same way they would treat a family member.

An agency nurse once told me that she worked at a facility one evening that was so short of regular staff, that she was among just agency aides—no staffers. Because none of them knew the patients, they were at a loss on how to help them. There were no regular staff people to even tell the agency help who the patients were who were missing wristbands. She saw disoriented patients, sitting out in the hall, not knowing their own names. Therefore, she couldn't administer medications to those patients. The patients had to wait until the next shift when that shift's nurse could identify them.

Nursing homes should strive to give incentives to aides in order to keep excellent ones. Many excellent nurse's aides never leave the sytem, but they leave their present facility to go to work at nursing homes that may pay 25 cents more per hour. Therefore, nursing homes should strive to give raises to excellent aides, rather than lose them, not be able to replace them right away, or replace them with bad aides.

Firing Staff

As for the bad aides on nursing home staffs, they should be fired. When I say nursing home staff never gets fired, I should qualify this statement. They usually don't get fired for bad work, abuse, neglect, or even stealing from a patient. If they get fired, they do for stealing from the facility. I knew an aide who gave good care to my mother. However, she was fired for making long distance phone calls from the nursing home's line. I also knew two aides who got fired because one had the other punch her out on her time card after she'd left. Sometimes, however, aides would be fired for abuse if the accuser had clout because she was a family member and a nurse herself. The staff listened to patients who had relatives who were nurses somewhere else. In one instance, an aide was abusing a patient by scrubbing under her nails until her fingers bled. This patient had a daughter who came to the nursing home every day to feed her lunch. Her daughter was a hospital nurse. Her daughter came to visit one evening, bringing her husband who was a doctor. When they witnessed what the aide was doing, she reported it to the nurse on duty, because the administrator had aleady gone home. Fearing for her mother's safety because the charge nurse had no clout to fire the aide, she bribed another aide by giving her $15 to watch over her mother during the evening shift, to make sure the bad aide didn't abuse her. The next day the daughter marched into the administrator's office and said, "If you don't fire this aide, I'll report you to the state." It worked.

Because some aides aren't trustworthy, you should label all your elder's belongings and give a list of them to the administrator. When you visit, make sure all belongings are there. Two hours after a visitor came to see my mother and left a plant, it was stolen. When another visitor left a bottle of nail polish for my mother, it was stolen. I reported the theft of the plant, but not the nail polish.

I can remember one untrustworthy nurse's aide who would take her food into a patient's room during her break and watch the patient's television. It was obviously against the rules. Strangely enough, she would even routinely flush her plastic forks down the patient's toilet, plugging it up.

It's not uncommon to hear aides shout at their supervisors and even walk off the job, only to return the next day and not be fired. I routinely saw nurse's aides tell nurses they refused to do certain tasks. (To be fair, I should note that some nurses shout and argue with their supervisors, too!) At one nursing home my mother was in, an aide was allowed to "write up" nurses and even family members, but nurses and family members couldn't complain about them and get results. Nursing homes are topsy-turvy. It's a wonder to me that nursing schools send their students to do internships at nursing homes. What will they learn there? Unprofessionalism and a poor attitude toward patients.

As I've said, many staff members at nursing homes spend their lives going from one to another. The aides (and nurses) often criticize other nursing homes they are familiar with for bad care, not realizing that the one they're at is just as bad. Or, they criticize their co-workers for a poor attitude or bad care, not taking a good look at themselves.

Working Conditions for Staff

The working conditions are bad for all nursing home staff, particularly aides. If, for example, an aide calls in sick at the last minute, and no agency aide is available, the other aides often pick up the slack. They take on more patients than usual, without getting paid a penny more.

At the last nursing home my mother was in, nurse's aides were actually encouraged to come to work even if they were sick. They would get bonus pay for every 30 days they worked without taking a sick day or being absent for some other reason. To someone making minimum wage or slightly above, he often couldn't afford to miss even one day of work. It might mean the difference between being able to pay his rent or not. But if he was sick, what did it do for patients who caught his germs? The patients got sick.

At the last nursing home my mother was at, another incentive for aides involved working a double shift to get paid double the normal rate, if a staff aide did call in absent. It was cheaper for the nursing home to pay this to a staff aide to work a second shift,16 hours total, rather than to have to pay an agency three times the rate of minimum wage for an aide.

However, overtime work for an aide who may be already tired wasn't always a good solution. (Paying an aide to come in on a day off would have been better.) For nurse's aides who often do lifting, even eight hours is tough, but extra money for a double shift is very attractive.

When an aide is tired, this often compromises patient safety. The aide may be even more scatter-brained or careless than usual. I actually knew an aide who worked a triple shift. She was a single mother and needed the money. By her third shift (graveyard), no one knew that she had started with the morning shift at 7 a.m., and she wasn't about to tell the graveyard shift nurse. (I would imagine there are state laws against it. If not, there should be.) Imagine how dangerously exhausted she was in dealing with the patients for 24 hours straight.

Although unions for caregivers are organizing in some places to raise wages and give healthcare benefits, this doesn't always improve care for patients. Yes, good aides may not leave facilities if wages improve. Some aides I've known go on to childcare work that isn't as strenuous. However, with bad aides, more money doesn't improve their cleanliness skills, safety skills in dealing with a patient, or their common sense. I suppose that with higher wages this may make it easier for a nursing home to threaten a bad aide with possible firing if he doesn't tow the line.

The job of a nurse's aide is not a glamorous one. He wipes people's rear ends, gives enemas, lifts and turns bedridden patients, changes diapers, empties catheter bags and commodes, cleans dentures, etc. However, if a facility trains an aide, and reinforces the training with regular inservices to review the basics, this may make an aide feel as if he is valuable and doing significant work. Inservices should help aides to review the basics such as keeping patients elevated in bed who need to be, hoyer lifting patients safely, washing hands properly, and wearing latex gloves, etc.

Some nursing homes give training so prospective aides can get certified. I knew of one nursing home that once waived the instructional fees of $600, so aides could get certified and later work at their nursing home. However, it stopped doing this. It's a pity that a nurse's aide, who most likely isn't properous, would have to pay for expensive training, only to start working at minimum wage.

The life of a nurse's aide is sometimes one without a bright future. Some aides say they want to become nurses, though few of them actually do end up going to nursing school. I remember one aide who told me she wanted to work as a mortician's assistant, bathing corpses and doing makeup. She said she was used to seeing corpses at nursing homes, and that there was "good money" in working for a mortician once one got certified through training. Most of us wouldn't want this job.

One outstanding aide, both in her skills and caring attitude, told me she thought the nursing home gave "lousy" care to patients. She said, however, that she didn't have the confidence to work at a hospital when I suggested that she should strive for better pay. She was in her 50s and had worked at nursing homes for 20 years. She eventually ended up leaving that nursing home, and went to another.

I met several aides (and nurses) who were honest and didn't defend the poor care at their nursing homes. Often, they told me in confidence that they wouldn't want to be patients there themselves, and that they were looking for jobs at other facilities, hoping there might be better ones.

If a facility is a good one, even though nurse's aides may be basically unskilled people, the institution will instill its philosophy and values in the aides. The institution needs to reinforce the belief that aide work is important work, and that each patient deserves the very best in care. I noted that even religious-affiliated institutions fell down in this area.

Yes, nursing homes have trouble finding aides who are consistent in the care they give. Yes, they may have passed their Certified Nursing Assistant (CNA) exam, and yet they didn't master the skills of cleanliness and other skills. And, yes, some can't understand or speak English very well. But, even with the latter problem, nursing homes must work with the aides to develop their skills. At one non-profit nursing home I knew of, volunteers gave English lessons to staff. That's probably why some aides were particularly devoted to the facility and stayed a long time.

My brother and I sometimes bought birthday and holiday gifts to some aides (and nurses), or even brought some pizza or takeout food to them when they worked double shifts. Why couldn't the nursing home do this? I always showed my appreciation to aides and nurses who performed well, praising them, saying kind words about them to their supervisors, and writing letters about them to the administrator. I showed an interest in them and got to know them on a personal level. Many had nice children that they brought as visitors to the nursing home on their days off. Their children were beautiful people, too.

I wrote a letter of reference for a nursing home nurse when she began applying for hospital jobs. As in all correspondence that you will read in this book, I included this letter I wrote, using fictitious names so as not to identify anyone or a facility.

Letter of Reference for Mary Smith, R.N.

Mary Smith has cared for my mother at Nursing Home Y for about a year and a half. During this time, I've come to know Mary very well, as I've spent many long hours keeping my mother company and being involved in her daily care.

During my mother's 15 years of illness and extraordinary medical problems, I've met dozens of healthcare professionals. I've observed that Mary's level of professionalism far exceeds that of anyone I know in the healthcare field. She always demonstrates deep respect, empathy, caring and compassion in dealing with patients and their families. In addition, her excellent communication skills in both ordinary and stressful situations for families is a rarity in today's healthcare system. She is both efficient and attentive to detail in treating patients. Going above and beyond for each patient is a daily routine for Mary, despite her having 40 patients. I've never known Mary to be overwhelmed by her workload, nor has she ever complained about her numerous responsibilities. In fact, Mary loves her work so much that she even phones the nursing home on her days off to inquire about my mother's condition and that of other patients, and to follow up on their care. (I learned about this from another nurse on the unit.)

I've noticed that Mary is a highly-respected nurse at Nursing Home Y by patients, families, and staff. She takes every opportunity to work along with her peers, and she very closely supervises and assists nurse's aides.

This is the only letter I've ever written recommending a nurse. I feel compelled to do so because of Mary's extraordinary skills, efforts, and leadership which deserve to be recognized. I can tell nursing is truly a calling to Mary.

Sincerely.....

Nurses aren't always treated fairly at nursing homes. At one nursing home my mother was at, the nurses stayed after their shift ended for as much as an hour without pay to write in their charts. They said there weren't enough hours in the day to do all the work. Nurses complain that governmental paperwork is excessive and that it calls for one resident care manager on each unit to do most of it, rather than have that nurse out on the floor caring for patients. Nurses say there's a need to lobby politicians in Washington, DC about this. However, even if governmental paperwork wasn't as extensive, that would mean that two nurses to 40 patients are out on the floor at some nursing homes. That is still inadequate. Incidentally, the state dictates the ratio of aides and nurses to patients.

As for nurses at nursing homes, it was interesting to me that the only male nurse I saw employed at three nursing homes had an administrative position. He was an assistant director of nursing. There were, however, some male nurses who showed up who were sent from agencies as substitutes.

Nurses in institutional situations feel they don't have time to give individualized care. For example, when my mother needed medication that was supposed to be given on a full stomach, she was routinely given it on an empty stomach. When she needed an antibiotic for her pneumonia to be given on a full stomach, it was given on an empty stomach. The reason for this was that the nurses didn't deviate from their routine of walking down the long hall at a certain time to give medication to patients. They figured they might as well give my mother's medication at the same time, since it was in the general time frame of when it was to be given. When I asked the nurses about her cancer drug, knowing it was recommended to be taken on a full stomach to prevent nausea, they said it wasn't true. I was familiar with this drug because my mother had taken it once before in her life. The upshot was that I told the nurses I would phone the doctor and ask for his opinion, and if he believed it should be given on a full stomach, he could write an order to that effect. He did just that. The nurses complied. As a family member you are often forced to go above the nurses' heads if you feel it's in the best interests of your elder.

As for the nursing home nurse's plight, to earn extra money, nurses sometimes work double shifts, which is exhausting, both physically and mentally. They walk up and down the halls pushing a medication cart, passing out dozens of medications. If medication errors are possible in working a single shift, I would imagine medication errors are more possible in a 16-hour shift.

Nursing Home Errors

It is estimated that 98,000 patients in hospitals die each year. Most of these deaths are due to medication errors made by nurses, but some are due to infections. In nursing homes, accurate statistics aren't available because the patient is in such frail health anyway, that it's often hard to pinpoint the exact cause of death. It's obviously even more important for nursing homes to be cleaner and safer than hospitals because elderly patients can't fight off infections, and they can't spring back from medication errors the way younger patients can. Nurses and aides are ultimately nurses and aides, no matter where they work. However, the institution sets the standards, and if an institution refuses to set standards for fear of alienating their employees and damaging their self-esteem by correcting their errors, then how are they helping the patients? Are they in business to make the patient even sicker and uncomfortable, and to die from infections and medication errors.

At hospitals, inexperienced, incompetent, or careless nurses can give the wrong medication or the wrong dose of it. Errors aren't readily caught. At nursing homes, where there's only one nurse out on the floor of a unit, there's even less chance of catching the error. Even at hospitals, if good nurses speak out to a supervisor against a nurse who made an error, the good nurses often pay the price. They often begin getting bad reviews and eventually get fired, if they speak out repeatedly. Or, if nurses report inadequate staffing levels to a government health agency, they fear retaliation by their supervisors. At nursing homes, the situation is worse. Nurses, if they want to keep their jobs, often become silent partners in poor care.

Sedating Patients

Another medication issue at nursing homes is the one of sedation. I remember two nursing home nurses told me that some patients take far too many drugs. One nurse told me some of her patients took as many as 15 pills a day. One nurse, in particular, told me that she felt bad that patients were so heavily medicated so as not to cause problems. She soon left the nursing home to go to work at a hospital. At any nursing home, you will see patients sitting in wheelchairs spaced out in the halls. One nurse told me that if patients could walk when they entered the nursing home, a week later they couldn't. What happens with ambulatory patients is that if they don't want to stay there, they try to walk out. The nurse then calls the patients' doctors to get authorization for drugs to tranquilize them. This is often bad for patients since they lose not only their coordination and strength, but their alertness. A nursing home will not allow patients to stay if their family members won't allow them to be sedated. The liability is too great. They could be injured, for example, in trying to escape. They could walk out the door and get hit by a car. The nursing home would then be sued. The nursing home doesn't have enough staff to sit with patients and keep them occupied. Since there's only one nurse on floor duty, and sometimes only three aides on each unit for as many as 40 patients (evening shift), often they won't even hear an alarm if an ambulatory patient tries to walk out the door.

What if a family member requests that his elder's doctor not authorize sedation? A nursing home can legally have their "house doctor," (who isn't on duty there, but is a consultant by phone), prescribe medication if a patient is out of control. My friend's mother was in such a situation at a nursing home. My friend's mother died because the sedation made her lose her coordination. She tried to get up out of her wheelchair, fell down and broke her hip, and never recovered. My friend sought legal advice because she specifically had her mother's doctor forbid sedatives. My friend found she couldn't sue because a nursing home ultimately has the authority with a house doctor's permission to sedate the patient if the staff feels the patient is a threat to herself or others. (Incidentally, even in an adult foster home, if they aren't given permission to sedate an ambulatory resident who tries to escape, then they won't allow the resident to live there. Again, the liability for them is great.) When it comes down to it, no one, no matter how much money you pay them, will ever care for problem people. In nursing homes, they call sedation "behavior modification." (In fact, nursing homes use many euphemisms. "Long-term care facility" is a euphemism itself for "nursing homes." And, the kitchen supervisor at a nursing home told me that cookies for snack time were "nutrition.")

If a patient escapes from a nursing home, the state inspector will count that as a penalty during her annual inspection. Nurses tell family members not to fear tranquilizers as being harmful. They often say that they are giving them in small doses. Each patient may react to medication in a different way. With elderly patients, often over a short period of time, tranquilizers make them weak, and they can't lift themselves out of a chair without falling down. Further, there is often a cumulative effect to taking tranquilizers over a period of time, making patients more mentally feeble.

Dying Patients

No one at a nursing home has time to sit with any patient, even if he is very ill or even dying. One of the things that bothered me the most at nursing homes was when I saw nurses walking past a patient's room when the patient was moaning. They wouldn't stop to investigate. If they didn't have time to sit with a patient, they perhaps could have gotten an aide to attend to him, or at least ask the patient what the problem was.

At the last nursing home my mother was at, it was a religious-affiliated facility. When patients were dying, one would think a nun from the convent on the property would be called in to sit with the patient, or even the chaplain who lived down the block. However, I saw many patients who had no families die alone. The nurse would place a damp washcloth on the patient's forehead and leave the room.

Even on the holiest of religious holidays, Christmas and Easter, it was disappointing to me that the nuns from the convent never came in to greet the patients and wish them a happy holiday. Again, the institution sets the standards for caring, and if nurses and aides see a lack of caring on the part of the administration, they often become indifferent, too.

Family members often put their loved ones in nursing homes during their final months or weeks of life, thinking they'll receive 'round the clock care. My next door neighbor told me that years ago she put her mother in a nursing home when she was in the final stages of cancer. She, like many family members I know, had to repeatedly remind the nurse that her mother needed her regular pain medication. My neighbor said the nurse would respond, "Oh, she's not due for medication until five minutes from now."

If you find your loved one is in his final days at a nursing home, tell the nursing home you will pay for a private duty nurse on graveyard shift to assist the patient. This is a good idea, too, if the patient has pneumonia. With one nurse to as many as 80 patients on graveyard shift, she can't possibly help a seriously ill patient. Perhaps one of their staff nurses could put in an extra shift. In reality, you shouldn't have to pay extra. They should be adequately staffed. But, since they aren't, you take the necessary measures to ensure care. You could even contact an agency about sending a nurse, with the facility's permission. Incidentally, if your loved one is ill, even during day shift, be prepared to spend your time there, keeping after the nurse to give your elder care. With so many other patients, she can't be checking on your loved one all the time. Pneumonia is common at nursing homes in the winter.

When a patient is dying, the nurses either have too many patients to attend to him and can't give frequent pain medication as ordered by the doctor, or they just resent being reminded and postone giving it. Yes, it's cruel and callous, but they don't like being told what to do by a family member, according to one director of nursing who chided me on more than one occasion.

How Staff Reacts to Complaints

Whenever I had valid complaints about lapses in the promised, basic care, the director of nursing would always remind me that staff didn't like me for complaining, and for reminding them what to do. After listening to her diatribe on a few occasions, I one day, replied: "I'm going to have to remind you about care if you're not providing the care you promised. I never ask for anything beyond the basic, promised care."

On a bright note, there were two nurses in one facility who told me that I'd taught them "so much about asking for care and attempting to get it." One said, "You are unique as a family member and advocate. I've never seen anyone advocate like you in my 20 years at nursing homes."

Many nursing homes need to remember that they are supposed to be treating a patient, and not focusing on how they feel about a family member. If one is a schoolteacher, for example, and doesn't like a child's parent, would the teacher ignore or mistreat the child in school? Sometimes nurses ignored or mistreated my mother because they didn't like me.

Right-to-Life

When I, for example, complained to the director of nursing that the graveyard shift nurse was not following doctor's orders, she again blamed me. The graveyard shift nurse was shorting my mother on her feeding tube formula, her nutrition that was life support. What was the graveyard shift nurse trying to do? Commit euthanasia? I had caught the graveyard shift nurse in the act, and reminded her about the proper amount to be given. She said she would give the proper amount. However, from this point onward, I counted the number of cans of food my mother had left before graveyard shift and again after graveyard shift when I came back in the morning. I found the graveyard shift nurse was still shorting my mother on formula. When I complained to the director of nursing, she didn't address herself to the problem, except to say that the nurse shouldn't be doing it and that the nurse didn't like me because I was telling her what to do. I then wrote a letter to the administrator clearly stating that care had dwindled to such a low level as to even deny a patient her proper level of feeding tube formula. I said I would report such flagrance to the state. (At this time, I was also making plans to take my mother home.)

After the administrator spoke with the graveyard shift nurse, the nurse had such bravado as to chew me out. When I was leaving one night, she woke up all the patients, including my mother, screaming at me for making "false accusations." (And, what does this teach the nurse's aides who were listening?) I told her of my evidence and she was stammering, making excuses that didn't make any sense. This nurse even had the audacity to say, "You know I love your mother," parroting the motto of most facilities that say they "love their patients."

When care sinks this low, a patient might as well be out in the street. Certainly, a family member who takes the patient home, can do much better than this. I reported this facility to the state after I took my mother home.

Nursing homes breed poor attitudes when the supervisors don't fire employees, and worse, condone their unprofessionalism. Attitudes of nurses, as I've discussed, often involve not wanting to treat patients whom they personally feel have no quality of life. Often, nurses who want to put patients "out of their misery" ask the doctor for morphine for pain when the patients have pneumonia. At the first nursing home, when my mother had pneumonia, she didn't seem to be in pain. We wanted to give her a chance to recover from her hospital ordeal where we suspected a medication error that led to her coma. The resident care mananger at this nursing home, who made it clear to us that she didn't feel my mother should be "kept alive," was able to obtain the order for morphine from my mother's doctor. We called the doctor and protested that she shouldn't be given morphine. She was already heavily sedated with anti-seizure medication. We felt that even with a small dose of morphine, her breathing would get more faint and she couldn't fight the pneumonia. The doctor understood our concerns and followed our wishes. He thought we'd asked for the morphine.

Some nurses at nursing homes should realize and respect the fact that a family member isn't trying to preserve life just for the sake of preserving life. Sometimes a family member is trying to give a relative a chance at recovery, even if the chance isn't good that she'll recover. My mother recovered from brain cancer, though the odds of her recovery were practically nil. One wonders if some nurses have any empathy and even the common sense to realize that life and death issues aren't black or white. Don't they realize that their attitudes might not be so cut-and-dried if it was their family member?

Nurses' Attitudes

Some nurses need to reflect and understand that patients and their families are human, and react in human ways during crisis. When my mother was awaiting surgery for her brain cancer tumor, 16 years before she died, the nurse told me that the night before her surgery she was concerned about "trivial things." The nurse said that she was surprised that my mother talked about how she was going to lose her hair, instead of worrying about the surgery. I told her that perhaps people who are faced with life-threatening surgery may be trying to focus on the trivial because they don't want to break down emotionally and tell you how scared they really are.

It's my hope that if some nurses don't receive adequate training in sensitivity, that in the practice of nursing, they will listen to patients and their family members and gain insight into this area.

Years later, when I placed my mother at the second nursing home after her head injury, I was very worried when my mother developed pneumonia. The nurse seemed offended when I expressed my worries. She said, "I don't understand your emotions." She was in her 40s, and had been practicing nursing for 20 years. Not only was she rude and insensitive, but, as I was to find, she was making a value judgment. She felt my mother was in such bad shape anyway, being semi-comatose, that I shouldn't be sad about her pneumonia. It was the attitude that, "She's better off if she dies." Would she have thought that a more normal attitude would have been that I should be happy? Ironically, about four months later, this nurse was stricken with cancer, a second time, and had to quit her job. She showed up one day at the nursing home with a bald head covered by a bandana. She had come to visit one of her nurse friends. She didn't see me, and I didn't approach her. A few weeks later, I heard that she died. I was sorry that someone so young as her had died. I began to wonder if in working at the nursing home and seeing people reach a ripe old age, though not in good shape, this nurse might have been envious that at least they'd had decades of life before reaching the end. She was probably wondering if her cancer would take her at a young age. Maybe when my mother had pneumonia, she was thinking that I was "greedy" in wanting her to live a long life, and that she was fortunate to have had so many years. At any rate, it's always dangerous when a healthcare professional makes comparisons. Each person has a different outlook on life and death. We should not try to evaluate what is a right or wrong reaction to a disease. We should just accept someone's emotions.

Oftentimes, patients are scared of dying and have a strong will to live. If a terribly ill patient does survive a nursing home, despite a lack of good care, even errors and abuse, some nurses assume they are receiving "excellent care" because the patient has lived so long. Most family members realize that some patients survive anything, and it's not necessarily due to what may or may not have been done for them.

Death From Poor Care

From what I saw, day after day, year after year, most patients in nursing homes die from poor care, before their illness takes them. A family friend who was a nurse and also once worked for the state as a nursing home inspector, told me this when I first confided in her about care issues. When nurses at nursing homes have the attitude that patients with certain conditions don't recover, perhaps they've never seen patients recover because a nursing home hasn't afforded them the proper environment to recover. It is largely an environment of germs, not just because the other patients are old and sick, but largely due to the unclean practices of staff.

I remember an agency nurse who substituted at the nursing home my mother was at, told me that he was surprised at how unclean his nurse colleagues were, in general. The day after he said this, a staff nurse came into my mother's room, and didn't take her shoes off to stand up on the sink counter to replace a light bulb. Even if she had, this still would have been unclean. The sink counter was used to place the sponge bath tub, towels, glasses of water, and medicine cups on. Since I had a bottle of Pine Sol ™ (that I brought from home and was often using), the nurse asked me if I'd disinfect the sink. If I hadn't been there, by the time she found a housekeeper to disinfect, an aide might have come in and placed something down on the sink counter. Further, one wonders if disinfectants can kill all germs.

There are so many unclean spots in a patient's room, and often the nurses set things down on contaminated surfaces. The sponge bath tub which is filthy is set down by the aides on the patient's tray table that he eats from. Nurses place spoons to stir medication not only on tray tables but on medicine tables where aides have placed dirty diapers while cleaning a patient. The point is, knowing that aides do unclean things, spoons and medication shouldn't be laid on bare surfaces without a towel being put underneath.

It doesn't help a nurse's aide's concept of cleanliness if some nurses don't practice cleanliness. For example,

I noticed a nurse emptying my mother's wastebasket, something the nurse's aides should have done. Afterwards, the nurse didn't wash her hands. She proceeded to crush my mother's pills to shoot them through her feeding tube. I gently asked her to wash her hands. It's unsettling that a layperson should have to correct a nurse. One wonders, too, how many unhealthy practices are committed when the family member isn't there. When the family member isn't there, the staff is probably even less careful.

Uncleanliness by nurses is also a problem at hospitals. When my mother was hospitalized, a nurse picked up a pill that had fallen on the floor. She proceeded to give it to my mother. I brought that to her attention, too. Nurses don't like to be corrected, no matter how nicely you speak to them. I avoided blaming her by saying, "Could my mother have another pill, please?" This works better than saying, "That's a dirty pill." If nurses come to work sick, as I've seen some do at nursing homes, ask them to wear a mask when they enter your loved one's room. (I even bought a box of masks for nurses and nurse's aides to wear. I put a sign in the room asking them to wear one, if needed.) If I saw a nurse with a cold, I'd say, "Do you need a mask?"

Often, nurses don't bother to wear latex gloves when they should. A nurse should always wear gloves in working with a feeding tube patient, that is, in administering formula and medication through the feeding tube. With a feeding tube patient, I observed that nurses never washed the pitcher with soap that they used to measure my mother's formula in. They merely rinsed it out with water. This is like cleaning your dirty dishes with no soap, just water. Worse, I saw a nurse swishing water around in the pitcher with her bare hand to clean it. Previously, she had touched the lid of the garbage can out in the hall that contained dirty diapers and that aides touched with their dirty latex gloves after cleaning up a patient. I don't know why a nurse would handle something that is supposed to be kept sanitary with bare hands, when she could have worn gloves.

At nursing homes, I've even seen nurses dispose of syringes in the wastebasket of the patient's room, instead of disposing of them in hazardous waste boxes. This violates law.

Other Problems With Nurses

A lot of nurses at nursing homes told me nursing decisions involve common sense, yet it's amazing how many times nurses don't exercise common sense. A lack of cleanliness, telling the patient's family that he won't recover right in front of him, and chewing out family members in front of patients, show a serious lack of judgment, besides unprofessionalism.

Some nurses at nursing homes would openly discuss the condition of other patients with me. For example, one nurse told me, "Can you believe that Mr. Smith wants a feeding tube for his wife who has Alzheimer's and stares off into space?"

Although I've complained in this book about nurse's aides giving "assembly-line" care in nursing homes, nurses often do, too. I remember at one nursing home, a new staff nurse entered my mother's room, and thought my mother was a man, because she didn't have much hair. This error wouldn't have occurred if the nurse had bothered to read my mother's chart and looked at her name. In all fairness, this happens at hospitals, too. Or, there are nurses who perhaps look at the chart ahead of time, but enter a patient's room and address her simply as "Ma'am." If they have such an impersonal way of dealing with patients, do these kind of nurses even like patients, or people, for that matter?

Some nurses in nursing homes have poor English skills, being from foreign countries. Since there is a shortage of nurses in the U.S., we will see more nurses coming here from foreign countries. These nurses are sometimes denied jobs at hospitals because their spoken English isn't good. While their written command of English may be good, how can patients, families, and doctors communicate with them, particularly over the phone, or in an emergency?

At nursing homes, I found that substitute nurses from agencies gave me valuable care information that my mother's staff nurses were afraid to tell me because they might contradict the institution's policies. For example, an agency nurse told me she thought my mother was alert enough to start eating by mouth. At the time she told me this, I had arrived at the same conclusion myself, but I couldn't get the nursing home staff to agree because the speech therapist there kept giving my mother a negative evaluation. (A speech therapist evaluates a patient's swallowing ability. I will deal with this swallowing controversy in depth in Chapter 4, "The Feeding Tube Fiasco.")

Postscript

In this chapter, I have brought home the point that in trying to get the care that a loved one deserves at a nursing home, one can't be faint-hearted in bringing care issues to the surface. You simply can't allow things to happen that further damage the health of a family member.

The reality is that patients go downhill in nursing homes, and when a patient starts to fail, the nurses often attribute it to the "disease process." However, in many cases, the patient deteriorates and dies from the uncleanliness or lack of care, not the illness that brought him to the nursing home. Medication errors, leaving windows open in cold weather, and infections due to the staff's uncleanliness lead to more health problems. The patient's resistance is often lowered by poor care. By blaming the patient's disease process for deterioration in his health, the staff is often refusing to see the cause and effect of poor care.

Chapter 3

Working With The Institution

Dealing With Management

In attempting to get the best care possible at a nursing home, you should know the resident care manager (RCM) of the unit your elder is in. She works day shift. She is usually one of two nurses on the unit. Although she doesn't work with the patients on the floor, she is supposed to do the paperwork, and therefore keep a care plan in place for the patient. She is also supposed to keep in touch with all the nurses on all shifts regarding each patient's overall care. She attends the quarterly care meeting for each patient and is in charge of fielding complaints. What we found was that sometimes a resident care manager had that job because she didn't like working with patients. A resident care manager who is a good one, has usually had experience out on the floor working with elderly patients and enjoys it. If a resident care manager isn't responsive to your complaints, then perhaps you should have your loved one transferred to a different unit. Or, an alternative is to speak to the social worker at the nursing home about care. Yet an alternative is to go the director of nursing. If all of them don't seem to have an answer, you could then go to the administrator. The latter could probably sit down with you, the resident care manager, and the director of nursing, if need be. I remember two such joint sessions my brother and I had with the whole crew at the first nursing home.

You talk to the administrator as a last resort. You don't want to make waves unless you've tried everything else. At a nursing home, social workers usually have no clout when it comes to care issues. The nursing staff often sloughs them off, feeling they don't know the realities of delivering care. The director of nursing is sometimes intransigent— too much of a bureaucrat. I caution you, too, in transferring your loved one to another unit. Nurses are often petty. They vent their bad feelings about family members to other nurses, so in another unit, your elder may not fare any better. The nurses may not like you right off the bat and not follow your wishes.

If you find you are getting bad advice in regards to the care of your loved one from the resident care manager, it may be because she either doesn't know much about the actual practice of nursing or because she just doesn't care. The nurse on the floor may not even like the resident care manager because the "RCM" doesn't fully know about the difficulties the nurse has in being out on the floor. Some RCMs are fresh out of nursing school, as with some other nursing home nurses, so it's the blind leading the blind. As I've discussed before, continuity of care at nursing homes is a problem. Although the RCM is supposed to pass along care issues that a family member has, to all shifts, somehow nurses on evening and graveyard shifts don't always hear about concerns. For example, if you find your loved one often has a soaked bed in the morning, you can assume she's not getting changed often enough on graveyard shift. Your best bet is to call up the graveyard shift nurse at 11:30 p.m. or talk to her before 7 a.m. because the problem is occurring on her shift. Tell her to make a note of this for all relief nurses on graveyard shift. By the same token, you can complain directly to the day shift nurse about a recurring problem on her shift, and ask her to make a note of it for the relief day shift nurse.

To ensure that certain care is being done, try to set up a schedule with the RCM for certain tasks. For example, if you get a doctor's order for four times a week of restorative aid, (more than what the nursing home offers), ask if it can be done at 9 a.m. Then, if you come in at that time, you can monitor that it was done. Otherwise, you'll be told it is being done, even if it isn't.

At one of the nursing homes my mother was in, we knew the RCM was checking off care that hadn't been done for our mother. There is nothing to prevent an RCM or nurse from doing this, unless a family member asks to read the elder's chart on a regular basis. For example, if the doctor orders that a bedridden patient should be gotten out of bed and into a wheelchair twice a day, the chart will state that it is being done. Even if you know it isn't happening, the chart may note that it is. The nurse's aide may check off in his report that he got the patient up in a wheechair. If he didn't check off that it was done, the RCM may merely say that he actually did it, but forgot to check it off on his report. In the years that my mother was in nursing homes, I perhaps read the chart once or twice. I didn't have to believe what I was told about care being done, since I was there to witness whether it was done or not. If you notify the state about care not being done, the state can levy a penalty fine against the nursing home, particularly if the care was ordered by the doctor or if its basic care.

In complaining to nursing home staff, it's best not to hit them every day with complaints, if you can possibly avoid it. Write the date and time that you found your elder soaked in urine in bed, for example, over a week's stretch of time. Present that paper to the RCM. She'll then have a week's overview, and can't just say there was one bad day of care. In reality, for all the money you're paying for minimal care, all the minimum should be executed.

Sometimes the RCM will try to get you off her back when you repeatedly complain about care. For example, she'll tell you the reason that your elder isn't receiving good care when everyone else is, is that you're around too much of the time making the aides nervous. If this is the case, you say that they need to monitor their aides so that you don't need to be around to ensure that care is being delivered. After all, if they consider you to be a nuisance, they are really considering the patient to be a nuisance. The patient would be complaining, too, if she had the ability to complain.

It's a vicious circle at nursing homes. No one really listens to anyone else. The nurse's aides complain to nurses that they have too many patients; the nurses complain to the director of nursing (DNS) that they can't handle the patient load; and when a family member complains about care, he is initially listened to, but nothing is remedied. If complaints persist, the staff usually verbally beats on the family member. A lot of nursing homes have between 120 to 160 patients, and even if just a small percentage of family members are there on a regular basis and complain, it's too much for the staff to handle.

One would think that with what a nursing home charges, it could offer more than three meager meals a day; one sponge bath a day; some music in a large activity room; ten minutes of range of motion exercises two or three times a week (if that); and a nurse delivering medication and treating bedsores that the aides most likely caused the patient to have from not changing his diaper as needed every two hours. Unfortunately, warehousing is the norm at nursing homes. The attitude is that patients go there to die, rather than to live in dignity for however long they have left.

I was told by a former nursing home nurse that there's not much difference between the "best" and "worst" facilities. I think she was right. This is because all seem to have routine problems, such as a lack of care, neglect, and even abuse. Management often "deals" with these problems by ignoring them and hoping they'll go away. Keep in mind, too, as this nurse said, that neglect is abuse.

At a nursing home, an elder gets group care. Unless the patient becomes ill with pneumonia, requiring suctioning out phlegm and giving oxygen, normally the staff spends a total of about one hour and 45 minutes out of a 24-hour period tending to each patient. This is what I observed day after day, year after year. This one hour and 45 minutes includes a nurse giving medication and aides bathing, changing, and feeding patients. Therefore, one can pay thousands each month for a private room and minimal access to a nurse and aides. If, for example, your loved one gets pneumonia, the nurse's care may involve one and one-half hours out of a 24-hour period. Each time my mother had pneumonia, I had to alert the nurse that she had it, and I had to insist that she treat her for it. At a nursing home, there is ready access to oxygen, a suction machine, and a hoyer lift. However, if a family member isn't there to request that the elder receive the type of care that involves the use of this equipment, what is the point of having this equipment available?

When a patient is sent off to a nursing home, make sure her doctor has filled out a sheet called "Physician's Orders for Life-Sustaining Treatment." However, this doesn't mean the nursing home will follow these orders, My mother's doctor filled out the form with instructions for the nurses that if my mother had no pulse, her heart stopped, and she was not breathing, she was "DNR," meaning "Do Not Resuscitate." If a patient isn't very alert to begin with and is bedridden, normally the family requests DNR and lets him die a natural death. To try to resuscitate him would only leave him in worse shape, since by the time a staff member discovered he wasn't breathing, chances are he would have lost oxygen to the brain. Consequently, he wouldn't likely recover, and would be brain-damaged. In my mother's case, we did ask the doctor, however, to stipulate on the form that she was to receive "Advanced Intervention," meaning that 9-1-1 should be called, and that she could receive, for example, oxygen, suctioning, medication, and IV fluids. He also stipulated that she receive antibiotics, feeding tube formula, and fluids.

It's interesting that even with these formal Physician's Orders, nurses don't always react to giving advanced treatment unless the family member is there insisting on it.

I was told in confidence by a family friend who is a nurse that the fact of the matter is, that if a doctor sends a patient off to a nursing home with DNR orders, this signals to a nurse that his patient has a poor prognosis and isn't expected to recover from his illness. Our nurse-friend said that unfortunately, nursing home nurses have too many patients, and that some end up picking and choosing who they'll help. The staff members may ignore a patient in my mother's condition, or at least, end up giving her less care than the other patients receive. I'm sure, however, many nurses don't believe this is right and treat each patient equally.

I wonder what a nursing professor would say about picking and choosing who receives care? I'm sure she'd say it's outright discrimination and unethical.

One thing I can say is, given the attitudes of staff, in order to get the best care for our loved one in a nursing home, it's helpful to have more than one family member advocating for the elder. It's important that all family members, in fact, present a united front. If family members disagree about whether to continue treating a patient for illnesses, the staff may slack off even more. They will take the attitude of the family member who thinks the patient is better off if left to die. My brother and I were always committed to seeing that our mother received care, giving her as much of a chance as possible to enjoy whatever time she had left. The staff did pick up on the fact that my brother and I often didn't get along over matters not related to our mother. This was dangerous and led the staffers to use this to their advantage. For example, when my brother complained about therapy issues, physical therapy, in particular, the physical therapist, instead of addressing himself to this issue, got off complaining about me. He falsely said I wouldn't listen to him when he told me that certain physical therapy wasn't feasible for our mother. It was very common for staff to divert the conversation over to "such and such a family member alienates staff by not listening," or "by complaining." Then, the conversation shifts to a complaint about the family member rather than to the care issue itself. In this case, my brother was subtlely discouraged from voicing his complaints. My brother should have backed me up, but instead felt badly and didn't fully pursue the care issues that he set out to address.

Another common tactic that staff members use is to start complaining about you if you complain about care. In fact, if you complain, they'll sometimes tell you that two staff members witnessed you doing something that you shouldn't have been doing. When they tell you this, insist on knowing who the staff members were. You have the right to know. If they tell you that they can't reveal the staff members' names, that's hogwash. They tell staff members the names of family members who complain about them. Therefore, it should cut both ways.

What family members often find at nursing homes, is that they pick their battles. If you care about your loved one, you insist on the staff keeping her clean, and you insist on safety issues, such as in transferring a patient to a wheelchair. You advocate for those. With the other care issues, you often pick up the slack, either doing it yourself or paying to have someone come in privately and do it. While it sounds wrong to do this, as you are paying for care, you realize that what is supposed to be done, and what actually does get done are two different things. You can't negotiate for everything. If you complain about too many things, they'll become even more hostile and tune out completely.

At nursing homes (and hospitals), whenever staff sees a family member doing care that they say they provide, but don't follow through on, or that they execute so poorly as to harm the patient, no one feels ashamed. One would think that an administrator, resident care manager, or director of nursing would have the pride to say, "That's our job. We should be doing it." However, that's not the case.

Throughout my mother's years at nursing homes, we did write letters to staff reviewing care issues. It's necessary for a family member to keep these letters in his file at home, so that down the road, if more critical issues arise, and you feel you need to contact the state with complaints, you have documentation.

It should be noted that often our letters to nursing homes complimented them for any good care that we noticed or improvements in care. At times, we forced ourselves to embellish on something ordinary that they did right. In other words, at nursing homes, good care could be referred to as "excellent."

Letters to nursing home staff should be kept factual with no sarcasm about bad care. Avoid presenting them to the administrator unless neglect is flagrant or there is abuse. Perhaps you could start by writing the letter to the resident care manager and copying the social worker.

When placing a loved one in a nursing home, it's helpful, (and nursing home social workers agree), that you outline basic care points. Following is a sample of "Family Care Concerns" that we drew up to be placed in our mother's chart. While many points seem obvious, they are noted because while in the hospital, prior to her nursing home entrance, these points weren't always followed.

Family Care Concerns

1) Blood draws/blood pressure left arm only. (Due to right mastectomy.)

2) Feeding tube precautions:
   A) Please advise aides to turn off the feeding tube before changing her diaper.

   B) Please advise aides to keep her elevated in bed, especially for at least a half hour after her tube feeding.

   C) Please coordinate wheelchair transfer times, so as not to interfere with feeding tube formula time or digestion times.

   D) Please run feeding tube slowly so the patient doesn't vomit.

   E) Please don't put dye in feeding tube formula.

3) Please have patient in her wheelchair twice daily for two hours.

4) "Head Injury Patient." Please make sure aides use extreme caution when transferring her into a wheelchair, changing her diaper, and pulling her up in bed. No hitting or jolting head.

5) Bedrails should always be used.

6) Skin breakdown concerns:
   A) Patient should be changed and turned every two hours.
   B) Please wear latex gloves.

C) Patient is allergic to diaper wipes. Please avoid cleaning patient up with wipes after urination. Dampen and soap terrycloth towels, instead.

7) Please don't roll patient onto her stomach tube, and keep tube free from urination areas.

8) No catheters, please. (Got bladder infection in hospital).

9) Restorative aid five times a week as per doctor's orders.

10) Constrictive hose to avoid clots in legs, and arm and leg splints as needed. Please advise aides about care in turning patient in bed when splints are on.

11) Family prefers bed bath, instead of shower or bath-tub bath, for the time being. Please dry patient well.

12) After shampoo, please use hair blower on low setting only, because of some bald spots. Please don't leave hair wet.

13) Please keep windows closed. Patient has had colds, sinus problems.

14) Avoid patient contact with those having cold or cough.

15) Patient has been very conservative about drug use. Doesn't even use aspirin unless necessary when ill.

Tests/Vaccinations

*Patient had TB test. Please no routine tests/vaccinations without notifying family first.

*Had tetanus shot in November. Doesn't need another.

Allergies

Allergic to bee stings.
Drug allergies: Dilantin, sulpha, amoxicillin

Patient has Blepharospasm. Eyes squint and blink and are sensitive to bright light. No medications, please.

Reminder

Patient likes to be called by first name

* * * * * * * * * * *

As for a sample letter to the resident care manager, documenting specific care problems including dates and times of occurrence, I provide the following. This documentation forces the staff to stop denying that care problems exist. However, this doesn't mean they'll be able to resolve them.

To: Jane Jones, R.N., Resident Care Manager

Dear Jane:

As a followup to our last memo dated Aug. 11, we would like to update you on care issues observed that should be addressed. In general, the staff remains friendly and courteous, and several aides, namely, John and Joe, have done an excellent job. After your emphasis on initial care problems occurring during the late night shift, we have seen a clear improvement on how our mother is being positioned in bed.

Nevertheless, four basic areas have yet to be dealt with satisfactorily, on a regular basis:

1) *Changing and turning the patient every two hours*
2) *Resulting skin breakdown and prescription cream application*
3) *Feeding tube precautions*
4) *Wheelchair operation during patient transfer*

While the listed problems seldom produce immediate emergencies, we have done our best to simplify the staff's duties to only these four tasks. Please find enclosed, notes that detail some of the examples from these four areas of care observed over the past ten-day period. Assuming that you share our concerns, we hope that you can suggest some approaches to improving the level of care. We will gladly make ourselves available for any meetings or recommendations you may have to help remedy these problems.

As you can imagine, the stress of dealing with a parent's illness is considerable. The continual effort of monitoring staff and assuming staff responsibilities as well, is an unnecessary challenge we would like to avoid. We look forward to your suggestions and further cooperation.

Sincerely....................

Friday, Aug. 15

A.M.
—*Blood drawn from the wrong arm, despite instructions and posted warnings.*
—*Aides unfamiliar with feeding tube precautions.*

Swing Shift
—*Aides can't set up folding wheelchair.*
—*Aide arrives alone, requesting family help for changing a diaper.*
—*Patient rolled over onto her side, on swollen left hand and fingers.*

Saturday, Aug. 16

A.M.
—Patient left lying flat on back, bed soaked in urine.

Swing Shift
—1:30-4:30. No diaper change until I used the call light.
—Aide wanted family assistance. Unfamiliar with two-hour dia-
    per change schedule.
—Could not set up wheelchair.
—No diaper change until 8 p.m. when I used the call light (Three
    and one-half hours without a diaper change).

Sunday, Aug. 17   Good Care Observed!

Monday, Aug. 18

Swing Shift
—Patient's left arm trapped under her side during diaper change.
    Patient opened mouth in pain.
—Aide left patient slumped in bed with diaper off center.
—Bed soaked in urine and skin rash appeared.

Tuesday, Aug. 19

A.M.
—6:30-9:30. No diaper change until I used call light.

Swing Shift
—3:30 p.m. —Aide knows nothing of wheelchair schedule. Leaves
    to get another aide to help. Doesn't return until 4 p.m.
    Doesn't know about two-hour diaper changing schedule.
—Nurse has no time to check skin rash. Asks me to apply pre-
    scription cream.

Wednesday, Aug. 20

A.M.
—Nurse too busy to apply skin rash cream. (I applied it on A.M.
      and Swing Shifts.)

Swing Shift
—Aide doesn't know about two-hour diaper changing schedule,
      feeding tube precautions, nor how to set up wheelchair.
—4:50-8:15. Aide changed diaper after several calls. Patient
      soaked in urine with skin breakdown. (Nearly three and
      one-half hours before diaper changed).
—Aide suggests family hire private help since he is too busy to
      come in every two hours. Aide left soiled linen in room.
—Patient changed again at 10:40 p.m. after I used call light.
      (Changed two hours and 25 minutes later).

Thursday, Aug. 21

A.M.
—6:20-9:20. No diaper change until I called aide. He wants me
      to help.
  Unfamiliar with how to position patient in bed.

Swing Shift
—3:30. No water for patient after 2 p.m. tube feeding.
      Aide called at 3:30. Arrived at 4 p.m. for wheelchair
      transfer.
—5:00 I had to search for aide to transfer her back to bed.

Note: I had to apply prescription skin cream on both shifts.

Friday, Aug. 22

A.M.
—I applied prescription skin cream (and also on Swing Shift).

Swing Shift
—Evening aide asks for me to help in changing diaper.

Saturday, Aug. 23

A.M.
—A.M. nurse tells me to instruct aides on changing diaper,
*   positioning patient in bed, and wheelchair use.*
—Aide left me with patient for 20 minutes with her sliding off
*   her wheelchair, until help could be found.*
—I was asked by nurse to apply prescription skin cream (and
*   again on Swing Shift).*

Swing Shift
—No response to 3:30 call for aide until 4 p.m. Aide wanted my
*   assistance in changing the diaper.*

Sunday, Aug. 24

A.M.
—6:30-9:30. No diaper change until I called.
—I was asked by nurse to apply skin cream.

What is obvious from the schedule, is that had I not been at the nursing home, my mother would have been neglected for many more hours, or care might have been skipped altogether. Many nurse's aides knew nothing about what to do for her.

What becomes all too clear at nursing homes is that as soon as aides have become familiar with caring for a patient, they quit, and there is a turnover of staff. Or, on days when an aide has the day off or is on vacation, an aide will arrive who knows nothing about the patient, and the nurse hasn't oriented him to the patient's needs.

Further, when a patient is transferred from the Skilled Unit to the Intermediate Care Unit, a new crop of aides must learn to work with the patient. Again, the nurses don't orient the aides, so a family member must be on hand to orient them.

Besides new aides, moving to a different unit, means a new resident care manager. It's almost as if the patient is moving to a new nursing home. When my mother moved from the Skilled Unit of the first nursing home to the Intermediate Care Unit, we had a care meeting with the social worker and the new resident care manager. We printed up a list of our mother's care needs, regarding R.N. and aide care. On this sheet, we also plainly stated that "Family members and our mother's physician should be promptly notified if our mother's condition should change." While one would think that this is a given at a nursing home, nothing should be assumed.

It seems hard to believe that there is often such little communication between nurses and nurse's aides. However, the nurses are struggling to manage their work load, and don't have time to work with the nurse's aides. Ideally, to alleviate a lot of care problems, the nurse should go over at the beginning of each shift with each aide what each of the patient's needs are. At some nursing homes, I found some aides who didn't even know the name of the nurse on duty. And, of course, the nurse was busy passing out medications for 25 to 40 patients and couldn't check up on whether the aides were even entering a patient's room at all. If an "Activities of Daily Living" sheet (ADL Sheet) was posted above the patient's bed, this sheet wasn't even read by the aides. For example, an ADL sheet might read, "Transfer patient to a wheelchair after sponge bath." However, there was no one to monitor whether the aide followed through. Most patients at nursing homes can't push the call light for help, if no one shows up to help them. They could sit in bed for eight hours or longer before someone shows up.

Instead of spending time helping our mother come out of her coma and increase her level of alertness, we were on hand at the nursing home to assist with routine personal care.

As for a skilled patient, it seems that the attitude of staff members towards her is, "Well, it's free to the patient, so the family shouldn't expect anything." Medicare and private insurance pay hundreds of dollars a day for a skilled patient. Often, the aides justify not giving sponge baths regularly, and not changing the patient's diaper, because they've been told by the resident care manager that it's free care. It's not uncommon for the nursing home staff to feel that the family should do the care or hire a private aide. It's as if they don't realize that the elder has paid into health insurance and the social security system through the years.

In the Skilled Unit at the first nursing home my mother was at, the resident care manager horsed around and came up with the most implausible explanations on how care was actually being given to our mother, but that we weren't noticing it. She said that patients often soak their entire bed in two hours before their next diaper change. And, she said that aides may have been turning our mother's body from side to side every two hours, but that we must not have been realizing that her body had been turned.

When the resident care manager finally stopped horsing around, we got her to post a time sheet for aides to sign in on when they entered our mother's room. The time sheet stated the two-hour intervals for changing the diaper and turning our mother. It was posted inside the doorway so the aides didn't forget to sign it if they entered the room. We found that no one cheated and signed in despite not providing care. It made the aides somewhat more accountable and reminded them overall to do their work.

In dealing with nursing homes, every once in a while, a followup letter should be written to staff noting improvements in care and yet, outlining basic care points that still aren't being followed.

The following letter was written to the resident care manager of another nursing home, and the social worker was copied. As you can see, many of the same care issues existed here, too, as in the previous facility. (Aspiration precautions mean that a patient with swallowing difficulties should be kept elevated, so that saliva or fluid doesn't go down the wind pipe after coughing, and get down into the lungs.)

To Ann Smith, R.N.,
Resident Care Manager

Dear Ann:

In general, we have been very pleased with the friendly and courteous attitude of the staff at Nursing Home X, and we have seen a clear improvement in the overall level of our mother's care compared to other facilities.

Our observations and recommendations focus on four basic areas where changes could be beneficial:

1) Aspiration Precautions
2) Changing and turning patient every two hours
3) Chair transfer schedule
4) Restorative aide schedule

Comments

1)— Patient is often slumped in bed and not pulled up with her head at the top of the mattress.
— She should be tube fed in bed with her upper body elevated per the speech therapist's sign to help minimize coughing and aspiration chances.
— Changing should precede a set feeding tube schedule so the process is uninterrupted. Family would like to be advised of the schedule.

—*Best feeding tube position includes the lower lift of the hospital bed elevating her legs and the patient on her back, but elevated.*

2)—*She appears to be checked on average every three hours for incontinence. She is frequently left in her wheelchair for up to four hours instead of two hours, thus diaper changing runs behind. By lowering the back of her wheelchair, her diaper could be changed while in the wheelchair.*

— *In bed while being turned, extra care needed when arm splints are on to avoid hurting her ribs and arms, etc. A pillow under her side and between her legs should not be forgotten.*

3)—*We would like to have her up in a chair by 10 a.m. and back in bed before noon. Then again for two hours in the afternoon and back to bed before changing and feeding.*

—*Please remind aides to transfer her with care to her wheelchair since she has sometimes seemed frightened and her head has been jolted. Also, the hammock clamps should be kept from pinching her legs. Washcloths, under the clamps, can be used as buffers.*

4)—*Patient has a history of blood clots and should receive her full five days of restorative aid exercise for one-half hour each day.*

—*We expect a substitute if the restorative aide is absent and family would appreciate knowing the schedule. (While family is present much of the daytime, we have yet to observe restorative aid sessions.)*

Reminders

A.) Please observe "Left Arm Only" precaution for blood draws.
B) Please notify a family member prior to administering any injections, drugs, treatments, enemas, suppositories, etc.

(Extra water is the preferred treatment for constipation.)
C) *Concern exists that Phenobarbital is hard on the stomach if not given during, or shortly after the feeding tube formula.*
D) *Can the patient receive a shampoo in bed until her cough subsides?*

We appreciate the opportunity to review the points identified above and are confident that attention to the indicated refinements will ensure that our mother receives the best possible care. Please do not hesitate to call us with any questions or concerns that may arise. Thank you.

Sincerely ....

* * * * * * * * * * * *

Many of our letters to staff focused on care reminders for aides that any aide should have known, simply by having gotten trained and certified as a "Certified Nursing Assistant" (CNA). However, we found we needed to repeatedly outline basic points on hygiene, in positioning our bedridden mother in bed, in hoyer lift safety, and basic comfort issues relating to the room. One would think that family members' letters would be a welcome reminder of what aides weren't doing that they should be doing, so that the nursing home could note pitfalls in care and correct them for the benefit of all patients. Such is often not the case.

Some of the following issues would concern a lot of family members. They can be used as family guidelines for care and as a checklist. I didn't present these to the nursing home staff, but from time to time, I brought up some of these points, as needed.

Hygiene Reminders for Aides

1) Change diaper every two to three hours to avoid skin breakdown and bladder infections.

2) When changing her diaper and turning the patient, be careful not to bruise her head or knees on the bed's side bars.

3) Always use gloves when changing diapers and giving sponge baths.

4) Record all bowel movements.

5) Don't use two diapers at a time to avoid changing the patient regularly.

6) With sponge baths, don't place your bare hand in the plastic tub to check water temperature. Hold your hand underneath the faucet.

7) Don't soak terrycloth towels in sink. Soak them in the plastic tub.

8) Don't wring terrycloth towels with bare hands before you work on the patient. Use gloves.

9) Don't take terrycloth towels from another patient's room and use them for our mother.

10) With a sponge bath, please use more than just two washcloths and one hand towel. Must use towels to rinse body. Must dry body well.

11) Clean armpits, and in between fingers and toes.

12) Use gloves when carrying out dirty diapers and clothes.

13) Don't wheel the dirty laundry bin into the patient's room to strip the bed.

14) Record all bowel movements as small, medium, or large.

15) Don't clean ears of the patient. Ask the nurse to do it.

16) Don't scrub the patient's face.

17) Use a mask if you have a cough or cold.

Hoyer Lift Safety for Aides

1) Two aides should operate the hoyer lift. (If one is unavailable, ask the nurse for help).

2) Don't allow metal slabs of the hoyer's hammock to push against the patient's head when transferring the patient. Use pillows to buffer head.
3) Don't allow the patient's head to be bumped when transferring her.
4) Release the tight metal clasps of the hammock once the patient lands in the wheelchair.
5) When the patient is lowered back into bed, make sure her head doesn't hit the bedboard.

Positioning Patient in Bed

1) Elevate the patient's back.
2) Alternate the position of the patient from right to left.
3) Patient is more comfortable if, when receiving a tube feeding, she is resting on her back, but elevated.
4) Never have the patient sitting on her knees when her back is elevated and she resting on her side. (I found my mother on many occasions with her body twisted to one side. Her body weight was completely resting on her knees.)

Miscellaneous Care Reminders for Aides

1) Don't open the window. (Aides forget to close it.)

2) Don't turn down or turn off the thermostat.

3) Keep blinds and curtains open.

4) If the nurse isn't available, turn off the feeding tube before lowering the bed. Afterwards, ask the nurse to turn the feeding tube back on and re-elevate the patient.

Some families find it too stressful to try to deal with nursing home care problems. They get frustrated in dealing with the staff who often turn hostile when unresolved problems are repeatedly brought to their attention. I had a wealthy friend who retained a healthcare management company to send one of its nurses to advocate for her mother at a nursing home. A healthcare management company may charge a few hundred dollars per hour. If a patient is at a nursing home, its nurse will review care issues with the staff. Of course, this becomes expensive depending on the regularity of visits you want the company to make and how much time they spend following up with the patient.

Knowing nursing homes as I do, the staff doesn't like outsiders coming in and telling them what needs to be done, be it family members or colleagues in the healthcare field. I learned that they didn't like nursing colleagues from elsewhere when my mother first became a hospice patient, but hadn't left the nursing home yet. The staff ignored my mother's hospice nurse who made weekly visits, just like they sometimes ignored doctor's orders or tried to get around them. The staff often feels they don't have to answer to anyone. I even remember overhearing a conversation with another hospice nurse who came to visit another patient. The hospice nurse and the staff nurse were discussing care issues. Apparently, the staff nurse hadn't bandaged the patient's surface tumor, as the hospice nurse had instructed her to do on her previous visit. (Incidentally, one can be a hospice program patient and also be living at a nursing home. This will be discussed further in Chapter 5, "Alternatives to Nursing Homes.")

At any rate, a healthcare management company might not have any better success than a family member does. For some, it may be worth a try, however, especially if one doesn't have the time to deal with the staff.

Most family members, even if they don't visit their elder regularly, do attend quarterly care planning meetings that the state usually requires a facility to have.

Care Planning Meetings

At quarterly care planning meetings, the resident care manager and the social worker attend. In addition, often the physical therapist attends. If you request the director of nursing to attend, she will, too. At these meetings, the staff can get defensive, but they try to be on their best behavior. No matter how complimentary you've been in the past, at the first sign of a complaint, they may say, "Can't you ever tell us of anything good we've done?" This was once said to us by the physical therapist in attendance. We politely told him that we often wrote to the administrator thanking her for all the "tireless work" she and her staff did. I suppose staff members often look at family members as being adversaries. Perhaps they think it's a family's job to make them feel good, since they rarely get praised by their supervisors.

In my decades of teaching and communications work, I can't remember being praised by an employer, and I don't expect it. If I'm lucky, a student or client says something nice every blue moon.

We'd often start out the meeting by focusing on the positive and my brother and I discussed what was being done right. Then we stated, "There are some points that still need addressing." We also said, "We know if your loved one was in a nursing home, you'd like to see that he was getting the promised care that he was paying for." We always brought notes to the care meeting—so we didn't waste our time and the staff's time—or we'd often print up a paper and photocopy it to distribute to all in attendance. This paper stated our concerns, along with improvements in care made since the last meeting. We'd sometimes even distribute this paper a few days in advance of the meeting.

At a quarterly care meeting, the staff often tells you that the next time you walk into your elder's room and you spot a care problem, to come and get them right away. However, this rarely worked for us since it was often hard to track down a staff person when a problem occurred. Being short-staffed, they were either busy with another patient, you couldn't find them, or they'd find some excuse not to come. For example, the social worker who was getting tired of my repeated complaints, once replied when I went to get her, that she was busy. She wasn't working. In fact, she looked like I'd interrupted her daydreaming.

Sample Letters to the Social Worker

Following is just one of the letters I wrote to the social worker about persistent care issues. This social worker demonstrated repeated callousness. She informed me that I was alienating the staff with my repeated complaints. My complaints were polite, but they were repeated because the problems weren't resolved. She had told me that if I didn't like the care, we could go someplace else. In trying to remain professional, I did her the courtesy of referring to her "kind and caring assistance" and by stating, "recognizing that you are a person of high standards." Neither statement could have been farther from the truth. Further, she had once told me that she had no social work degree, and that, in fact, she never even studied it in college. (This didn't surprise me.)

In my letter to her, I mention aspiration precautions. These are things I will discuss at length in Chapter 4, "The Feeding Tube Fiasco." Aspiration involves the feeding tube patient getting fluid in the lungs. The patient can choke on feeding tube formula, either resulting in death or pneumonia if the patient is kept flat on her back while the formula is pumped into her stomach. Further, you will note that I complained that my mother smelled of urine under her armpits due to the fact that the aide used the same wash-cloth to clean under her armpits that she used to clean her urinary area. She even cleaned her urinary area before clean-ing the upper part of her body. This doesn't follow proper procedure.

This is the letter:
To Jane Doe, Social Worker

Dear Jane:
   My brother wrote a letter to you before I reported to him of our noontime conversation today. I agree with him on several points, especially the need for your nursing home to find some way of monitoring its staff, without putting the embarrassing and frustrating burden on the family to report basic care prob-lems. As I said last summer, it's very awkward and unfair to put family in the line of fire, drawing hostility and countercharges from a number of aides whom we've reported.
   I realize that you might not be fully aware of some of the nurse's aide problems I most recently spoke about to nurses. Recogniz-ing that you are a person of high standards, I'm certain you would agree that some of the routine practices I've observed on the part of aides are unacceptable. In fact, they would present health and safety problems for any patient which you would feel badly about. Please consider the following:

* *Blowing Stench. This involves leaving dirty diaper pads, dirty diaper wipes, dirty towels, and dirty latex gloves in my mother's room, often right on the heater, on counters and tables, on the floor, or even in her bed. The last time this occurred was particu-larly embarrassing. My mother's elderly friend came to visit and reported to me that she'd found a diaper on the heater, filled with feces. Of course, it's a fire hazard, in addition to being smelly.*

• *Someone Else's Feces On My Mother's Shower Chair. An aide rolled in a "poopy" shower chair for my mother to be transported down to the bathroom and bathed in.*

• *My Mother Smells Of Urine And Sweat After Her Sponge Baths. Surprisingly, most recently, her underarms smelled of urine after her sponge bath. Whenever sponge baths aren't done properly, I always pick up the slack, and redo them myself, rather than bother a nurse by complaining. (However, after I redo the sponge bath, I usually do bring it to the nurse's attention for her own records.)*

• *Room Window Left Open In 50-Degree Weather With Mother in Her Room. This is particularly frustrating in that I have a sign on the window reminding people not to do this. The last time this happened, the aide returned three and one half hours later. Fortunately, I returned about 10 minutes after she left the window open.*

• *Forgetting Aspiration Precautions. You, yourself, put a sign above the bed as a reminder, but as you've noted, it's not being followed.*

• *Slamming The Already Brain-Damaged Side Of My Mother's Head Against The Metal Part Of The Hoyer Sling. On one occasion, her eye was nearly poked out, too. Many aides don't even bother to get a partner to operate the lift, even though they are inexperienced at using it.*

• *Bed Remade After Her Sponge Bath With Wet and Dirty Drawsheets. Here again, rather than alienate an aide, I always remake the bed myself, and then later report the problem to the nurse.*

• *Neighboring Patient Left Naked On Top of Her Bed With the Door Wide Open. This went on for a half-hour until I came back from an errand and was able to summon the nurse.*

Please be aware that my mother's nurses have repeatedly brought these problems to the attention of the remiss aides. Either they don't care, or they just don't get it.

I would sincerely appreciate your taking care of these and other general issues without further engaging me in any discussion or involvement with aides.

I'd like to say one last thing in closing, in case you haven't considered it. The cost of nursing home care is overwhelming. It's a real sacrifice for us, and yet we always make a point of paying on time or even ahead of time, feeling that we must support those who support us. We've always loved our mother very much. Widowed young, she raised us as a single parent. We believe she fully deserves the promised comfort care—delivered in a humane and responsible way—without further hassles.

As always, thank you very much for your kind and caring assistance.

Sincerely..........................

I should explain that I hadn't intended to write the social worker a letter, in addition to her receiving one from my brother that day. However, she unexpectedly showed up at my mother's room to inform me that I was alienating the aides with my numerous complaints. She wasn't addressing herself to my complaints, so I documented them in the letter. This letter led her to call a meeting with both the nurse and the aides in my mother's unit to discuss the care issues that I pointed out that were obviously flagrant, as you can see. However, in reality, they weren't anything new or unusual for a nursing home.

My brother's letter was equally courteous and made compliments that really weren't deserved, particularly in the first paragraph.

In the second paragraph, my brother refers to a "physiatrist," who is a physician who specializes in physical therapy. In the next to the last paragraph, I should note that the facility refused to follow doctor's orders that aides should sit my mother up on the edge of the bed to strengthen her back muscles. The staff didn't change its position on this, saying that it was a safety issue, even though two physicians ordered it, including her internist. We feel the facility didn't want to take the time to do it. My brother and I ended up doing the task ourselves, sitting our mother up on the edge of the bed daily.

Here is my brother's letter:

While this morning's meeting was cancelled, we appreciate your efforts to quickly clear up any difficulties involved with our mother's care. As we've stated before, much of her stable condition can be attributed to a clean, well-organized facility with excellent nursing care and an extremely high level of dedication on the part of administrative and supervisory staffs.

Her family doctor and visiting physiatrist have been impressed with her health despite her overall condition, and their consensus included the view that uncommonly frequent family companionship, an above average amount of restorative aid, stimulation from oral feeding, and the family's monitoring of daily care, have been beneficial. While these activities haven't been encouraged by your facility, the results for the patient have been positive. Fortunately, we are glad to see a continued commitment from the facility to be flexible in sharing a mutual interest for the best possible quality of patient care.

In preparation for our meeting, I think it may be helpful to clearly define our viewpoint, realizing that I may not thoroughly speak for Charlotte. Nonetheless, it seems inevitable that the unreliability and inconsistency of work performed by aides in the healthcare field, is the major remaining challenge we are all struggling with. Your facility appears to invest more in trying to solve this problem than any organization we can imagine.

However, mistakes are made, and not admitted by those responsible. Even if Charlotte's observations are 80 percent erroneous, from a facility standpoint, I am sure that you would consider the remaining 20 percent to be unacceptable.

From a patient's perspective, the unnecessary family presence for monitoring care and inefficiencies it produces, could be easily solved by the installation of a video camera. A less practical solution could be a third party "quality care" observer, to point out weaknesses in care and indicate where corrections may be called for. Since I doubt that your policies would permit such solutions to be enacted, it would be our hope that you can suggest another mechanism for regulating and assuring patients' families that standards of aide care are being met.

Lastly, regarding the doctor's order for sitting the patient up briefly, on a daily basis, he certainly does not see a safety concern. Accordingly, however, we would be willing to sign any form releasing your facility and its staff from any responsibility for an accident that might occur in the process. If aides are uncomfortable working with Charlotte, maybe someone who didn't find her presence intimidating, could spare the 60 seconds.

Again we thank you and your colleagues for trying to work with us to ensure the best care on the patient's behalf, without making it a daily ordeal.

Sincerely ....

* * * * * * * * * * * *

The Bottom Line On Care

Without engaging in arguments with the facility's staff, the bottom line on care is:

1) Your loved one is spending his life's savings at a nursing home. Can't he at least be kept clean, safe, and live and die with dignity?

2) What would a staff member want if his loved one was a patient there?

3) Cleanliness and safety standards are set by the state, and the nursing home needs to follow them.

4) If the nursing home doesn't monitor its staff and doesn't advocate for the patient, then the family member must. You are compelled to report problems.

5) Presumably, the staff went into the healthcare field to serve patients, so they must serve them, and they should care about the care issues.

6) You are asking for no more than what the facility promised—basic care.

Many staff people who work at nursing homes seem to subscribe to the belief that if you repeat statements about giving "excellent care" enough times, the statements will be accepted at face value.

Even if a staff member truly believes the care is excellent, is there no room for improvement?

What helped me when the care concerns I'd voiced weren't listened to, but sloughed off, was to come up with pat answers to the institutional jargon.

Examples:

Social Worker: You're the only one who complains.
Answer: Don't you feel there's any room for improvement?

Nurse: We give excellent care.
Answer: Shouldn't you let the patient and/or family member be the judge of that?

Resident Care Manager: If you don't like it, you can go
    someplace else.
Answer: I'm not asking for anything that wasn't promised.
    You are required by the state to give this kind of
    care. I'm trying to work with you rather than get the
    state inspectors involved.

Social Worker: You've alienated the staff with your com-
    plaints.
Answer: That doesn't surprise me, but you've unfairly put
    the burden on the family member to monitor care,
    because you don't monitor your staff. It's your re-
    sponsibility to monitor whether each patient is get-
    ting the promised care, either by putting a camera
    in each patient's room or having a supervisor moni-
    tor your nurse's aides to ensure each one is kept clean
    and safe. How do you ensure that patients who have
    no family get the care they are paying for?

Director of Nursing: The staff doesn't like you.
Answer: They don't have to like me, but they have to give
    the patient the care she deserves and pays you for.

A major reason that things are chaotic at nursing homes
is that aides are allowed to do practically anything without
reproach. At one nursing home we were at, aides were
allowed to insult nurses and even write up complaints
about them. Worse, an aide was allowed to write up a false
complaint about me. She said I called her stupid when I
asked her to read the sign above my mother's bed about
having her elevated. She perhaps feared I'd complain about
her, so she felt she needed to complain about me. Administrators are so fearful that aides will leave, they'll often accept any behavior from them. Instead of allowing aides to
write up supervisors and family members, they simply need
to be told they'll be fired if they can't act appropriately.
Somehow in healthcare, staff never seems to realize that

patients are customers who pay their salaries. After the aide wrote me up, stating falsehoods, the resident care manager reprimanded me in front of the aide. I plainly refuted the charge and told them we were paying thousands of dollars a month for care, and I intended to see that care was not only done, but that it was done properly. When I mentioned how much the cost of care was, they looked aghast. The resident care manager was 26 years old, and probably didn't even own a house. She had no concept of the cost of anything. In fact, at another nursing home, a nurse in her late 50s thought the monthly cost of care was $2,000. When I told her it was three times that much, she said, "This care isn't worth that." (Rather unprofessional of her to say that, even though she was right.)

Staff could do so much to remedy problems at nursing homes by not fostering an adversarial relationship with family members. Instead of telling nurse's aides that a particular family member complained about this or that, they should say, "Family members commonly complain about such and such." The reason for this approach is that all patients' families usually have the same complaints. From meeting other families, we learned they were disturbed about the same issues we were.

Staff should also tell aides that if a family member spots them not wearing latex gloves in giving personal care to a patient, the family member has every right to ask them to wear gloves. You are not "supervising" their aides by asking them to do something they forgot to do. If you don't alert the aide to the mistake, he'll infect your elder before the supervisor has had time to correct him. If you do report him, he is mad at you for tattling. I always risked getting flack from the professional staff for dealing directly with the aide, but in a situation of uncleanliness or lack of safety to the patient, you can't reach a nurse in time before the deed is done. It always seems to go back to the fact that the professional staff would rather endanger the patient than possibly hurt the aide's feelings. If the staff really cared about the patients, they'd thank a family member for alerting them to problems, rather than be fearful of losing incompetent aides.

Years ago, I read about some disability rights attorneys suing two nursing homes in the San Francisco area, claiming they provided shabby care that violated federal anti-discrimination laws. The suit was on behalf of several patients and their relatives who made use of the Americans With Disabilities Act. It required equal treatment for the disabled. The suit charged that leaving patients unattended for long periods, failing to turn them in bed or bathe them, using improper chemical and physical restraints, falsifying their records, and deceiving their relatives, violated their rights. Unfortunately, this kind of treatment is business as usual at nursing homes. I and my friends would often compare notes about the nursing homes we placed our elders in. In my mind, this lawsuit really drives home the point that the most vulnerable members of our society who are old and disabled and can't speak for themselves are victims of the worst kind of discrimination.

Dealing With The Ombudsman

We've known families that were just as diligent as we were in trying to work with nursing homes to see that their family members got the care that they deserved. Some of them resorted to going to the ombudsman to complain. In reality, they fared no better than us. At best, the slack is remedied for a couple of weeks, and then it's business as usual. Sometimes you'll see ombudsmen visiting the nursing homes, and they'll stop into elders' rooms and introduce themselves. They'll ask you if you have any complaints. Often, I'd speak informally to them without lodging a complaint or showing them correspondence I'd written to the nursing home staff. At one nursing home, we saw ombudsmen come and go in a matter of every six months. Some facilities don't even have ombudsmen to cover them, since it's a volunteer job. Ombudsmen are like anyone else in the healthcare field. Everything is relative to them. They think, yes, there are problems with keeping patients clean, though "This facility isn't as bad as the rest." Their attitudes were often that you weren't going to find any better facilities. In other words, they took notes, but they really didn't address themselves to specific problems. They concluded that since the facility wasn't as bad as the rest, it was good. Ombudsmen may be a start in resolving problems for some people, but as a hospital nurse once told me, you try to contact the State's Long Term Care Office and see if you can't talk directly to someone with more authority who inspects facilities.

Complaints can be made confidentially to ombudsmen, if you wish. As for family members who did complain regularly to ombudsmen, the staff always seemed to know who had complained, not only by the nature of the complaint, but by the fact that so few family members ever showed up on a regular basis, that they could figure out who complained. Of course, some family members walk down the hall with ombudsmen and it's obvious to the staff that they've lodged a complaint. I even once overheard a nurse saying to an aide that Mr. So and So's family must have complained because the ombudsman was investigating such and such.

Incidentally, as I mentioned before, we avoided going to the ombudsman to complain, but always tried to work with the staff to remedy problems, so as not to alienate staff more. We found that in the healthcare system, professionals are often vindictive, and ignore the patient even more if complaints are formalized. When problems persisted, we did write letters to the resident care manager of the unit or the director of nursing, just to have a paper trail, so that if something catastrophic happened, we would have adequate documentation of long-standing problems that weren't resolved.

An ombudsman once told me that she tries to "persuade and negotiate" with the nursing home. It's obvious, however, that nursing homes don't listen well to ombudsmen, unless they present a pattern of complaints. In serious cases of abuse, the ombudsman contacts the State Licensing Agency of Long-Term Care Facilities or contacts the Attorney General's Office. Certain violations can lead to the loss of license to operate and loss of Medicare and Medicaid certification and funding. To contact an ombudsman, you can contact either the State's Long-Term Care Office, the State's Agency on Aging, the State's Human Services Department, or the Governor's Office.

If you decide to contact an ombudsman over routine care issues, document your complaints, such as how often you found the neglect occurring, and specifically when you found the neglect occurring (i.e. when you found your elder soaked in urine.) You can also complain to the Senior Services Division of your county.

I remember an ombudsman tried to get the administrator of the "absolute best" nursing home in town, where I'd placed my mother, to allow a "Family Council" to be established. This nursing home was run by the clergy. It was the concept of safety in numbers where common concerns of all families could be discussed. The ombudsman said the social worker could join the weekly meeting. Of course, the administrator never got back to the ombudsman about this. I believe all nursing homes should be required by law to have ombudsmen set up Family Councils. Otherwise, nursing homes can hide behind statements like, "You're the only one who complains." If you hang around a nursing home as much as I did, you get to know other families, and you realize you're not the only one with particular kinds of complaints as the management would like you to believe. The management doesn't want to hear about what families think of the care. Does the nursing home ever send out surveys or queries to family members? Essentially, what the nursing home believes is that they don't have any problems, only that the family member is a problem. And, they say that if you don't like it, you can go someplace else, but " we're the best." It also amazed me that if you got a staff member to admit the care wasn't what it should be, her attitude was that they were better than the bad ones. This lack of logic, unfortunately, is all too common in healthcare. Comparing yourself to something that is perceived as being worse, makes little sense. If, for example, a school that you send your child to, tells you they have some bad teachers, but that they are the best school because they don't have as many bad teachers as the others, would you be comfortable sending your kid there?

If only nursing homes showed the same vigilance every day of the year as they do when the state inspector visits annually. For those few days a year, during day shift when the inspectors are around, things seem to work. Of course, the administrators always instruct staff on what and what not to do around inspectors. The resident care manager also has a watchful eye on the aides.

All family members that I got to know through the years my mother spent at nursing homes complained that staff didn't know what goes on behind closed doors. As I previously discussed, there was the case of the woman who was pulled up in bed by the nurse's aides and whose head was hit against the bedboard, thereby causing her a stroke that led to her paralysis. The daughter who later questioned the administrator, a member of the clergy, said the administrator never fully investigated how the accident happened. When the daughter called in the state to investigate, the administrator merely kept repeating that they had the highest rating of any nursing home in the area. Often, it's as if the administrators are in total denial of mistakes made. Nursing homes that don't document, fully investigate, and report patient accidents or injuries to families and the state, incur fines and could be shut down. However, if anything is done, the wheels turn very slowly. With an elderly person, it's hard to prove what really happened unless a staff member speaks up and reports another staff member. The staff feels that by believing they give excellent care and saying they love their patients, they owe nothing more. As for the daughter of the patient, the last time I spoke with her, she had filed a lawsuit against the nursing home.

Dealing With The Administrative Policies

Nursing home administrators will tell you when you bring safety issues to their attention, that accidents are investigated. They miss the point. You are speaking about preventing accidents, and they're talking about what will happen should an accident occur. I have given the example of one nursing home my mother was at, where they didn't have a hoyer lift. They lifted my mother out of bed using a bedsheet, and transferred her into a stretcher type of wheelchair that elevated her back once she got into it. When I told the administrator that transferring a patient using a bedsheet was unsafe, he changed the subject and blamed me, the family member. He said I shouldn't be in the room at the time she was being transferred, because the aides would get nervous with me looking on. As far as an accident being investigated, I said to him that he was missing the point. I wanted to prevent an accident. I said they should have a hoyer lift. This nursing home was the most expensive in town. It was not only lacking in wheelchairs, hoyer lifts, and shower chairs, but it didn't have enough linen.

The bottom line is, administrators don't care if you bad-mouth their nursing homes to the state or to your loved one's doctor. They don't care who you bad-mouth them to. There's a shortage of nursing homes, and they usually have enough business with hospitals quickly throwing out elderly patients.

In my mind, quality of life is often determined by the level of care an elderly person receives, and the caring attitude of those around them. In a nursing home, the staff's attitude toward the patient and its neglect and justifications to not give required care, diminish a patient's quality of life. The staff talks about how the patient should be allowed to die right in front of the patient who oftentimes is at least semi-alert.

A family member sometimes wonders what a patient gets for his money at a nursing home. Even when you're visiting nursing homes to select one for your elder, the promotional literature they hand you, doesn't spell out their daily services. I believe they don't specifically state their services because they know those services are sporadic and that they don't deliver on the care they verbally say they provide.

At nursing homes, more and more, they are raising their fees according to the level of care needed by the patient to where one feels they are charging a base rate for room and food, and everything else is extra. Essentially, you are paying thousands each month for just room and food. About two weeks before we transferred our mother out of one nursing home and placed her into another, we received notification that the present nursing home was raising its fees.

The following letter, written by my brother, to the administrator raises questions as to how the level of care is defined.

To : John Doe, Administrator

Dear John:

In reviewing your letter dated Nov. 1, we noted that two separate rate increases have been planned, beginning next month. New pricing based upon the patient's level of care raises a couple of questions relating to our mother.

It would be helpful to receive a clarification of the differences in the care provided for Levels 1, 2, and 3. Specifically, I would appreciate the opportunity to read a summary of the actual care functions to be performed at each level. While there are several that my mother doesn't use, it would be important to make sure that we are not passing up some assistance that would be beneficial.

You can have the summaries faxed to my attention. Thank you again for your past help and for your response to this request.

Sincerely.......

A bedridden person is defined as needing the most extensive care (Level 3), because turning and lifting the patient is required, and he is totally dependent for care. However, with this level of patient who pays more because of his condition, often less is done. For example, a bedridden person usually wears a hospital gown, and doesn't need to be fully dressed with pants, socks and shoes, etc., as does an ambulatory patient needing this assistance. A feeding tube patient pays more for a nurse to fill a feeding tube bag with formula. However, the patient isn't eating food and doesn't require assistance from an aide to feed him. Therefore, there are so many gray areas of level of care. We took our mother out of this nursing home, not because of the fee increases, but because we had already planned to do so due to poor care. Two weeks after the administrator's letter notifying us of fee increases, my mother, who'd been on the waiting list at another nursing home, was accepted. Therefore, we transferred her.

What you're paying the nursing home for, is often for care you're not getting, but are supposed to get. In the case of a bedridden person, the advantage one initially sees of having her in a nursing home is that the aides will do the lifting and turning of her heavy body. However, if this isn't done on a regular basis, there is often no advantage to having a bedridden patient at a nursing home. She merely sits unattended to in bed. Particularly if a patient is heavy, an aide won't lift her and will leave the patient alone, unless the family member is there to assist with the lifting. One often initially feels that at least the patient will get his diaper changed and his heavy body turned during the night every two hours as promised, so a family member can go home and sleep. This is usually not the case. On graveyard shift, the nurse and the aides have twice as many patients and are even less prone to attending to them. Therefore, a patient may only be changed once or twice at most in an eight-hour period.

Most people would say that the more a family member is willing to do for a patient in a nursing home, the staff gets used to having you do it, and they do even less. However, the reason a family member often does as much as she does, is because after repeated complaints of neglect or poor care, the care still isn't being done. So, at that point, you either accept what little is done, or you transfer a loved one to another facility and see if it can do any better. Or, you can take her out of institutions and find care alternatives.

At the last nursing home my mother was at, one day I overheard the director of nursing tell a substituting agency nurse that I did most of my mother's care. In reality, I did 99 percent. She said it matter-of -factly as if it was just fine for them.

The reality is, no one likes to lift a heavy, bedridden patient, not even at a nursing home. Some foster homes won't do it, and often home health aides won't. They may say they do, and you pay for it, but it doesn't get done, at least not on the regular basis as needed. Therefore, if you want lifting and turning done on a regular basis, you have to do most of the care yourself, either getting assistance at a nursing home, or you find some foster homes that do it, as stated in Chapter 5, "Alternatives to Nursing Homes."

The nursing home mentality is such that low standards and low expectations for patients is the norm. Eating is considered an activity, as is sitting in a wheelchair. They are defined as such on the ADL sheet. At home, activities might mean reading to an elder or having him listen to music.

If there were more hired help at facilities, perhaps there could be more real activities for patients. I knew a terrific nurse at a nursing home who, after eight months, got fed up and left. On the rare occasion that no patient was ill and that she'd done all of her work well before the end of the shift, she took the time to go into a patient's room and read to him.

Even though it would be nice to have activities at a nursing home, if it is short-staffed, at least the cleanliness and maintenance issues should be the priority.

If any care is executed, it is often done halfway. If and when a diaper is changed, if the bedsheet underneath is soaked, the bedsheet isn't changed.

My brother and I often wondered what would happen if the nursing home told aides to check the diapers of incontinent patients every hour instead of every two hours. Since aides took "every two hour" diaper changes to mean every three, four hours or more, we wondered if telling them to change a patient every hour would get them to change the diaper every two or three hours.

I often walked in on aides in the early morning, who two minutes after they entered a room, had skipped giving a sponge bath as required, and were merely putting on a fresh diaper on my mother. They had intended to put on a fresh gown and get her up in her wheelchair without so much as even wiping up her soiled skin. Rather than report them, I would say, "My mother needs a sponge bath as scheduled. I will help you give her one." If a family member is not around to check up on them, it's no wonder care isn't done. Again, no one bothers to figure out what goes on behind closed doors. The answer is often nothing—no care. If you complain about an aide, the aide often turns against you, and makes countercharges that the management asks you to answer to. It's really unbeliev-able. We pay their salaries, and they treat us like that.

If aides knew that spot checks were going to be done on their patients for cleanliness while they were doing personal care and that they would be fired on the spot if they were caught cutting corners, perhaps they might be more motivated. Spot checks would also curb dumping garbage and dirty diapers into a patient's wastebasket with-out carting them off. Spot checks could also alleviate the problem of piling dirty linens and clothes on the floor (which is unsanitary), and not carting them off. The only time I didn't see those common occurrences is when the state inspectors came for their annual inspections. Other-wise, nurse's aides wouldn't be reminded to avoid these unsanitary practices.

If there was a special R.N. coordinating patient care by the nurse's aides, spot checks could be implemented. The R.N. could even make sure that patient's windows weren't left open. If nurse's aides were perspiring from lifting pa-tients, they'd sometimes enter rooms and turn off the ther-mostat, or if they wanted to air out a room with odors, they'd open the window and turn off the thermostat. They'd forget to turn the heat back on. A spot check by a nurse could alleviate these problems, too, so a patient wouldn't be left in a cold room for several hours.

If I'd walk into my mother's room and find an aide changing my mother's diaper and wiping her rear end, it wasn't uncommon to see my mother turned over on her side with her legs dangling over the edge of the bed. If she had started to fall, her fall couldn't have been broken with-out her or the nurse's aide being injured. With spot checks by a nurse, she could even reinforce proper methods of turn-ing a patient. She could note common problems aides have in working with patients, and then give inservices review-ing basic care problems. Aides often forget to even lift bedrails back up after working with a patient. Mobile pa-tients, in particular, could fall off the bed.

One thing that becomes clear in seeing what goes on at nursing homes, is that from a family member's perspective, it doesn't pay to have minimal standards for care. Minimal standards become no standards at all in a very short time. For example, even at some private nursing homes, they give bedridden patients sponge baths every other morning, instead of once or twice a day. Even a sponge bath a day is certainly minimal if one is incontinent. Usually a bedridden person who urinates on herself needs a sponge bath every morning and evening. If, however, the rule is a sponge bath every other day, then a patient often won't even get that. It's in the best interests of a nursing home to have adequate aide care and enough aides to keep patients clean, otherwise the nurse will have more work in treating and bandaging skin wounds due to poor aide care. One nurse told me that when aide care is bad and patients get skin breakdown, it's difficult to give skin treatments on top of passing medications to 40 patients.

In an attempt to prevent skin breakdown, at one nursing home, fungus powder was used on my mother's rear end. This is done by the staff for its own convenience, certainly not for the health of the patient's skin. If she urinated and wasn't cleaned up in a timely fashion, the fungus powder would act as a skin barrier, the aides thought. The trouble with this was, that one aide in particular, who was not cleaning my mother up for hours at a time, dumped layers of fungus powder from the back end to the front of the diaper. Besides not helping her irritated skin, fungus powder certainly wasn't good if it got into her internal body parts. Worse, this aide borrowed a neighboring patient's bottle of fungus powder to use on my mother. How unsanitary.

Spot checks by a special nurse who coordinates aide care would also reveal common problems such as dumping dirty sponge bath water, tainted with feces and urine down the sink, rather than in the toilet. As I mentioned previously, if enough towels were even used to begin with, dirty towels wouldn't need to be re-dipped into a sponge bath tub. By dumping dirty water into the sink, this could contaminate the sink for nurses who use it. They fill glasses of water and sometimes flush feeding tube bags in the sink.

Other routine care issues that we encountered from time to time involved an aide who always threw my mother's gown on the floor while giving a sponge bath. After the sponge bath, instead of putting a new gown on my mother, she would ask me if I wanted my mother to wear the dirty one again.

In giving sponge baths, some aides would drip water onto the floor creating a hazard for visitors and staff. They would never even notice. Dirty washcloths would not only be thrown on the floor, but even left in my mother's bed with sheets unchanged.

Sometimes aides would reuse terrycloth towels. I sometimes used rolled up terrycloth washcloths and placed one in each of my mother's palms. Nurses tell you to do this, so a brain-injured patient who contracts her fingers doesn't dig them into the palms of her hands. (Actually, wrist splints or arm splints are better so the fingers don't curl as much.) Believe it or not, after some aides gave my mother a sponge bath, they would sometimes take a damp or dirty washcloth that they had already used and roll it up in her palm.

After sponge baths, powders become a hazard, too. Often, aides get carried away using baby powder after a sponge bath to freshen up the patient and avoid dry skin. I'd find powder all over the floor. In fact, one of my friends who had a parent in a nursing home elsewhere slipped on powder on the floor. He broke his hip, became bedridden, developed lung problems from lack of exercise, and he died of pneumonia. Her father was alert and had been walking well. She sued the nursing home. Often lawyers won't even take the case of a nursing home patient, since a monetary award is minimal in compared to the costs of trying a case. Unfortunately, an elderly patient who is spending money being cared for in a nursing home and isn't being a "productive citizen" earning money, is often seen by the court system as not being very valuable.

Other lapses in care that one routinely witnesses involve aides handling food. I saw aides filling glasses of water with ice for each patient. They would scoop ice into glasses with their bare, unclean hands, rather than bother to use a spoon.

When my mother was strickly getting nutrition through her feeding tube, she would sometimes get diarrhea. You would wonder how someone who wasn't eating real food, just formula, could get diarrhea. I found diarrhea was common at nursing homes. If one patient had it, it spread fast among patients on the same hall. If an aide didn't wash her hands and use latex gloves in doing personal care, she was transferring germs from one patient to another. In particular, there is danger when a patient who has swallowing problems gets diarrhea. If she gets diarrhea, she could get stomach flu, vomit, and aspirate from vomiting.

If personal care is terrible at nursing homes, what is even more disheartening is the attitude of administrators. As I previously discussed, at one of the best-rated nursing homes in town, the administrator actually capitalized on poor aide care. He was into double dipping. My mother was allowed free skilled care by Medicare and her insurance in that facility, when she left the hospital. The care was so bad, we thought of hiring a private aide to relieve me when I wasn't there. We told the admnistrator that since aide care wasn't as a rule getting done, despite our insistence, I and another "family member" would have to do it. He actually suggested that we could hire one of their aides on his day off and the nursing home would get a cut of the aide's private work. You would think that the director would be so ashamed of their care and be afraid of getting reported to the state. Can you imagine suggesting that they get more money to fix their problem? At this time, we learned of a "better" nursing home, and we put our mother on the waiting list there. We ended up finding our own private aide, the daughter of a nurse-friend, and we paid her. However, we told the staff that she was a family member, and that she wasn't getting paid. We figured that the staff would end up doing absolutely nothing for our mother, if they knew we were willing to pay for outside help, as many families resorted to doing.

At this same nursing home where bedsores were especially prevalent because of poor aide care, the nursing home billed the patient's insurance for special visits from a dermatology nurse to recommend treatments. How about just keeping the patients clean?

Strangely enough, the next nursing home we put our mother in, didn't allow private aides to be brought in. Their rationale was that private aides weren't needed because they did their jobs well. (In reality, this wasn't the case.) But, they also cited another reason. That is, that their aides would feel badly because a private aide would likely be paid more money than what they were paid. So, why didn't they pay them more money, so they weren't unhappy and didn't leave the facility?

After listening to the contorted thinking that goes on in institutions, it's enough to make a family member scratch her head, to say the least.

One does empathize with the plight of some aides who are honest about doing their very best, even though their skills are lacking. Nurse's aides do get a raw deal at nursing homes. Besides poor pay and too many patients, they are often not assured of regular work. At nursing homes that take a lot of short-term rehab patients who leave and return home, if they are low on patients for a few days, some aides get sent home. Then, the aides are short on making ends meet.

As I previously discussed, often if aides need money, they exhaust themselves by working a double shift. Then they'll go home to sleep for a few hours and be back for their regularly scheduled shift. Although a family member sympathizes with these aides, your first concern is whether your parent, under these circumstances, is getting even less care, due to the aides' exhaustion.

One nursing home my mother was in, hired many Russian aides. Sometimes I heard Russian spoken over the intercom. I wondered how the aides could do their job, follow the routine, and observe safety precautions, if they didn't know English well enough. Perhaps they could pass the nurse's aide certification written exam, but that didn't mean they could adequately function on the job.

Due to the shortage of nurse's aides, in the rare event an aide does get fired for something flagrant, she goes to another nursing home and gets hired. If she gets fired there, it's not uncommon for her to come back to the first nursing home and get rehired. Or, you see agencies send aides to nursing homes where they once worked, but got fired at.

Many aides offer substandard care. Many are poor, and aren't in good health themselves. At a hospital, all staff, whether they work with patients or not, are required to have chest x-rays. This is often not the case at nursing homes. Caregivers at nursing homes are hired and come to work hacking away. Who knows what lung problems they have? During flu season, many nurse's aides can't afford flu shots and many nursing homes won't provide them for free. They catch the flu, come to work sick, infect other aides, and end up infecting patients who die. Doesn't the nursing home think it's more economical to provide aides with free flu shots, so they don't end up short of healthy aides and have to hire agency people or pay other staff aides overtime to fill in? Does it make economic sense to kill off patients with flu germs? Those elderly patients who've had flu shots can end up getting the flu anyway, being around sick aides.

According to the way the staff thinks at nursing homes, no patient is an ideal one. Nurse's aides feel that a patient who is "totally dependent" or bedridden, is hard to lift, turn, and change diapers for. However, they don't like mobile, disoriented patients who are often placed at nursing homes because they are combattive.The patients can punch and hit, regardless of the medication they take to sedate them. Like nurses who talk in front of the patient about her condition, nurse's aides will sometimes talk about how the patient is a "vegetable" or a "nuisance." Connect the dots. The aides hear nurses being so blunt, so they pick up that kind of talk.

As I've noted, working conditions for nurses aren't really any better than for nurse's aides. With as many patients as nurses have, a patient often is in distress for hours and even dies in her room without someone knowing about it until hours later. Nurses feel they don't have time to treat illnesses or deal with a dying patient. Twenty-four hour care at nursing homes is an impossibility. One nurse and a few aides can't possibly monitor a few dozen patients. They can't possibly know if someone is sick in his room until it's too late, unless a family member visits and notifies them. If the nurse does know someone is sick, most of the time, she'll postpone responding, and let the illness fester, perhaps getting sidetracked with other duties. Or, often the nurse doesn't care enough to treat the patient. The nurse is just one nurse out on the floor, with as many as 40 patients. She gives multiple medications to each patient; deals with patient injuries from falls; does bandaging for skin breakdown; writes in the patients' charts; phones the doctor for medication; and phones the pharmacy, etc. In reality, nurse's aides see a patient no more than once every three or four hours, if that, but they do see the patient more than the nurse does.

An excellent nurse at a nursing home told me in confidence about something she found disturbing that the director of nursing instructed her to do. The director of nursing instructed this evening shift nurse that if the graveyard shift nurse was late in getting to work, as she sometimes was, she should leave work anyway, before the graveyard shift nurse got there. (Why not fire the graveyard shift nurse, you ask?) If the excellent nurse did leave on time, that would mean four aides on duty for 80 patients with no supervisor. The only other nurse in the building was at the opposite end, taking care of her 80 patients. In a patient emergency, even if an aide miraculously happened to be in a patient's room at that very time, the aide would have to run clear across to the other side of the building and search for the only other nurse on duty. That's one nurse to 160 patients. As I've said, there really is no 'round the clock care at nursing homes because of the inadequate staffing levels. A patient might as well be at home with the family member sound asleep. Of course, if a patient has pneumonia and is dying, even on day shift, one nurse can't help. One would think that a nursing home would call in an extra nurse to help an ill patient or a dying patient who can't be transported to the hospital, and whose family would expect the nursing home to take care of for the money she pays. (The patient's Medicare and insurance company doesn't want to foot the bill for the hospital because she's already at a facility.) Sadly, if a patient has pneumonia, the nursing home doesn't want to do anything.

If the patient leaves the nursing home to receive treatment like surgery, often the hospital discharges the patient prematurely. Nursing homes have been known to ship the patient back to the hospital later that same day. How can an elderly patient survive this back and forth treatment. It's the, "You take care of her. No, you take care of her." The patient often can't survive this shuffling around.

As for pneumonia, my mother did receive a pneumococcal vaccination every winter in the nursing home. However, it never helped her, because her pneumonia always originated from colds she got from ill staff. Once she got the cold, the nurses ignored it. (When I took my mother home from the nursing home in her weakened state, the last eight months of her life, she didn't get pneumonia. At the first sign of a cold, I gave her a cold remedy, because I knew she couldn't blow the mucous out of her nose and that it would seep down to her lungs. The nursing home would just allow the cold to develop into pneumonia, and then not want to treat the illness.)

In my mother's case, she could still receive feeding tube formula during her pneumonia. However, when I was finally given permission to feed her by mouth, pneumonia would set my mother's health back. While she was being treated for it, weak and not alert, she was not able to eat by mouth. Consequently, during her three weeks of recovery, she'd lose the progress she'd made and the momentum in exercising her throat muscle that she'd made. It was a real chore to get her stronger so she could be alert enough again to eat by mouth. The feeding tube issues will be discussed in Chapter 4.

Besides delaying treatment until a patient gets full-blown pneumonia, once a nurse at a nursing home gets around to calling the doctor, the doctor often delays in getting back to the nurse. I often had to remind the nurse to make a second call to the doctor in an urgent situation. She would get busy with other tasks. With pneumonia, the delay is often lethal. Sometimes, before the nurse got through to the doctor, the pharmacy that the nursing home dealt with would be closed. Of course, pharmacies make emergency deliveries to nursing homes late in the evening, but often the nurse wouldn't be motivated enough to call the pharmacy until morning. By then, the pneumonia was worse.

Sometimes if a patient is very ill with pneumonia, the physician will order a respiration therapist to visit the nursing home and do suctioning of mucous. Physicians often realize that nursing home nurses will not suction a patient on a regular basis if she has pneumonia. If a patient is very advanced in her stage of pneumonia, this professional suctioning may be needed. The nurse often delays in calling the respiration therapist once she receives the doctor's order. At one nursing home, a Catholic nurse who had just received her degree from a Catholic university's nursing school, delayed calling the respiration therapist after she received the doctor's order. Why? She wanted to waste time questioning me about why I wanted to save my mother's life.

Little is done at nursing homes to help prevent lung problems in bedridden patients. Not only does getting them out of bed and into a wheelchair help their lungs, but regular aide care in changing their diaper and turning their bodies helps them exercise their lungs. Beyond this, bedridden patients can very simply have the backs of their beds kept elevated. Nurses and aides can even pat patients' backs and try to loosen any congestion on a regular basis. Unfortunately, a lot of nursing homes don't bother with any of these tasks on a regular basis. Another method I used with my mother was to help her cough by laying her flat on the bed, turning her on her side, and patting her back. Then, I'd re-elevate the bed.

(Incidentally, I always thought, from what my mother's doctor told me, that bedridden patients were very prone to pneumonia. Therefore, I was afraid of taking my mother home and not being able to deal with pneumonia. However, I now believe that pneumonia isn't inevitable for some bedridden patients if they are given the proper care of being turned in bed regularly, gotten into their wheelchairs, and not exposed to sick caregivers. The nursing home, I believe, does much to cause pneumonia for a bedridden patient just by not giving her the proper care. As I've said, during the last eight months of my mother's life when I took her home, she made it through winter not getting pneumonia in her cancerous and weakened condition. She got pnemonia every winter at the nursing home. Therefore, one wonders, as I now do, what is the purpose of putting bedridden people in a nursing home? They are more prone to germs and poor care which causes them to become infected and get ill, thereby needing a nurse. At home, they often don't need a nurse, if cared for properly. Of course, once a patient does get sick in a nursing home, and requires a nurse, help isn't on the way. The nurse either responds too late or doesn't want to respond.)

If family members must be around to notify nurses of illness, they shouldn't have to notify nurses of obvious physical changes in a patient. For example, my mother had a large, ugly sore on her scalp. Having little hair and a bald scalp in many places, one could easily see a large, bloody crust of pus on her scalp. There were a total of five nurses in a three-day period who saw it. No one gave it any attention until I finally asked one nurse to do something about it. She had had this sore once before at the nursing home. A nurse who had since left the nursing home identified it as psoriasis. This latter nurse told me she'd seen other patients at the nursing home get it. She felt it was due to nurse's aides not rinsing a patient's head well after shampooing it. Before my mother entered the nursing home, despite bald patches on her head, she never had this problem.

When I asked the nurse to call the doctor, she got an order from him to treat the sore with those over-the-counter shampoos for psoriasis. When the doctor said she needed a shampoo each day for two weeks until the psoriasis cleared up, the nurse told him she didn't have time to shampoo her every day. While this may have been true, I decided to do it myself, since the alternative would have been to have a nurse's aide shampoo her. Even if the nurse's aide did follow through, which is doubtful, she would leave her head wet wrapped in a towel, and leave her hospital gown wet from the shampooing.

Nursing home staff is often angry with family members who complain. They must realize, however, that they choose to work in nursing homes and are free to leave themselves. Most

nurses told me that their pay at nursing homes was com-
parable to what they'd get at a hospital. However, they said
their benefits weren't good. If nursing home nurses were
angry, it was often because they felt they had too many
patients. Although hospital nurses may have only five patients, they are required to give advanced care to those patients, not just pass medications. At nursing homes (and
hospitals, too) nurses often don't realize that they are prone
to making mistakes if they have a poor attitude about a
patient or family member, or are angry about too much
work to do.

   I caught medication errors at nursing homes. What bothers me is the times errors may have occurred that I didn't
catch. At nursing homes (and hospitals) nurses speak of
"human error" as if it's not preventable. Is it more appropriately "human carelessness"? What I observed at nursing homes is that medication errors were sometimes made
because the nurse felt she knew the patient and had her
drugs committed to memory. One would think that knowing a patient over a long period of time helps a nurse not
to commit errors. I thought nurses always checked charts,
but they don't. If a doctor orders a change in medication,
unless a nurse reads the chart, she won't know about it
unless the nurse on the previous shift tells her (which she
should, but doesn't always.) Or, the nurse would obviously
know about it if the doctor called in the order at the time
she was on duty. When the nurses didn't read my mother's
chart, this resulted in two kinds of medication errors.
Once a nurse brought in an extra dose of anti-seizure medication in the afternoon. My mother only took it twice a day,
morning and evening. Another time, a nurse didn't read
the chart and therefore didn't know that one of her drugs
had been discontinued, and another had been substituted.
In both these types of medication errors, the drugs wouldn't
have killed my mother, but they wouldn't have helped her
condition. For example, an extra dose of anti-seizure medi-

cation will sedate a patient more. In hospitals, medication errors are more likely to cause death, because the patient can get someone else's medication, with the nurse not being familiar with patients. If errors don't cause death, they can cause severe illness, injury, or a coma, particularly in an elderly person who can't spring back as well as a younger one. As laypeople, we've come to know that nurses don't have to admit medication errors, and if someone else suspects an error, he'll keep quiet. If I ran over a nurse with a car and said, "It was human error," people would be appalled that I didn't confess to it being human carelessness. Professional errors are not to be excused as human error, either. They are due to carelessness.

Nurses at nursing homes, as a rule, don't appreciate having family members around even if they come to do their work for them. They don't like having family members around who can spot errors or uncleanliness that leads to infection. Some nurses would rather have a patient get sick without family members there to prevent an error, than have a family member spot the error and correct it. I often thought that nurses went into the field because they liked to help people. Sometimes, in the healthcare field, helping people is the farthest thing from the employee's mind. If you read a nurse's chart for a patient at the nursing home (or hospital) it often reads like a gossip sheet. What they write in reports about a patient or even a family member is something they might not say to your face, and may not even be true. It may be totally self-serving, just to cover themselves. If a family member complains about care, a nurse might write in her report that he was angry and rude. (Further, I've read doctor's charts when they slip out of the exam room at the clinic, and they often contain observations that have nothing to do with the patient's condition or well-being.)

Nurses are sometimes unprofessional in other ways. Again, one wonders about the extent of their training. At two nursing homes my mother was in, nurses would walk up to family members telling them to go and see a doctor, because they might have such and such a problem. I not only overheard this, but I was the victim of it twice myself. Two nurses at different nursing homes told me they thought I looked like I had a thyroid problem. As doctors and some nurses will tell you, thyroid problems can't be diagnosed by looking at someone. When I was first told by one nurse that I may have a thyroid problem, I was upset. I felt I had no symptoms of fatigue or weight problems. I didn't have a bad skin color, nor did I have a lump on my throat. When I called the doctor's office to speak to the nurse, she said that the nursing home nurse was unprofessional. I wondered if these nurses who walk up to family members like this, would walk up to strangers in a store and remark about their health. When I saw the doctor, I found I didn't have a thyroid problem.

As for other nursing issues, if the nursing home doesn't have air conditioning, as if often the case, nurses should make certain that in hot weather, patients receive extra water to keep them hydrated. This is, of course, unless the patient's doctor has restricted water intake. In some nursing homes, patients die of dehydration when it's hot.

If a patient is bedridden, she can gain twenty or twenty-five pounds very easily even just taking feeding tube formula. This happened to my mother. Unlike in your own home where there is no scale that you can weigh a bedridden person on, nursing homes have scales that you can roll a wheelchair onto, with the patient sitting in the chair. Sometimes nurse's aides have trouble weighing patients using this method. You can get the nurse to assist an aide. The wheelchair slides over a platform. (The aide has presumably weighed the wheelchair ahead of time with no patient in it.) When the patient is wheeled over the platform scale, the weight of the chair is subtracted from the total weight. The problem is, the weight of the patient may be off by a few pounds, depending on how well the patient is positioned in the wheelchair. If you question your elder's weight, have her re-weighed by the nurse.

No matter how hard you try to communicate well with staff, and keep on their good side, again, nursing home personnel don't like having family members around for any length of time beyond a short visit. Deep down, they know this isn't the type of care they would want for themselves. They don't want people around asking questions or asking for help for their elder. You walk a very tight rope, but if you feel your elder deserves care, you must ask for it.

Advocating for Physical Therapy/ Occupational Therapy

Unless your loved one has a good chance of being rehabilitated, physical therapists at nursing homes often won't strain themselves to get a patient walking again. In fact, one of my elderly neighbors left one of the best-rated rehab facilities in town. He was told they couldn't help him and that he'd never walk again. Two months later, he could walk a block, after he went home and his family worked with him.

If your loved one has been discharged from the hospital and is given the prognosis after a stroke, for example, that he can walk again, you will probably seek a rehab facility. However, I've seen some short-term rehab patients enter long-term care facilities just to be rehabilitated. This is especially true if the patient wants to recuperate at a religious-affiliated nursing home that offers rehab, but isn't a rehab facility, per se.

Sometimes private, non-profit nursing homes have extensive physical therapy wings with all kinds of equipment and even a sauna that go unused. They remind me of a hospital rehab facility. Why do they have these? Because wealthy benefactors have gifted them. At one such facility that my mother was in, the physical therapist either sat around reading the newspaper, using the exercise bikes and treadmills himself, or even once in a while, wheeling patients around the building in their wheelchairs. He seemed to care little about his job. He said that since the facility was a long-term care facility, not a rehab one, that hardly any patients came through who could use the equipment. We knew that saunas stimulate movement in paralyzed legs, besides helping with circulation, and my mother's doctor was willing to authorize this care for her through her insurance. However, the physical therapist said it was too much trouble for a patient in my mother's condition to be wheeled to the sauna and hoyer-lifted into it. When my brother and I said we would wheel her ourselves and stay with her while she was in the sauna, he still made excuses. He said that someone "comatose" like my mother wouldn't benefit from it. When we said our mother wasn't comatose anymore and that she was eating food, was very alert and understanding us, he said, "She probably doesn't even taste what she's eating, and besides, it's just soft food." He further implied that she slept so much of the time that she didn't have any quality of life. Unprofessional, to say the least, but typical of the negativity and callousness that we were all too familiar with at nursing homes. Our mother wasn't in good enough physical condition to have her transported by care ambulance to a sauna at a physical therapy clinic. And, the administrator at the nursing home wouldn't go above the physical therapist's head, so we didn't pursue the idea, but still advocated for other care issues. You'd think that this physical therapist might have wanted to do something for somebody to earn his keep. Interestingly enough, a few weeks after our conversation with him, the daughter of an elderly patient who was a hospital nurse asked for the use of the sauna for her mother. Her mother was immobile, too. With her mother's doctor's order, she wheeled her mother to the sauna and got assistance from the physical therapist. It was evident to me that patients who had family members in the nursing field were often listened to more than we were.

What disturbed me the most, was that the staff, even at this religious-affiliated facility where the slothful physical therapist was, didn't try to help us, knowing how much we were trying ourselves to help our mother. Of course, no one ever suggests anything that may improve the patient's comfort, because they are afraid that a suggestion might mean more work for them. At this nursing home, the physical therapist said splints weren't used. We had learned that splints should be used in moderation, but that exercise was much better. However, this physical therapist told us that "too much" range of motion and splints were "torture." I don't think this physical therapist would find anyone on this planet to agree with him. The nurse later told us that splints weren't used at this nursing home because there was no one to put them on and take them off. (It only takes two minutes to put them on and another two minutes to take them off, but chalk that up to an extra task, in the eyes of the staff. They spend more time telling you why something can't be done, rather than just doing it.)

It boggles your mind when you stop to think about how some healthcare "professionals" including physical and speech therapists, give you self-serving explanations on why they shouldn't give care or therapy to your elder. They never give you the other side of the argument. If range of motion isn't done often, arms, legs, and all extremities get contracted, and contractures are very painful. Feet can "drop" (a dropping of the anterior portion of the foot), because splints aren't used at least some of the time. And, if leg splints aren't used at all, an immobile person can get painful sores on his heel. Comfort care isn't given if it means more work for staff. In order for my mother to get comfortable splints for her legs, since the nursing home wouldn't help us, and her insurance wouldn't pay for a

physical therapist from the outside to come in, we talked
her doctor into authorizing a visit from a physiatrist, a
physician specializing in physical therapy. If a doctor can
prove to an insurance company that more specialized help
is needed, he can authorize this. We also told the doctor
that we wanted this specialist to come to advise us on
whether we could get our mother to stand up, using a standing frame that the nursing home already had.

Standing frames, when used during the first year of being paralyzed, aid in preventing atrophy of the leg muscles.
They improve range of motion, help improve circulation,
and lessen contractures. They help maintain bone integrity
and reduce swelling in lower extremities. Further, they
strengthen the cardiovascular system, help kidney and
bladder functions (movement helps patients void), and
they help prevent bedsores.

Standing frames are quite expensive for bedridden patients—a few thousand dollars or more, and insurance
won't cover them. A standing frame is not only for paraple-
gics, but it can be adapted with additional support for quadriplegics in wheelchairs.

We knew the physical therapist wasn't willing to help
us with a standing frame, but that perhaps a physiatrist
could make visits when my mother was at the point where
she was strong enough to stand. The physiatrist visited two
years after my mother became bedridden. She said a standing frame for our mother was premature because her legs
had become so contracted at the knee. She said that my
mother could benefit from the nursing home's tilt table.
Her body could rest against a tilted board with her feet
pushing against the small board at the bottom. She also
said that sitting her up on the edge of the bed and putting
a stool underneath her feet would help with the problem
of "foot drop." My mother's legs were so contracted that
she would have needed to wear full-length leg splints for a
year to straighten out her legs, rather than ones from the

knee down, as most leg splints are. You cannot wait two years before significant physical therapy is done on a bed-ridden person. During that time, the nurse's aides mercilessly bent my mother's legs at the knees, when positioning her in bed. Her knees and femur bone became weak, and her ankles became crooked and weak. We felt leg-length splints would be too much of an encumbrance for my mother, particularly as she spent so much time in bed. We wondered how the aides would be able to move her around in bed with them on. We figured it would be hard to remove these splints as often as they needed to be, in order for the aides to change her diaper. Therefore, we decided against them. However, we didn't want her feet to drop more and more, and we felt that putting her on a tilt table would help her legs somewhat. We needed the nursing home staff's help, however, to position her on a tilt table, and we also wanted help in sitting her up on the edge of the bed to strengthen her back muscles. The physiatrist said it was remarkable how, after two years, her back muscles were still so strong that her torso wasn't leaning backwards or off to the side when she sat on the edge of the bed.

Despite the physiatrist's order, the physical therapist and administrator said it wasn't feasible for my mother to either be put on a tilt table or helped to be seated on the edge of the bed. My brother and I ended up doing the latter task ourselves. It should be noted that the physiatrist's order wasn't even reponded to by the physical therapist. He just ignored it like the doctor had never placed the order, until we followed up on it with him. He just stated on her chart, after we questioned him, that those activities weren't feasible for our mother. Here again, we could have gone to the ombudsman, but if the administrator sided with the physical therapist, as she did, we probably would have been told that if the management didn't think it could safely help a person in our mother's condition, then it couldn't take the chance.

With the physiatrist's help, even though we felt the leg-length splints were impractical, we were able to obtain some expensive leg splints for below the knee that my mother could wear when she was up in her wheelchair. We, of course, had to put them on ourselves. They would help to prevent further foot drop, though they wouldn't be able to straighten out her legs. The nursing home mentality is such that for a bedridden patient, it doesn't matter if their feet drop and their legs contract at the knee, because they'll never be able to walk again anyway. However, leg-length splints are indeed needed to keep the legs straight. If legs are kept straight, then a caregiver can help a patient stand and pivot, even if the caregiver bears the patient's weight.

It was made clear to us that the nursing home didn't want its staffers to put stress on their backs to move our mother into a seated position onto the edge of the bed. In reality, this is no more strenuous than turning a patient in bed to position her on her side, or pulling her body up in bed. Since my brother and I would assist and even watch our mother while she was on the edge of the bed, we'd be doing most of the work. Further, we were also prepared to give a written statement that the nursing home wouldn't be held liable by us if our mother slid off the edge of the bed. Since they didn't want to help us, my brother and I helped her to the edge of the bed ourselves a few times a week. It not only strengthened her back muscles, but it helped her sense of balance and facilitated bowel movements.

It made little sense to us, too, that in giving the patient some restorative aid at this nursing home, immediately after her workout, they would position her and re-bend her knees. The common sense thing would have been to keep the back of the hospital bed slightly elevated so that the patient, on her back, could still keep her legs stretched out with a pillow under each calf supporting the leg. This is a good position to be in for a while, alternating with the side to side positioning.

In reality, the restorative aid done on our mother's legs at this nursing home was largely useless. This nursing home, more than the others, had aides who would bend her knees to the point where if she was positioned on her side, her legs would jut straight out, away from her body. If they positioned her on her back, they would bend her legs at the knees to where her ankles were practically pushed up to her rear end. The point of bending the knees, for example, is so the body won't slide down the bed, if the patient is well-elevated. However, one doesn't need to exaggerate the bending of the knees to achieve this end. We placed a sign above my mother's bed with an illustration showing the pillows placed under each calf, not under the knees, when she was on her back.

While we gave up on the idea of getting our mother to stand with a standing frame, because she was way too contracted, if you're serious about looking into getting a standing frame for your elder, rather than walk into a therapy equipment store and talk to a salesman, do some professional inquiry. We called the rehab center at a local hospital and asked to speak to a physical therapist. The therapist actually invited us in to talk to him. We described our mother's condition, and we asked about standing frames that were available.

If therapists at nursing homes—whether a physical, occupational, or speech therapist—adopt the attitude that nothing is worth doing for a patient, why are they there? The majority of patients at nursing homes aren't very functional, so is a therapist going to find an excuse not to do anything? Besides unprofessionalism, there's a real lack of common sense in finding excuses not to do anything. There is always something that can be done for someone. If nothing else, a therapist can at least give ideas to a family member on how he can help his elder by doing exercises.

For bedridden patients, little is done as far as physical therapy in any nursing home. (It should also be noted that in the hospital, before my mother arrived at the nursing home, no physical therapy was given to her. The hospital's physical therapist said it was against their policy to do range of motion exercises with an immobile patient. All the hospital physical therapist did was to demonstrate for me on how range of motion exercises—called restorative aid at nursing homes—are done. It's a mystery to me why they'd deny a patient this therapy.)

At any nursing home, the norm is ten minutes of range of motion exercises two or three times a week. In reality, even this minimal requirement isn't met. Range of motion is supposed to be done by a restorative aide. He is usually a nurse's aide who does restorative aid exclusively, working only part-time.

At the first nursing home my mother was in, (not the one with the slothful physical therapist), the restorative aide, if he came at all, would only do range of motion exercises on my mother's arms, not her legs. When he came, he would spend just two minutes bending her arms back and forth at the elbow. For example, you take each arm at a time, gently bending. With the legs, you gently bend each one at a time, back and forth at the knee. With arms, you can also do circular motions at the shoulder, with each arm stretched out. With legs, you can also do circular motions at the hip, with each leg stretched out.

For bedridden people, two hours a day of range of motion, done at eight intervals (15 minutes each time) would be good, so a patient doesn't get as stiff as he normally would. If a body is stiff with muscles contracting, it is harder for the caregiver to move the patient around in bed. With restorative aid, initiated as soon as the person becomes paralyzed, his body will have a chance of staying more supple. In this case, the caregiver doesn't ruin her back changing a diaper and turning the patient.

Since nursing homes always tell you in the beginning that they'll do what the doctor orders, one way of trying to get more restorative aid from them is to do something our mother's doctor suggested. If the nursing home says it gives restorative aid three times a week, get a doctor's order for five days a week at ten minutes each. If nothing else, if they aren't following through on the promised three days a week, maybe you'll get the promised three days, if it's now supposed to be five days. Again, as silly as it may seem, you try to figure out how they'll respond.

At the first nursing home that was the rehab facility, the physical therapist had recommended leg splints below the knee for 10 to 12 hours a day and arm splints for the same length of time. (The doctor later told us that exercise was important, and that splints, at this point in time, could be used only two hours a day.) The physical therapist told us it would take four weeks to get custom-made arm and leg splints. After four weeks, when the splints arrived, it was obvious the splints weren't custom-made as they were very loose-fitting. We concluded that perhaps they were intended for a different patient, or even used by a previous patient. (In fact, when we showed the splints to the physiatrist two years later, she said the splints were very old-fashioned and hadn't been used for patients in 10 or 15 years.) Further, we later learned that a patient should be fitted for leg splints by an orthotist, not a physical therapist. My mother, at the time she got her first splints, was a skilled patient, so Medicare and her private insurance were picking up the tab for her expenses. We should have, in retrospect, asked the nursing home's accountant for the bill they sent them. It would have been interesting to see if the nursing home had billed them for new splints. It should also be noted, that at this time, we paid an R.N. friend to make an hourly visit each day to our mother in the skilled unit. She helped us with restorative aid. She laughed when she saw the splints.

At a nursing home, particularly in the beginning, you have no reason to question what a professional is telling you about your elder's healthcare. The physical therapist prescribes splints for 10 to 12 hours a day, and you go on his recommendation. In retrospect, the physical therapist probably knew the range of motion exercises weren't going to be done adequately, so he just figured the patient would be better off in splints. They don't do what's in the best interests of the patients. They merely do what's easiest for them. They don't supervise their restorative aides.

With the help of our R.N. friend, we gave about two to two and one-half hours of restorative aid a day to our mother. No exercise is ever too much, according to a doctor, done at different intervals. Contractures look awful. As a patient becomes more contracted, often you see their knees and ankles turn inward, besides their arms and legs bent.

I also did restorative aid on the wrists, fingers, ankles and toes with circular motion.

Nursing homes often suggest pain killers for immobile patients. At the rehab facility, the resident care manager— who had no practical nursing experience, except for what she'd gotten as an intern in nursing school—suggested pain killers because my mother was immobile in bed. My mother showed no sign of pain. She wasn't grimacing or moaning. I suggested to the RCM that if she suspected my mother was in pain, rather than drug her with more medication, (she was already sedated with the anti-seizure medication, Phenobarbital), why not see that she got the restorative aid she was promised?

Occupational Therapy

At one nursing home my mother was in, I noticed that some patients had some very comfortable-looking hand / wrist and arm splints. After the restorative aide there had so vigorously tried to stretch out my mother's contracted left arm like she was ripping it open at the elbow, my mother's arm and hand became permanently deformed-looking. My mother had been crying out and gritting her

teeth while the aide was doing this. I told the physical therapist who was in charge of her work that if this was the way
they handled restorative aid at this nursing home, I'd do it
myself. The aide was a mental case, totally oblivious to my
mother's cries of pain and horrified expression. (No, she
wasn't fired after I reported her to her boss.) Thanks to this
aide, my mother's left arm and hand took on the appearance of an upside-down walking cane. Her right arm and
hand were also contracted. I spoke to the occupational
therapist at this facility to inquire about what could be done
for my mother, not in the way of rehab purposes, but for
the purpose of preventing further contractures that could
lead to skin breakdown and infection. (My mother's fingernails were digging into her palm.) Incidentally, occupational therapists usually work with the elderly to help them
with daily skills, such as dressing themselves and brushing their teeth. The occupational therapist was helpful and
said that we should check with my mother's doctor to see
if my mother's private insurance might cover her evaluation for these splints, based on the fact that they would aid
in maintaining proper hygiene. Because we worded the
request this way, my mother's doctor was able to get her
insurance to authorize new arm splints, even though she
wasn't a rehab candidate, after having been bedridden for
three years.

Interestingly enough, this occupational therapist used
to work at the rehab facility where my mother was first at.
There, my mother had received her first arm and leg splints
which didn't fit her. This occupational therapist told us
she'd left that facility because she was told to bill Medicare
patients for one- hour visits, but was instructed to give only
15-minute visits. Fraud! This is a good reason to attempt to
find out when visits by therapists will be made and to be
present at them.

In reality, it's not only therapists connected with nursing homes who should be monitored, but therapists with

other healthcare organizations, too. (I will also discuss this at length in Chapter 4, "The Feeding Tube Fiasco," dealing with speech therapists). While most therapists are honest, you want to be on hand to ask questions and make comments.

Shortly after the occupational therapist gave us the good advice about how to obtain splints, she left the nursing home. Since the nursing home didn't replace her, my mother's insurance paid for an occupational therapist to come from the outside. She worked for a healthcare association. It became evident to me that she was fudging on time, spreading out visits to fit splints, and trying to make things look really technical. I wondered why she was making multiple visits, and why she didn't bring all sample splints with her in one visit, instead of three visits. I talked to the former occupational therapist who'd come back to visit the nursing home after she'd quit. I mentioned the strange behavior of the occupational therapist sent by the association. She said this wasn't the usual way of doing things and that I should report her to her supervisor. When I did complain to her supervisor at the association, as is often the case when you complain in healthcare, the supervisor was indignant, raised her voice over the phone, and denied that the occupational therapist was wasting time. However, I was firm with this supervisor and asked her to send another occupational therapist. This other one worked out well.

We had a choice of the type of arm splint we could get for our mother. When a patient is in a nursing home, in particular, get the simplest splints available. Get any type of splint that is easy to apply, and that is soft and comfortable. Inflatable arm splints, which you must blow up, are impractical. No nursing home staff member will take the time to do it. Worse, the staff often can't figure out how to inflate them. Further, the splints shouldn't be worn in bed, because it's too hard for the aides to change the diaper of a patient and turn her when she's wearing splints. The splints could injure her ribs when she's being turned. The aides won't take the time to remove them and fit them back on properly, either. The splints should be used only while the patient is in her wheelchair, a few hours a day.

In dealing with therapists in general, remember that if your family member is in a nursing home, her insurance company often limits her to using those therapists, unless the nursing home doesn't have the particular therapist she needs. This is providing the nursing home or therapist it contracts with will accept the amount of payment the insurance company is willing to give. And, often, if you want to pay a therapist privately, because you don't like the therapists at the nursing home and want to hire your own, an outside therapist may not want to do this. It often depends on whether the organization he works for allows him to go to facilities that have their own therapists. (More bureaucracy and policies that don't make sense to a layperson.) Even an independent therapist often feels badly about being privately hired by a family when a facility can provide its own therapists. In addition, the nursing home administrator might not even allow you to bring in an outside therapist he hasn't authorized. We ran into all of the above problems at one facility or another.

At any rate, a therapist should never write an elderly, infirm person off. Some do, because they feel the elderly person doesn't have much potential. There is always something that can be done for an elderly person who is ill.

Keeping In Touch With The Doctor

If your loved one is in a nursing home, chances are the doctor may forget about her. Usually, states require that a doctor makes two visits a year to a nursing home patient. He often doesn't, anyway.

I watched a prominent retired surgeon die at a nursing home without his physician ever visiting him. He was ambulatory and had memory problems. His elderly wife could not get the middle-aged couple who took care of him in their home to continue helping him after two years. Since his own physician wouldn't make visits to the nursing home, the nurses had the young "house physician" (who consulted with the nursing home), visit him.

Don't let your elder's physician forget about him once he's gone to the nursing home. Oftentimes, for example, a patient such as my mother will leave the hospital in bad shape, heavily medicated. The nurses at the nursing home are often inexperienced and don't know much about certain medications. My mother remained drugged for far too long, many weeks, without us knowing whether it was safe to have her anti-seizure medication reduced by the doctor. It didn't really dawn on us that it might be better to reduce that medication. We didn't figure this out until after my mother began having lung problems with her heavy medication and inactivity. Also, if a doctor recommends a vitamin supplement, such as iron or potassium, there again, he may not discontinue it, and the nurse won't question it. Nurses don't often have the time or take the time to contact a doctor over possibly benefitting the patient with a reduction or discontinuation of a medication. Therefore, the patient continues taking supplements for months, for example, that she may no longer need. Keep in touch with the doctor yourself about the benefit of pills over a period of time, and ask him to talk to the nurse about reducing or discontinuing the medication.

Nurses often do contact doctors about getting an order for a sedating drug for a patient who is restless and causing trouble for them. The doctor will authorized the medication, unless the family member has specifically instructed him not to authorize sedation. But, as discussed before, nursing home administrators will not allow a patient to stay there if they feel he needs sedation and the family won't allow it.

Make it clear to the doctor that if the nurse has contacted him about a drug other than one to treat a physical condition, that you should be contacted first, before he gives his authorization for it. Write him a letter to this effect and tell him that all on-call physicians should be alerted to it in the patient's chart. (The benefit, of course, of having a loved one at home is that you're dealing directly with the doctor through a private nurse.)

Other medication problems we ran across at nursing homes had to do with on-call doctors' errors. For example, when my mother's doctor wasn't available, and his colleagues were on-call, some preventable errors were made. The on-call doctor prescribed a medication that had sulpha in it that my mother was allergic to. Nurses should always question an on-call doctor about a medication by going over the patient's drug allergies. (Even one's own physician can be careless in not asking about drug allergies.) Further, if an on-call doctor is assisting, the nurse should make sure the doctor knows her total condition. For example, an on-call doctor didn't know my mother couldn't swallow pills, and that most of her medication came in liquid form. He prescribed a drug that was delivered in tablet form, and that couldn't be crushed into liquid form with water without losing its potency. Fortunately, a nurse on a later shift caught the error and told the doctor my mother needed the pill in liquid form.

At nursing homes, you do have the right to refuse x-rays for your loved one. We gave instructions to my mother's doctor that if she had a recurring cough, it should be treated with antibiotics. With all the germs at the nursing home, my mother would get coughs, and I'd instinctively know if the cough was a dangerous one by the way it sounded. Rather than give her unneeded x-rays, have to wait for an x-ray technician to come, and for the x-ray to be read by a radiologist, I instructed the nursing home and my mother's doctor to proceed with antibiotics.

Billing Problems

Chances are, you will spend time disputing nursing home bills. Sometimes the errors are honest mistakes or due to carelessness, but sometimes they are even due to double dipping and outright fraud.

At the first nursing home, when my mother was covered by Medicare and her private insurance in the skilled nursing unit, we asked to see what the nursing home was billing Medicare and her private insurance for, as we were finding some interesting little charges on our bill. As a skilled patient, virtually everything was covered by Medicare and my mother's private insurance at that time, unless we specifically asked for some extras that weren't needed. For example, as I previously mentioned, Medicare and her insurance wouldn't pay for her private room, so we had the nursing home bill us the difference between a private room and a double room. (Incidentally, by law, a nursing home patient can't be reassigned to another room without one's permission.)

In reviewing one of her insurance bills, we found that the nursing home had billed for a resuscitation device. She didn't have a resuscitation device because she entered the nursing home as a "DNR" (Do Not Resuscitate) patient! (This was the same nursing home that had given her used splints and had probably billed her insurance for new ones. We didn't check that bill.)

Never take a nursing home bill at face value. At the first nursing home, we spent hours questioning all bills. The bookkeeper there was clearly double dipping. She would often tell us that my mother's insurance wouldn't pay for such and such. We were initially told by my mother's insurance rep that all of her feeding tube supplies and formula were covered. However, the bookkeeper was billing us for drain sponges, that is, gauze used around the feeding tube site. We noted that she had also billed the insurance for this. What we finally realized was that the bookkeeper was billing both of us, just in case the insurance didn't pick up the tab. If it did pay, the nursing home would get paid twice! An accountant friend of mine who used to work in the healthcare field, said that an institution deals with so many insurance companies and isn't always clear about what each does or doesn't cover. Therefore, she says, that sometimes bookkeepers in healthcare facilities end up double dipping. She doesn't condone this practice.

We sometimes hear of institutions committing Medicare fraud. When your loved one is a skilled patient and is covered by Medicare and her insurance, ask the nursing home to see the bill that they send Medicare and her insurance. You want to make sure your loved one is getting all services and supplies they are being billed for.

When your elder is in a nursing home as an intermediate care patient who has already exhausted her skilled benefits, the institution nearly always asks for advance payment of one month. It's collecting interest. When we voiced our concerns at one nursing home, the nursing home told us that if we didn't want to pay in advance, we didn't have to. If given this choice, don't pay in advance. I would guess that when you moved your elder out of there, they'd be slow in refunding your money.

As for billing you for supplies, realize that the nursing home often marks up supplies a lot. At the first nursing home, we were billed 85 cents for one Q-Tip ™. Maybe the nurses there were too busy recording charges for supplies so they didn't have much time to give care.

As far as personal supplies, such as toothpaste, bar soap, toothbrush, etc., tell the nursing home you'll provide your own. It's cheaper. You should buy diapers in bulk at a discount store. At one nursing home, they marked up disposable blue pads five times the medical supply store's price. These disposable pads line the bed and buffer it against urine that seeps out of the diaper. For supplies not covered as part of the room fee, price them elsewhere, if you feel you're being billed too much for them.

You also aren't obligated to pay for supplies that you don't want your loved one to have. The resident care manager, at the first nursing home, had wanted to charge us $200 for a foam mattress that she cut up to fit the back of my mother's wheelchair and the seat of it. She didn't even ask for our permission before cutting it up. I had a foam cushion at home for the seat. Further, the doctor had told us my mother needed the firmness of the wheelchair's back to exercise her lungs and breathing. Therefore, we didn't need to spend the money. I'm guessing that it was a foam mattress that the nursing home didn't need and the RCM wanted to unload it on someone, just like they did with the loose-fitting splints.

As for drugs, some large nursing homes have a pharmacy on site with a pharmacist on duty, sent by the pharmacy they contract with. The pharmacy on site stocks commonly-used drugs, and its parent-pharmacy in town delivers drugs that aren't on hand. Other nursing homes merely get deliveries for all drugs from the pharmacy they contract with. You should realize that at a nursing home, you aren't obligated to get over-the-counter medications from the pharmacy it deals with. Over-the-counter medications are marked up substantially. Tell the nurse to call you if your loved one has received a doctor's order for Tylenol ™, for example, so that you can buy it yourself.

You should not only question the nursing home bill, but the bill from the pharmacy that the nursing home contracts with. Your pharmacy bill will sometimes have errors.

As for laboratory work, blood tests are done by facilities the nursing home contracts with, such as a nearby hospital. A lab technician is sent to draw blood. You will receive a statement from the lab about the insurance being billed. With blood tests, hospital labs often double bill the patient and the insurance. My mother's blood tests were covered 100 percent by her insurance, yet the lab statement often asked her for payment. Perhaps the nursing home didn't supply the lab with insurance information. (As for the blood draws, despite a sign above my mother's bed that blood wasn't to be drawn from her right arm, her mastectomy side, the lab technicians never bothered to observe the sign. On one's mastectomy side, there is always the chance of infection at the site and swelling of the arm with no glands under the arm. Lab technicians are often careless, as nurse's aides are. One can see some lab technicians at hospitals who don't even wear gloves when they draw blood.)

There are usually no billing problems with dentists who contract with the nursing home. You will get a bill from the dentist. It's a good idea to check it, nonetheless.

Security Issues

I've read newspaper accounts of patients' families setting up a camera in their loved one's room to confirm their suspicions of aides abusing patients.

Even in spending 14 hours a day, seven days a week at nursing homes for nearly four and one-half years, I'm certain that I didn't catch all the instances of abuse, or even a fraction of them. Further, one must classify even rough handling of a patient as abuse.

My brother and I considered putting a camera in my mother's room at two nursing homes she was in, to prove that she wasn't getting the promised care on a regular basis. Surveillance cameras do document the time, so one could, for example, easily note the time span between patients getting changed and turned, besides whether sponge baths were being given, etc.

If nursing homes truly cared about their patients, they would want to install cameras in each patient's room with a central monitoring system at the nurse's station. Not only do nursing homes don't want to go to the expense , but I'm sure they're afraid of what the camera might document. Yes, cameras would help to alleviate any neglect, abuse, or theft problems, but by the same token, nursing homes would feel that they wouldn't be able to get aides to work there because they wouldn't want to be followed by the camera. If nursing homes installed cameras in each patient's room for checking abuse and neglect, someone would have to review the camera film, since nurses are not often at the nurse's station to watch what goes on in a particular room. Realistically, in this case, the camera would have to be used only as a means of doing spot checks, perhaps on certain patients and aides.

I remember an upsetting incident at the "absolute best nursing home" in town. A family member said she saw an aide hit a patient in a nearby room. She dialed 9-1-1 and the police came. They questioned the aide but didn't haul her off. Instead of the nursing home temporarily keeping the aide off the floor, and perhaps giving her a job in the laundry room or kitchen until they investigated, they switched her to another unit to work with the patients. I suppose she was never charged with anything because it was difficult to prove and perhaps the visitor who dialed 9-1-1 didn't want to pursue the incident, for some reason. I did know this aide and I knew she neglected my mother by not giving her sponge baths or changing her diaper on a regular basis. Whether she was capable of hitting a patient, I don't know.

If you feel that the nursing home may be an unsafe place, may not be delivering care as promised, you don't have an alternative for care, or you need to know for sure just how bad the problems are, you can install your own surveillance camera. You would let the administrator of the nursing home know about your plan, along with the ombudsman so that the nursing home couldn't come up with some other reason to dump your loved one out of the nursing home. (In some states, these cameras may be prohibited in nursing homes.) You and the ombudsman would explain that the camera was necessary to remedy lapses in care or problems with safety. If you did get a camera, you could get a cabinet to conceal it from the aides. The camera should have a clock system whereby you could also monitor when care was being delivered. We contacted a security systems company by phone, and it suggested that we buy a camera from Circuit City and install it ourselves. You can use your own television screen. It's a wireless camera, battery-operated with a timer. It has sound and night vision, too, costing a few hundred dollars. We didn't end up getting the camera at the two nursing homes with care problems we'd considered it for. Rather than get a camera, we were able to transfer our mother out of them. With the last nursing home, we simply decided we'd had enough of poor care and abuse, so I finally took my mother home.

What nursing homes should consider, too, is that if they installed cameras, besides monitoring their staffs and being able to check on seriously ill or dying patients, they could also monitor outsiders. At nursing homes, anyone can virtually enter through a front door or a side door, and not be questioned. Around 11 p.m., all doors are supposed to be locked and a door buzzer is used so the main door can be unlocked by staff for family. However, this is not good security after dark and before 11 p.m. At one nursing home, I noticed that sometimes the side and back doors that were automated would malfunction and wouldn't lock. On many occasions, if I left past 11 p.m. and checked to see if the door locked behind me, I found it didn't. The nurses didn't know why when I reported it. Or, more commonly, the aides would leave the facility to go on break, prop the locked door open with a newspaper, so they could re-enter without ringing. Any outsider could walk in and hide somewhere in a large facility with so few staff on duty.

Other Facility Problems

The state wouldn't have to look hard to find reasons to severely penalize a nursing home, if it wanted to, or shut it down.

The kitchen is a breeding ground for germs, alone. Many people who work in kitchens at nursing homes have just as bad cleanliness skills as nurse's aides. As one would expect, most of the kitchen help is paid minimum wage or slightly above. As a routine at one nursing home, for example, I saw kitchen workers take rubber floor mats that they stood on and place them on the drain counter to wash them. Afterwards, clean dishes that came out of the dishwasher would travel on an automated tray along the same counter. Further, spoons and utensils that would fall on the floor, would be used without washing them. The workers would soak dirty dishes in bins before placing them in the dishwasher. The bins had previously been used for dumping garbage.

I first noted horrid housekeeping problems in my mother's private bathroom. The housekeeper cleaned my mother's sink with the toilet bowl brush and the toilet bowl cleaning fluid, after she cleaned the toilet with them. She then cleaned the bathroom floor with the toilet bowl brush and toilet cleaning fluid. Common occurrences involved housekeepers throwing buckets of dirty mopping water down the kitchen sink of the nursing unit, instead of using the floor drain. Further, the housekeepers would first wipe down the dirty bathroom sink with a rag and cleaning fluid, and then proceed to use the same rag to clean the countertop, the patient's tray table, and the top of her medicine table.

Housekeepers in nursing homes, therefore, are constantly spreading germs. Consequently, I brought my own bottle of Pine Sol ™ to the nursing home to go over all the spots the housekeeper "cleaned."

There is very little attention to cleanliness at nursing homes. In the medical supply room of the "absolute best nursing home" in town, carpentry work was being done. There were sawdust and chips of paint over all the medical supplies that were supposed to be kept sanitary, such as my mother's opened box of feeding tube bags and her cans of feeding tube formula. Nothing had been covered. People are cleaner than this in their homes, without having sick people there.

One wonders if the laundry at nursing homes is really clean. When washcloths are used to wipe up feces and urine on patient's bodies and often thrown on the floor, can they ever get completely clean in laundry rooms where workers may forget to even use detergent? Or, sometimes the hot water system fails at nursing homes. Was the washing machine water really hot? I believe that the same type of washcloths to wash one face should not be used to wipe up urine and feces. Can't different washcloths be used by the facility to clean up urine and feces? Their "clean" towels were often stained with brown spots.

On the other side of the coin, sometimes towels smelled of chemicals like they hadn't been rinsed. At the first nursing home, I often brought fluffy bath towels from home for my mother.

At two nursing homes, when pillows became soaked with urine, they were not replaced. If anything was done, a new pillow case would be slipped over the dirty and wet pillow. (Often pillows would become soaked if my mother was positioned on her side and the pillow buffered her side. Or, a pillow would become soaked if it was placed in between her knees, when she was on her side, to prevent sores.) If my mother's hoyer lift hammock became soaked with urine, it was never washed. The aides hoped the urine would just dry. I ended up washing it.

When You're Ready to Try Another Nursing Home

If you've done everything you can to work with the institution, and you're thinking of transferring your loved one to another nursing home, try to be methodical about it. Before you transfer your loved one, write up a sheet of pros and cons on each nursing home, comparing the two as we did.

A sample of the Pros is as follows:

Present Nursing Home

- Proximity for family and doctor
- Larger, quieter room
- We already know the management
- Graveyard shift has better staff to patient ratio

New Nursing Home

- More restorative aid
- Perhaps better personal care
- All patients transferred to wheelchairs two times a day
- Less staff turnover
- Non-profit (less costly)
- More activities

Of course, you never really know for sure whether the care is going to be any better at the other facility until your parent is actually there.

Following is a letter my brother wrote to the administrator of one nursing home when we decided to transfer our mother out of it:

To: John Doe, Administrator

Dear John:

This will formally advise you of our plan to transfer our mother to Nursing Home Y. Although there have been definite improvements in the care received during the course of her stay in the intermediate unit, our hope is that she will receive adequate care in a new facility without the need for family to monitor staff's schedules.

While we have been very satisfied with a number of your personnel and regret giving up a nice room, one suggestion might be constructive. As I requested from you last week, a patient's family would benefit from a listing of the actual services and care to be reasonably provided on a daily basis. This may help to avoid some unrealistic expectations and alleviate some of the criticisms that seem to be prevalent with the substantial costs of nursing home care.

The transfer of our mother to Nursing Home Y will occur Nov. 18. Thank you again for your help over the past months and please pass on our appreciation to your assistant administrator.

Sincerely......

The letter was courteous, but, especially in the beginning, the aide care was horrid, and some of the nurses who openly chided me for "keeping my mother alive" were despicable.

After we left this nursing home, we sent copies of correspondence about its shabby care to the State's Long Term Care Office. More significantly, we also sent copies of the correspondence to hospital discharge personnel who had an agreement with this nursing home to send them patients. Later, we found that the hospital had gotten so many complaints about this nursing home, that it cancelled its agreement with the nursing home. The latter really hit the nursing home in the pocket book.

I'd like to close this chapter with what would strike a person as being an oddly sad story. I knew of a family member whom I feel made a bad mistake. The family member had her mother at a non-profit, religious-affiliated facility. She asked the administrator, a cleric, to assume guardianship of her mother, in case she preceded her mother in death. She didn't know the administrator well, and apparently had no relatives. I feel this is folly, as you need an outsider looking out for your elder while she's a patient in the nursing home. I believe there was a real conflict of interest here when the cleric accepted the plan.

Chapter 4

The Feeding Tube Fiasco

To Feed Or Not To Feed By Mouth

The sad fact is that if someone arrives at a nursing home with a feeding tube and isn't very alert much of the time, it's doubtful a speech therapist who specializes in swallowing problems will even give the okay for a family member to feed the patient by mouth. My mother was diagnosed as having dysphagia, that is a swallowing disorder. Even if a family member requests to be able to feed the patient "recreationally," that is, give a few spoonfuls of food to the patient for her enjoyment, not for nutritional purposes, the nursing home will often deny the request. This was my mother's situation at all facilities she was at, and the situation of many other patients we've known. The belief of healthcare professionals is that someone who lacks alertness can choke or aspirate while eating. The latter means that liquid, food, or even saliva can go down the wind pipe and into the lungs, causing pneumonia.

It's disheartening that even quality of life issues such as this aren't permitted to be decided by family at a nursing home. Many people I've met who once had loved ones on a feeding tube in a nursing home, and later took them home, can tell you how their loved ones were prohibited by a speech therapist to eat, and later began swallowing and eating at least pureed food.

A feeding tube isn't to be confused with receiving nutrition through an IV. It is surgically implanted into the stomach. It's also known as a G-Tube, from the word gastrointestinal.

We probably never would have had a feeding tube surgically implanted in our mother's stomach at the hospital
had she been in a coma at the time. However, she was very
alert, was talking somewhat, and was making gestures,
when we had the feeding tube implanted. The doctors, at
that time, expected her to recover. Her swallowing difficulty didn't start until about six days after her surgery for
her cerebrovascular accident. In the days after her surgery,
she was eating and swallowing well. The blood had been
removed from her brain after she fell and hit her head.
However, six days after her surgery, she got a fever and it
was discovered she had contracted a bladder infection. The
doctor thought her swallowing difficulties were temporary
and due to her infection and her weakened state. However, after the infection was cleared up by an antibiotic, she
still had trouble swallowing. When she first had trouble
swallowing, she was coughing up her food. She pocketed
her food around her gums. She was evaluated by a hospital speech therapist who told us that she shouldn't be eating by mouth. She suggested a feeding tube, though not a
permanent one, just a nasal gastric tube. Feeding tube formula would run through a tube inserted up her nose, delivering nutrition down her esophagus to the stomach. This
formula contains most of the nutrients someone needs to
survive, but one wonders how healthy it actually is. Further, one wonders if this type of nutrition causes other
health problems.

Apparently, clear liquids, such as water and juice are the
hardest for someone with swallowing impairment to swallow, along with solid foods. Soft foods, such as mashed
potatoes or cream of wheat, are often given to people to
rehabilitate them for swallowing. In my mother's case, the

speech therapist deemed that it was even dangerous for her to attempt to eat soft food. What we later were to learn, is that speech therapists always err on the side of caution. We were concerned that she was pocketing her food, but we wondered if she was disoriented from her heavy medication, and that this was causing her swallowing difficulties.

The doctors still seemed to think that my mother's swallowing difficulties were temporary and that the feeding tube running up through her nose would suffice on a temporary basis. While she had the nasal gastric tube, we were discouraged from testing her swallowing ourselves by giving her even a spoonful or two of food. (In retrospect, perhaps we should have done this.)

Before a patient even gets a nasal gastric tube, ask the doctor if a temporary solution might not be an IV. The hospital can give a patient an IV that contains all necessary nutrients. For some patients, this might work better on a temporary basis than a nasal gastric tube, and might buy some time so that the patient's family can keep testing the patient for swallowing on their own. We didn't pursue this because we felt intimidated by the evaluation of the speech therapist. (We found out about this temporary IV, a few years after my mother became ill, from a friend whose father had a swallowing problem after a stroke.)

My mother, perhaps disoriented from the heavy medication to keep the swelling down in her brain, pulled her nasal gastric tube out, requiring the nurse to reinsert it. When someone is disoriented, she can have her wrists strapped to a wheelchair or hospital bed to prevent her from pulling out her nasal gastric tube while the formula is running. However, in a hospital situation where nurses either forget to strap the patient's wrists or an aide removes the strap just to change the patient's diaper and forgets to re-strap the wrists afterward, a nasal gastric tube becomes a problem. One aide, for example, had asked the nurse to

stop the feeding tube formula from flowing only temporarily, so she could change my mother's diaper. When that
was done, and the formula was started again, the nurse
forgot to strap her wrist and my mother pulled out her tube
again. In a hospital (or nursing home situation) the convenience of the staff members comes first, and they aren't
expected to commit to memory a patient's special needs.
Therefore, what may be in the patient's best interests isn't
always considered. The staff members felt they couldn't
remember to keep my mother's wrists strapped, nor could
they continue to reinsert her nasal gastric tube if she pulled
it out. Therefore, they recommended that my mother have
a stomach tube surgically implanted. This seemed like a
radical solution—all because no one wanted to take responsibility for strapping her wrist while her formula was running. However, the gastroenterologist, a doctor who did
feeding tube surgery, believed it was more advisable with
a disoriented patient to do this. In retrospect, I think this
was a mistake. For the feeding tube surgery, my mother
needed anesthetic. She was already weak from her brain
surgery, and things didn't improve after she had the feeding tube surgery. She seemed to get worse.

It should be noted that the doctor sutured in a rather
awkward tube, a "peg tube," that didn't work well from
the beginning. Most feeding tubes are replaceable without
surgery, as we later learned, and could be changed if they
clogged up after six months or so, with a nurse reinserting
a new stomach tube. This sutured-in tube could only be
replaced with another surgery. The gastroenterologist sutured in this tube so it couldn't be pulled out by my mother,
nor could it be accidentally pulled out if a healthcare worker
was turning my mother and changing her diaper in bed.
The peg tube looked like a rubbery hose and turned into a
shriveled up mess after six months of use. It looked like an
intestine. Actually, it kept clogging even when it was rela-
tively new. The gastroenterologist said it would last a year.

It lasted a year and four months, but it was a constant hassle. That is, the formula wouldn't always flow freely and the nurse would sometimes have to stop the flow of formula. She would then push water with a syringe through the tube to get it to run more efficiently. (This happens with replaceable tubes, but not as much.) In a hospital or nursing home setting, a nurse starts the formula and leaves the room. The formula flows from a plastic bag held by a tall pole, much like an IV—but it is plugged into the feeding tube. If the tube should become clogged, the nurse doesn't know about this, having left the room, until she returns about an hour to an hour and a half later. If the patient receives medication through the tube before the formula starts, the medication is given on an empty stomach if the formula should stop flowing right after the feeding starts. Therefore, you don't want a tube that clogs up, and doesn't deliver the formula on a timely basis.

If a feeding tube is implanted, it should be one that doesn't need to be surgically replaced. The ones that don't need to be surgically replaced are also not the rubbery one's which clog easily.

It should be noted, too, that the gastroenterologist who did the feeding tube surgery at the hospital was anti-feeding tubes! If so, why would he do feeding tube surgery, you ask? It does seem nonsensical, doesn't it? Apparently, he had told my brother and I that his grandfather had a feeding tube and never regained his swallowing ability. After ten months with the tube, his grandfather who lived in a nursing home, said he wanted to die because he couldn't eat. I wonder if he never regained his swallowing ability because he couldn't find a speech therapist who would work with him, and his family was prohibited from feeding him? This is what often happens to institutionalized patients.

In the hospital, about a week after my mother had feeding tube surgery, she had seizures, and fell into a deep coma.

I believe she'd gotten weaker and weaker, and perhaps there was a medication error, as I discussed in the Introduction of this book.

As I also discussed in the book's Introduction, my mother reawoke after five months in a coma at the first nursing home. After this, my mother's level of alertness varied. The nursing home staff, who spends about 35 minutes each eight-hour shift with a patient, is not around the patient enough to notice periods of alertness. This was the case with my mother. Further, if a speech therapist visits, it's hard to schedule a visit when the patient is alert, because periods of alertness are hard to predict. To increase periods of alertness with a brain-injured patient, both speech and physical therapy should be offered. However, what we found was that we were not allowed to feed our mother, and thereby she wasn't allowed to be stimulated by the powerful stimulant of food. If one receives stimulation, one's level of alertness increases.

After five months of going downhill at the first nursing home, where she got her lung embolisms and nearly died, miraculously, my mother began to come out of her coma. We were hopeful she'd eat again, and that we cold have the feeding tube removed. She was showing periods of alertness, even talking. This was truly a miracle because in having had the lung embolisms—largely due to a lack of adequate physical therapy, not being transferred to her wheelchair to breathe deeply, and not being turned in bed regularly—she lost more oxygen to her brain and suffered more seizures.

When she became alert, we would bring our mother a cup of ice ceam, without the staff's knowledge, as there was no speech therapist's order for her to eat by mouth. From the hospital, she arrived an "NPO" patient, meaning that she couldn't eat by mouth, and she was a "tube feeder."

An important point to understand about feeding tube patients and institutional policy, is that there is a difference between a patient who arrives at a nursing home with a feeding tube and one who arrives there without a feeding tube, but later develops swallowing problems. In the latter case, the staff can't force a patient to get a feeding tube, and will keep feeding the patient by mouth until the patient aspirates and dies. Sometimes Alzheimer's patients lose their ability to swallow in the late stages of their disease.

If your elder arrives at a nursing home with a feeding tube, most nurses will tell you that you aren't even allowed to feed your loved one without a speech therapist's order. If you're lucky, however, one may say, "Go ahead and feed her, but I don't know about it." We weren't fortunate enough to come across a staff member like this.

My brother and I would sneak in ice cream which is supposed to be easier for patients with swallowing difficulties to swallow than most foods. It's soft and melts in the mouth. We were told this in the hospital.

When my mother first came out of her coma, since she wasn't alert all the time, we didn't want to schedule a speech therapist's visit and have her sleep through the visit. Therefore, we continued giving her food for a couple of weeks, hoping to stimulate her enough so she might be awake when the speech therapist came to evaluate her.

I should say that I'd go home at night and eat dinner, feeling extremely guilty and sad that I could sit down and eat, but that my mother wasn't allowed to.

We paid a private nurse we knew to come in and help us stimulate our mother with activities, like reading to her, doing exercise, and having her listen to music. It should be noted that although nursing homes do little for patients, they often don't like private nurses to come in to help, and some have policies against hiring them. For example, some don't want a private nurse giving medications because of the liability. However, the private nurse wasn't hired by us to do nursing duty, but to do activities with our mother.

And, we told the staff she was a "family member" which wasn't true.

This private nurse agreed with us that our mother seemed alert enough to swallow and she fed her ice cream, too. At this time, we asked my mother's doctor to authorize a visit by the speech therapist that her insurance would pay for. Therapists won't visit unless they receive a doctor's order. The first speech therapist, a part-time employee at the nursing home, came by when my mother was alert, and said my mother's swallowing was "excellent," and that there was "no chance of aspiration." She said she should be allowed to eat, starting with soft foods. She also said her colleague, a full-time employee of speech therapy at the nursing home, would complete the evaluation in two days. The second speech therapist had a different evaluation. (We were to learn from an out-spoken therapist a few years later, that it isn't uncommon for speech therapists to disagree since it's an art and not a science. She said that ten speech therapists lined up in a room will disagree over a patient's swallowing ability.)

At any rate, the second speech therapist paid a visit when I wasn't present. Later, she told me that it would be dangerous for my mother to be allowed to eat since she was slow to swallow her ice cream as she tasted it. I responded, "Perhaps she was savoring her food, because she hadn't tasted food in several months." I should mention at this point that it's advisable for family members to know exactly when the speech therapist is visiting so they can be present. Speech therapists are afraid of losing their license or being sued if a patient chokes while they are evaluating a patient, so they don't go out of their way to test them. I was to learn a few years later that if, for example, I'd been present and said that I would do the feeding in front of the speech therapist, then if my mother choked or aspirated, the speech therapist wouldn't be liable. I learned this a few years later when I saw a patient in a nursing home who didn't have a feeding tube, but was losing her ability to swallow. The speech therapist was called in for an evaluation, and I noted she had the nurse do the feeding, so she herself wouldn't be liable.

You see, at nursing homes, it's as if everything is kept a secret. A speech therapist, for example, won't tell you to be present at the evaluation so you can feed your family member, and she won't be liable if something adverse happens. However, that's the gist of it.

I was also to meet a nurse a few years later at another nursing home who confirmed this. She was a retired hospital nurse and her mother arrived at the nursing home with a feeding tube. Her mother was somewhat alert, but very weak. This retired nurse told me the way she got the speech therapist to agree to allow her mother to eat was by feeding her herself in front of the speech therapist. Then she said, "See my mother can swallow, so start her on eating by mouth now." Her mother had two things going for her. She not only had an aggressive daughter who tested her swallowing, but the daughter was a nurse and knew how to talk to the speech therapist. Just by virtue of the fact the daughter was a nurse, the speech therapist probably felt she couldn't dispute the issues.

As for my mother, because of the second speech therapist's evaluation, she wasn't given permission to be fed by mouth, not even by us, not even "recreationally." The latter was all we were asking for to begin with.

We went to the nursing home administrator to discuss the matter, and ask if we could feed our mother ourselves, so the staff wouldn't be liable, on just a recreational basis. The administrator happened to have a master's in speech therapy, and he said that because of the second evaluation, he wouldn't allow her to be fed even by us.

The administrator even read aloud to us the speech therapist's notes in my mother's chart, that said that she didn't recommend that she be allowed to eat. In reality, the speech therapist had agreed with me on one thing when she spoke to me after the evaluation. I told her my mother didn't have much quality of life, so even if my mother ended up aspirating as the speech therapist felt she would, why not take that chance and give her the opportunity of having some quality of life? She said she knew how I felt, and she agreed with me about the quality of life issue, and eating and taking a chance with aspiration. I said to her that I'd like to take the chance of feeding her anyway. She, of course, wrote in her chart that I said I'd feed her anyway, but she didn't report the fact that we had the conversation about my mother's quality of life, and that she did agree with me. She even told me that if I was going to go ahead and feed my mother, I should observe the techniques on how to safely feed her. She demonstrated these techniques. She also repeated gossip in her report, that is, that the nurses "reportedly" thought I had unrealistic expectations for my mother. When you read a speech therapist's chart notes, I would imagine that it might differ from what she's told you verbally, obviously to protect herself from liability issues. This speech therapist was fresh out of school, just like the other nursing home staff members at this facility. As a layperson, I can fully understand how the staff may not want to assume liability for their nurses and aides feeding patients by mouth who have feeding tubes. However, family members should always be allowed to feed their loved ones on a recreational basis. If the elder does aspirate from eating by mouth, then I could understand why a facility might reconsider having given its permission.

In retrospect, we knew that there were a lot of empty rooms at this nursing home, and I now have the suspicion that had we said to the administrator that we'd moved our mother out of the nursing home if she wasn't permitted to eat by mouth, he probably would have changed his mind to let us feed our mother ourselves, absolving the staff from its liability of feeding her. However, as is often the case in the beginning, you end up trusting and following the professionals' judgment when they say it's risky. The administrator said that if liquids or food went down the wind pipe and settled in her lungs, she would get pneumonia. He said that for the limited amount of eating that she would do— in eating soft foods that wouldn't add up to much nutrition— it wasn't worth the risk. What we later figured out, however, was that there are always two sides to every argument and that you're never given both sides. If you don't get the patient to practice swallowing with foods, for example, you also run the risk of having the patient's throat muscle atrophy. Then the patient could even choke on saliva. Or, she might not be able to be rehabilitated in the future. Again, the nursing home never considers what's in the best interests of the patient.

Nursing homes seem to continue classifying their patients as comatose, even when they awaken from a coma, and they have periods of wakefulness and alertness, but are totally dependent as far as needing care. My mother came out of her coma, and some medical doctors would either classify her as in a permanent vegetative state, semi-comatose, or just lethargic. She couldn't have still been in a coma, as she was able to eat, understand, respond a little, and do some talking. Her doctor agreed with me in calling her lethargic. Perhaps she didn't have hardly any strength to lift her limbs due to the length of time she'd been on a feeding tube, without being allowed rehabilitation for swallowing nor even having been given physical therapy.

I believe that nursing homes prefer to continue classifying a patient as comatose because that justifies their warehousing of the patient. Even when the patient is awake, and has expressions of being tuned in, the staff of nurses and therapists will ignore the patient and even say in front of her, "She won't recover." It's been proven that even patients in deep comas are aware of people present, but they can't decipher what they are saying. When my mother awoke from her coma, she turned to me and said, "You are very nice," as if she'd been tuned in for months, aware that I'd been caring for her.

As her family, my brother and I were prepared to feed our mother only when she was fully alert. We weren't asking or depending on the staff to take on any risks of liability. We felt that depriving our mother of real food and leaving her feeling less than full with artificial feeding tube formula, may even lead her to aspirate. You salivate more when you're hungry. If, indeed, you do have swallowing difficulties or aren't alert enough to swallow well, you can probably aspirate on an excess of saliva caused from the feeling of being hungry.

One of the reasons that we didn't insist with the nursing home administrator that our mother be allowed to be fed by us, was that we had put her on the waiting list at another nursing home that was supposed to be the highest-rated one in town. We thought that in a short period of time, our mother would be able to eat at this other nursing home, and that the speech therapist there would see it our way. However, we were in for another disappointment once we got there, two months later. The idea that someone can get pneumonia and even die from eating soft food is a possibility, if he isn't alert when he eats. However, I have always felt that since not being able to eat greatly diminishes one's quality of life, you take the chance of feeding a patient, even on a recreational basis, when he is alert.

The nursing home we took our mother out of was a rehab facility, and yet the staff didn't want to rehabilitate her for swallowing. The next nursing home, the highest-rated in town, was perhaps even more of a disappointment for its speech therapy. In the first five months there, we asked for three speech therapy evaluations, and all three proved worthless to us. We had been sneaking in food to our mother, and knew she had swallowing ability, but we couldn't get the speech therapist to agree with us. The speech therapist was not on staff at the nursing home, but contracted with it. She said we could get a second opinion (amounting to a third visit) from a speech therapist that she knew—most likely a colleague-friend that would probably side with her, we thought. We went ahead with the third visit, anyway, that proved fruitless. The following is a letter that I wrote to my mother's doctor after five months at this new nursing home. It had been a year since my mother's head injury. Doctors say you'll see the most improvement in the first year of recovery, and that's why it's necessary to receive adequate physical and speech rehabilitation in that first year's time. We felt our mother hadn't been given that.

To: John Smith, M.D.

Dear Dr. Smith:

After you spoke with my brother yesterday, I felt you needed to be updated on my mother's condition from someone in the unique position of knowing just what her level of alertness is. The nursing staff, with 40 patients to a unit, spends about a total of one hour and 45 minutes in a 24-hour period with each patient. Therefore, they don't see as much in the way of changes in a patient as family members do. As you've been told, the two speech therapists who recently saw our mother here, chose to visit her at times when she was barely alert, despite our specific requests with designated times.

I, for example, average 14 hours daily with my mother. I feel I'm your best source of information. Since about February, I've seen positive and at times, dramatic changes in her alertness. If I hadn't witnessed these changes, my brother and I wouldn't have wasted your time, our time, and the speech therapist's time in asking for a one-hour evaluation. My mother is alert much of the day, sometimes saying a few words in both Italian and English (not confusing the two), smiling, laughing, and understanding everything. She rarely coughs, but when she does, it's a dry, healthy cough. I've noted she sometimes lifts her left leg when she's uncomfortable or fearful of falling off her wheelchair. She sometimes moves her neck to follow me around in the room and to watch me outside the room.

She must have a good swallowing reflex. As evidence, I have walked in on her laying flat during tube feedings on various occasions, which is not supposed to be done. I have also witnessed aides cleaning her mouth with water-logged toothettes. When these things happen, although she coughs a lot, she hasn't aspirated, as one might expect. She has also been positioned awkwardly with her body bent over, bed elevated, and neck against her chest, making it difficult for most people to swallow. Nevertheless, she hasn't aspirated. You can bet these events are occurring when I'm not here, too. She has even vomited, but not aspirated, so she must have good swallowing ability. Of course, I work with the nursing staff to get problems resolved. The staff is somewhat receptive to my suggestions, and on the whole she receives better care here than at Nursing Home X. I'm sorry my mother had to waste away at Nursing Home X and nearly die there from lack of care.

Despite limited time with each patient, two nurses and three nurse's aides have reported to me that my mother says a few words to them every once in a while. My mother's friend who spends eight hours a week with her also reports many of the changes I've witnessed.

As my brother told you, we were extremely disappointed with the lack of professionalism that went into recent speech therapy evaluations by the speech therapist who contracts with this facility. Besides alerting her to designated times when my mother was most alert, we asked to be present at the evaluations. The most recent report from her associate that sits on your desk was done without my notification. Amazingly, to date, I don't even know the speech therapist's name. We weren't sent a report by her. We do know that she was female. Upon my investigation, I learned from a janitor here that "some strange woman" had

*entered my mother's room and "placed wet towels in her mouth."
She not only chose to come at an offbeat time without contacting
us, but she didn't even check with the charge nurse. (I would be
concerned that my mother would aspirate, if someone stuck wet
towels in her mouth. Both speech therapists did this. At the previous nursing home, the speech therapists did not. It concerns a
layperson about techniques used with a patient who may not be
comprehending very well.)*

*To date, my mother has seen four speech therapists, including
two at the previous facility. The first speech therapist at Nursing
Home X told me (while I was present at the evaluation), that my
mother's swallowing was excellent. She also said that my mother
should be started on soft food trays because there was "no chance
of aspiration." Two days later, another speech therapist who saw
my mother said that she didn't swallow her ice cream immediately and therefore, she was a high aspiration risk. She also admitted to me that my mother should "perhaps" be fed anyway,
since she didn't have much quality of life, otherwise. She showed
me techniques on how to safely feed my mother.*

*I do believe my mother's swallowing ability is okay when I am
present during the therapist's evaluation, as I was during the
first. I'm able to prepare my mother for the evaluation and stimulate her alertness, besides introducing the therapist.*

*My mother's alertness has greatly improved since that of the
first swallowing evaluation when her swallowing was "excellent."*

*This facility has given us permission to bring in our own speech
therapist when we feel we are ready for another evaluation. These
next few weeks, I will work on getting my mother's alertness and
communication skills to a better level. Perhaps then, we can call
in another therapist.*

*I'll be contacting you. Thank you very much for your assis-
tance and patience.*

Sincerely.......

In this letter, I refer to the two speech therapists who evaluated my mother at the new nursing home who used the technique of placing wet towels in a patient's mouth. At the previous nursing home, they at least tested her with food. It should be noted that most doctors and nurses I've talked to have never witnessed a speech therapist's evaluation. An agency nurse I met at one nursing home, who was outspoken, told me what she thought of speech therapy evaluations, when I asked if she'd ever witnessed one. She said that when she witnessed speech therapists   putting wet towels in patients' mouths and rubbing their gums, she thought she wouldn't want this to be done to her.

Some speech therapists take a terrycloth hand towel, pry open the patient's mouth and rub their gums with the towel. I know I wouldn't want to swallow my saliva after someone did this to me. I would "pool" my saliva, as a speech therapist calls it, just as my mother did. That's why she flunked the test, according to these speech therapists' reports. If a patient isn't able to decline this technique, perhaps it shouldn't be used. Worse, it was probably frightening to my mother because she was wondering what was going on, as I did to.

I can even remember a conversation I had with the director of nursing at this nursing home. I was practically in tears asking her to please give my brother and I permission to recreationally feed our mother. She sided with the speech therapist, and she said emphatically, "She will aspirate." It is unprofessional for anyone to make definitve statements such as these.

Having had enough with speech therapy evaluations, we continued to sneak in food to our mother to practice swallowing with her for another six months. While we weren't accomplishing much since we couldn't sneak in large plates of food, just snacks of ice cream, it was better than nothing. During this time, since she hadn't received swallowing rehabilitation and her original feeding tube had sprung a leak in its rubber, she had to go to the hospital and go through the uncomfortable experience of getting a new feeding tube. This did not involve another surgery, however, because she was not getting another peg tube. She already had the incision in her body from the other feeding tube, so the feeding tube site was already there. She was getting a replaceable feeding tube that was the kind that didn't need to be sutured in. In this procedure, however, the doctor did need to stick another tube down her throat, to check placement for the new tube. My mother's lips got all black and blue because she'd didn't want the doctor sticking the tube in her mouth. Just the ordeal of going back to the hospital all in one day, on a hot summer day, and having to fast for one day, on top of the discomfort and fear, was something that could have most likely been avoided. I believe it could have been avoided, if she had been able to begin swallowing therapy 11 months before, when she came out of her coma.

Our subsequent letter to the doctor asked him to give his permission for us to feed our mother, despite the fact that the speech therapists wouldn't agree to it.

To: John Smith, M.D.

Dear Dr. Smith:

Our mother's general condition has remained stable with no coughing since her brief recouperation from the stomach tube replacement.

Further, we know that she can swallow soft foods on a daily basis without adverse reactions, because we've been testing her without the nursing home's knowledge of it. Not talking much, her only interests seem to be family visits and eating real food.

We are requesting that you lift the ban preventing her rec-reational feeding. We are convinced that eating something would be important in her remaining time. If this course of action should unexpectedly trigger a health problem or contribute in any way

*to worsening her condition, we want to assure you that it is ex-
clusively a family decision for which you and the nursing facility
had no responsibility in causing. As family members, we will do
the recreational feeding. Please communicate the recreational feeding instructions to the nursing staff. As always, we appreciate
your cooperation and understanding.*

Sincerely ....

About five months prior to this, we discovered my
mother's cancer had spread to her other breast. We wondered why she shouldn't be allowed to eat if she had cancer and possibly a limited time to live. (As it turned out,
she lasted four more years, and didn't even die of cancer.)

The doctor, prior to this last letter, knew we had been
feeding our mother all along, but didn't want to get involved in speech therapy business. He followed the speech
therapists' recommendations. However, because of our insistence over a long period of time, and our mother's cancer, he did put through an order to lift the ban on feeding
our mother by mouth. The nursing home was willing to
follow the doctor's order and go above the speech
therapist's head, only if the director of nursing witnessed
that our mother could swallow without coughing or spit-
ting. The trial session worked, and the director of nursing
said she could swallow well. As I've said before, nursing
home staff members can refuse to follow a doctor's order if
they feel it conflicts with their policies.

If every healthcare person would try to work together
for the benefit of the patient, rather than waste valuable
time disagreeing with colleagues and family members,
maybe the patient would receive better care and a better
quality of life. I've been told that at some nursing homes, a
family member is always allowed to feed his elder
recreationally, despite swallowing difficulties.

In the beginning had we known that it would be an up-
hill battle getting a speech therapist to ever give permission for

even recreational feeding, we would have taken our mother home where we could have done as we pleased. However, speech therapists don't tell you that they rarely give permission for a patient in my mother's condition to eat. They often keep saying that maybe later on, she'll be more alert, and they can feed her.

At first, because speech therapists are supposed to be the professionals, you trust them. Although you're not comfortable with their assessment, you have a lingering doubt. You feel, "What if they are right? What if I might kill my mother by letting her aspirate?" At first, you feel you must err on the side of safety and work within the system to get her eating again. As we learned, it takes too long to work within the system and convince staff that one can eat. The patient loses valuable rehabilitation time, and loses the chance to fully recover later on.

I've always felt that if my mother had been allowed to eat when she first came out of her coma and was talking and answering questions, she would have had the energy and been sufficiently stimulated to make more significant progress in her general alertness. Since she wasn't allowed to be stimulated with food the first year, her potential for alertness was greatly diminished. She not only became more physically weak, but mentally lethargic. When you're physically weak in my mother's condition, without eating real food, you can't lift limbs, nor even have the energy to talk. Even when it's witnessed that a patient can swallow, sadly the nursing home staff looks at a patient afterwards and probably thinks that even if she'd been given the chance to eat before, she wouldn't have made progress anyway in her general condition.

When we put my mother into the hands of hospice, the final year of her life, two nurses told us that people in my mother's condition do recover from head injury. And, these nurses said that if she'd received the proper care, rehabilitation, and stimulation with food during the first six months to a year after her head injury, she would have stood a 50-50 chance of recovery.

Feeding tube formula renders one weak. It's not energy food. One becomes weaker and an elderly person often becomes too weak to lift her limbs or even talk without the benefit of real food. In my mother's case, after just a year of feeding tube formula and no rehabilitation, she got so weak that she got cancer again. One not only gets weaker, one sleeps more, and one's organs start to fail from inactivity. Her doctors agreed that she never would have gotten cancer again, having had slow-growing tumors in the past, had she not been reduced to a lethargic state. However, we found that doctors often know no more than speech therapists about whether or not a patient can swallow.

We took so much flack from two speech therapists when we disagreed with them. Initially, the nurses sided with the speech therapists, without even witnessing that my mother could swallow. The institutional mind is such that no one questions accepted beliefs. One speech therapist told us that if we didn't like her assessment, we could transfer our mother to another nursing home. It often boils down to defensiveness, on the part of the person who works in healthcare. What is in the best interests of the patient isn't fully considered. And, if often boils down to a power struggle between doctors and healthcare personnel who used to be considered their subordinates. Good nutrition is obviously essential, and most people would agree that while feeding tube formula can keep one alive, it doesn't provide the nutrition that regular food can. Good nutrition is also essential for healing pressure sores (bedsores). My brother and I even wondered, too, if the discomfort of having a feeding tube in one's body, the discomfort of having only liquid formula in one's stomach with medications, and the frustration of not being able to eat by mouth, could perhaps cause a brain-injured patient to contract her limbs more. What about the psychological effects?

While I'm sure there are some patients who really need feeding tubes, others are mistakenly dismissed by speech therapists as not being able to swallow safely under any conditions. When I look back at the facts, the speech therapist at the new nursing home was clearly unprofessional. She once made the statement in front of my mother that she would never recover from her stroke. Any professional who uses the word "never" is really not professional. As a family member, review what a healthcare professional says. Trust your instincts. If something doesn't make sense to you, that's because it probably isn't accurate. Look at all sides of the issue by weighing the pros and cons to your loved one's health. Remember that healthcare professionals look at what's best for them as far as liability issues. After taking my mother through the healthcare maze for 16 years, I have come to the conclusion that the healthcare system is among the worst of bureaucracies, particularly at nursing homes.

The mark of a good nursing home is really in how flexible it is in accomodating family members' wishes. After all, elders there don't have much time left for living, so they should be treated well. The mark of a good nursing home is also in how it reviews its policies when it realizes that the best interests of the patient haven't been served. After we proved our mother could swallow, I doubt whether the nursing home revised its policy on letting family members feed a patient recreationally with a doctor's order. I thought it was unprofessional, too, that the speech therapist, was actually reviewing my mother's chart after the director of nursing allowed her to eat. After that, my mother was no longer her patient, so she had no business reading her chart. She apparently told a nurse how shocked she was that my mother could swallow food. One wonders just how many patients in her 30 years of practice she'd written off, and who because of her evaluation, never got the chance to eat. You wonder, too, if professionally, she felt any regret or shame about her defensiveness in dealing with us. She, nor anyone else at the nursing home, ever came up to us and said they were glad my mother was eating. After my mother was allowed to eat, two of the nurses came up to me out of the blue and said that patients who have had massive strokes like my mother sometimes do swallow well, even though they aren't very alert. However, they never had the courage to say this to me before. It would have been very valuable for me to have heard this long before, even though I wouldn't have revealed that a nurse said it to me.

The Double Standard For Feeding Patients

In a nursing home, you'll witness a lot of patients coughing up food. The staff doesn't deny these patients with bad swallowing the opportunity to eat. Why deny a feeding tube patient the same pleasure and necessity? After my mother was allowed to eat, I said to one nurse that there were a lot of bad swallowers at the facility. She nodded her head. Two other nurses who became friends with me said that if they had a mother like mine, they'd want her to eat, too. I guess there were some staff members who actually recognized that feeding tube patients shouldn't be written off. One of my nurse-friends there said that my mother probably swallowed better that most patients there.

The physiatrist who saw my mother after she was allowed to start eating made the observation that my mother wasn't drooling as some brain-injured or impaired people do. In bringing up this point, I remembered even seeing brain-injured patients who drooled who didn't choke on food, and who seemed to have prospered for the few years they were at the nursing home. Consider very carefully whether you want to follow a speech therapist's recommendation and discuss all angles with the doctor.

It also doesn't make sense that a nursing home won't vigorously insist and ensure that aides follow feeding tube precautions, nor monitor them. If an aide lays a patient flat while the feeding tube is running, the patient could choke and die from formula getting into the lungs. Somehow the nursing home won't assure you that that won't happen, but by the same token, they'll deny a patient the opportunity to eat by mouth saying that that's a danger.

Further, in a nursing home, statistically, few residents are allowed to eat solid food, according to one nurse that I knew there. Most eat soft food that looks so unappetizing, or mechanical soft food, the latter being food that can be mashed up with a fork such as pasta and scalloped potatoes. It's pretty obvious that when patients are drugged considerably, they are diminished in their muscular ability. They can't keep their balance if they walk. By the same token, they lose their ability to swallow well. I used to express my concerns that if my mother wasn't allowed to eat food, her throat muscle would atrophy, and she'd choke on her saliva, aspirate, and get pneumonia that way. However, the nursing home staff would deny this. However, it's true, and it's common sense. One nurse, who became my friend, told me in confidence, of course, that I was correct in my assumption. One also loses one's taste buds in being denied food for a long period of time.

Common sense is often not used at nursing homes. The swallowing issue aside, I'll give another example of nonsense. I once told a nurse one winter that with some patients being ill, I didn't like to wheel my mother around the nursing home halls. The nurse responded that it was actually okay, since patients "become immune to those germs." I was stunned that she didn't reply that many frail patients die as a result of being in such an environment of germs. This nurse, incidentally, had been a nurse for 30 years.

As for speech therapists, it should be noted that at some nursing homes, there are staff therapists. At others, they contract with a speech therapist. Regardless, if you don't like the evaluation of the speech therapist, and you wish to pay for a private one that you choose, we found that we couldn't find one who would agree to come to the nursing home since the nursing home "already had one." We suspected that a private speech therapist feels that he doesn't want to go out on a limb and disagree with what another has said. After all, it's a liability issue. They feel they can lose their license if there's controversy over whether a patient is fit enough to swallow safely.

In addition, my mother's insurance stipulated that all visits by speech or physical therapists ordered by the physician would be covered only for therapists on staff at the nursing home or those authorized by the nursing home. Therefore, one often runs through an insurance maze of bureaucracy when trying to get authorization fo feed a patient in my mother's lethargic condition.

Further, your elder's insurance won't pay for any future visits by a therapist unless you can convince her doctor that she has shown improvement in her condition or alertness. As for the speech therapy visits, in my letters to the doctor, I stated that my mother had shown improvement in her alertness level, and therefore she was ready to see a speech therapist again.

Things to Consider About Swallowing

The longer you wait to start feeding by mouth, chances are, the harder it will be to ever get beyond the stage of recreational eating, to your elder eating half a meal, and then an entire meal.

The speech therapist told me that she'd like to see my mother more alert and coughing less before she attempted to feed her, after placing towels in her mouth. I believe this isn't always a practical solution. Alertness can increase as you feed a patient regularly, and she will probably cough less as she gets used to swallowing again. This is what I found with my mother. Not allowing her to eat for another few months, in between the speech therapist's visit, did her no good.

When the speech therapist checked for a gag reflex, I was told my mother didn't have one. I disagreed with the speech therapist on that point, and she said that maybe my mother had a gag reflex some of the time.

While I wouldn't go trying to get my mother to gag to test her swallowing, I would just feed her with food I knew she could swallow. I observed my mother coughed well, when she was laid flat. She had a good, dry cough, not a broken up one. That was a good sign, too. She was alert, as she would suck a toothette dipped in water, rather than just bite it as some non-alert patients do.

You need to consider what a speech therapist tells you and discuss it with the doctor. Then you can make your own decision. You may want to leave the facility if your elder isn't allowed to eat with you feeding her. I'm not condemning speech therapists. I'm merely saying that their advice didn't work for us, and wasn't practical in our eyes for our mother. I'm sure many speech therapists have been wonderful and have helped many people.

A patient becomes more alert by stimulating her even with a few ice chips which can be equivalent to saliva. If a person isn't choking on saliva, then he could tolerate an ice chip. I think a family member,who is around the patient more than any healthcare person can better determine his level of alertness and can decide when the best time for him to taste something by mouth is. A healthcare person will simply say that he's never alert, and that may be true when she is there, but that doesn't mean he isn't alert at other times.

After my mother was given permission to eat recreationally, I complained to my mother's doctor that the aides were still laying my mother flat in her bed by mistake during the tube feeding, as often happens at nursing homes. She would cough, but not aspirate, as is the danger. The doctor made the comment that she must have a good swallowing reflex if she wasn't aspirating from this.

At the nursing home, besides the disadvantage of not being allowed to eat by mouth, one who has swallowing difficulties is also told not to brush one's teeth with toothpaste. One gets plaque, gingivitis, or can lose teeth or get rotted teeth. One can get infections in one's mouth. The infections can poison the patient's body, the patient gets weak, and can die. There are so many disadvantages in not being allowed to eat and brush one's teeth, that the risk of aspirating from food is sometimes a choice that family members consider.

If you do decide to allow your loved one to eat by mouth, consider, too, that at home, there's always food available. If you have your elder at home, you won't need to transport food to the nursing home. The patient at home can get the food hot, not cold from the trip over to the nursing home. In my mother's condition, we never knew if she'd be awake at a certain time, so sometimes when she did wake up at the nursing home and could have eaten, we didn't have food with us. The smell of food is probably one of the most powerful sensory stimulants for all people to wake up to, even lethargic people. Since smelling encourages swallowing, have the patient smell things.

A speech therapist will tell you that the signs of aspiration are: runny nose, coughing, throat clearing, labored breathing and choking. My mother would sometimes cough during feeding, but she didn't aspirate. If a patient holds food in her mouth for a minute, a speech therapist will tell you this is a bad sign. In my mother's case, she may not have liked the food, but didn't want to spit it out. Or, perhaps her taste buds were shot from not eating for a long time, and from medication taken, so she wasn't able to recognize the taste of food. (Incidentally, I also found that my mother sometimes coughed continuously during tube feedings to where I'd have to stop the formula feeding. It was a moist cough. A nurse once told me that coughing by spinal cord injury and head injury patients was common. The point is, one never really knows when coughs are dangerous.)

As a rule, for my mother, I didn't worry if she coughed a dry sounding cough when she ate. She was getting used to swallowing again. A "broken-up" cough (moist cough) may signal that the patient isn't swallowing food well or that she's not swallowing her secretions well, according to what speech therapists told me.

Speech therapists and nurses will often scare you about feeding your relative. After we'd finally gotten permission to feed our mother, I was scared to death when she coughed while eating, fearing that this might be a sign of aspiration, as the staff had warned. When, in fact, every time she coughed, she never aspirated and never got pneumonia. If staff members saw her face was red after she'd eaten, they'd question me and ask me if she'd coughed. I was always so afraid that she'd lose her privilege to eat, that I'd always lie and say she hadn't coughed. My point is, don't get alarmed if a patient coughs, but maybe you should be concerned.

Speech therapists and nurses are afraid that liquids/ foods will get into the lungs of patients who have swallowing difficulties and cause pneumonia. A nurse can check the breathing of a patient with a stethoscope after he eats to try to determine if he's aspirated. She can also check the temperature of the patient for a few days after to see if he's developing pneumonia. I never asked the nurse to do this, but you can.

Feeding Tube Dangers

Perhaps the most compelling argument that a patient should be allowed to be rehabilitated for swallowing in a nursing home, is that a feeding tube can be very dangerous if feeding tube precautions aren't followed. In reality, the way nursing home staff feels, it's okay for a patient to aspirate and even die because an aide didn't follow feeding tube precautions. However, it won't let a feeding tube patient run the risk of aspirating from eating real food. Many times I caught aides in the act of not following feeding tube precautions. Each time when I reported it at nursing homes (and even at the hospital), the staff acted as if it was inevitable. It's very ironic, isn't it, that a nursing home doesn't care if a patient aspirates and even chokes to death due to an aide leaving a patient flat while the feeding tube formula is running. However, you must fight a battle before you get permission to let your elder eat by mouth. It's quite possible that in some cases a feeding tube patient will apirate from an aide's error before she aspirates from taking swallows of food by mouth.

Even if you decide not to allow your loved one to eat by mouth you should try to have a feeding tube patient at home for a very important reason. In the four years plus that we had our mother at nursing homes, and even when she first got her feeding tube at the hospital, nurse's aides constantly forgot that a patient must be kept elevated in bed when the formula is running. Otherwise she can aspirate and die. The idea that a patient can aspirate if she doesn't swallow well, when eating by mouth, is true. However, since nurse's aides at nursing homes often forget to keep a patient elevated during a tube feeding, I feel the risk is perhaps just as great to the patient in having her tube fed. In institutional settings, a patient should be allowed to be rehabilitated for swallowing as soon as possible, since, from what I observed with my mother, she was often being laid flat in bed during her tube feeding. Yes, we constantly reminded nursing staff that aides were negligent in keeping my mother elevated. They would come in to change her diaper and not realize that she was hooked up to the feeding tube. You wonder how someone can't notice a pole with a feeding tube bag next to the bed. I guess this goes back to the fact that nurse's aides often look like they are in a stupor traveling from patient's room to patient's room. Some are exhausted. They have too many patients, and it becomes like a factory of assembly-line care. Even those aides who routinely worked with my mother, never bothered to even look at her and notice a feeding tube was running. It wasn't just the aides who irregularly worked with her or an agency aide who goofed up. It was most all of them. Even when I posted signs above her bed that she shouldn't be laid flat, nurse's aides didn't notice them. No matter how many times I mentioned this at quarterly care meetings, the problem was never resolved. It truly amazed me that something so crucial to a patient's well-being was brushed aside.

The solution to this, with some patients, is to schedule a tube feeding while she is sitting in a wheelchair. However, my mother received tube feeding three times a day, so at least some of those times, it wasn't practical for her to be out of bed. For example, one of her tube feedings was at 5 a.m. when she needed to be in bed.

Another solution was for me to be at the nursing home with my mother during her tube feedings so that I could remind aides not to lay her flat. This worked some of the time, but not at 5 a.m. when I wasn't at the nursing home.

(Strangely enough, some aides who finally got the idea and kept my mother elevated, didn't understand that if you elevate a patient's back too far forward, she falls over. This happened to my mother. It is also bad for a patient with a feeding tube to be elevated too far forward because of the circular plastic button at the stoma, the entry site of the tube. It pierces the patient's skin. When a patient's body is bent too far forward, this circular button really hurts the patient. Some formula can also leak from the tube site because of this pressure against it.)

It should be noted, too, that a patient who has received the feeding tube formula, has a full stomach and could cough up the formula and choke if he is laid flat within a half hour or so of having finished the formula. In a nursing home, since there is no individualized care, and often no set schedule for aide care, if an aide comes in to give a sponge bath or change a diaper shortly after the tube feeding has finished, just from the motion of moving the patient around in bed, this could cause the patient to cough up the formula and choke.

If an aide comes to change the diaper of a patient whose feeding tube is running, often he doesn't want to go to the inconvenience of finding the nurse to shut off the tube. He may end up changing the patient anyway. Sometimes, he stops the feeding tube and disconnects it without using the proper sanitary precautions. He'll have dirty hands and doesn't even wear latex gloves.

I always waited an hour after my mother's tube feeding had finished before I subjected her to any activity.

With a feeding tube, restorative aid on the legs should not be done until an hour after the tube feeding formula has stopped. Range of motion on the legs, for example, puts pressure on the abdomen and a patient could feel sick with a full stomach.

In a nursing home, where an aide changes a patient whenever she has time, it's not always possible for an aide to even know when a patient was given her last tube feeding. Consequently, a patient can vomit from movement and aspirate. This is yet another irony of feeding tubes. With the bureaucracy of nursing homes, a patient can aspirate not from eating by mouth, but from feeding tube formula being administered dangerously because of the disorganized and careless institutional system.

It should further be noted, that it's a sign that a patient can swallow well if he can vomit and not choke to death or get pneumonia. While I'm not advocating to induce vomiting, I suspected my mother could adequately swallow, despite the speech therapists' evaluations to the contrary, when she vomited her tube feeding all over the bed one day, and didn't choke or get pneumonia. This happened on more than one occasion. You'd have thought that this was enough proof to get the staff to wonder about my mother's swallowing abilites. However, even after these incidents, I needed to get the doctor's order, and the nursing home still wouldn't agree until they witnessed that I could feed my mother without choking her.

Another problem was the care of the feeding tube at the nursing home. When nurse's aides rolled my mother around in bed to change her diaper, they didn't move her replaceable feeding tube so that she wouldn't be rolled on top of it. If they rolled her on top of it, and it came out, a new tube would have to be reinserted by the nurse. Sometimes aides didn't even realize that the tube had been jerked out. If it is left out for several hours with no one noticing it, the tube site closes up and the patient has to go through the ordeal of going to the hospital and having a new surgical procedure done. (I'm not referring to the sutured-in peg tube, but the type that can be replaced by the nurse.)

My mother's tube was accidentally pulled out twice by aides, but it was discovered. It's somewhat uncomfortable to have a nurse put in a new tube.

Besides this discomfort, my mother experienced pain, inflammation, and bleeding of the tissue around the tube site when the aides rolled her body onto her tube. This can also cause internal bleeding. It was frustrating for us to constantly have to remind the staff that aides were rolling her body on top of her tube and that this jerking of the tube was causing all kinds of tissue bleeding and swelling around her tube site. Yet, aides persisted in doing this.

At this point, the solution to taking care of the irritation was to reduce the tissue swelling by applying silver nitrate to the skin. This was painful in itself, causing stinging. I told the staff and my mother's doctor that it didn't make a lot of sense to cause her pain twice, first in jerking the tube, and then in using silver nitrate to reduce the swelling of the tissue. To make matters worse, I asked the nursing staff not to use silver nitrate unless I was present because I wanted to comfort my mother. One nurse who didn't like me because I had complained too much about care issues, took it out on my mother and applied the silver nitrate when I wasn't there.

Even when I asked the doctor for a doctor's order that it be applied "only in the daughter's presence," and the assistant director of nursing okayed it, I found out that the nurse had not even followed their orders. I found the used silver nitrate sticks in my mother's garbage can. The graveyard shift nurse wasn't even using the silver nitrate sparingly, but in great amounts, to shrink the tissue at the tube site. This caused my mother extreme discomfort. My mother was moaning hours later and her skin was burned around the tissue. I then asked the doctor to discontinue the nitrate sticks altogether, which he did, with the assistant director of nursing apprised of the order.

The graveyard shift nurse wanted to go against this order, too, but she couldn't. I had asked the assistant director of nursing to give me the remaining silver nitrate sticks so the graveyard shift nurse couldn't find them. The graveyard shift nurse took apart my mother's closet to see if I'd hidden them there. She couldn't find them, but she obviously wanted to use them against the doctor's order and the assistant director of nursing's order. Even rummaging through my mother's belongings was a state violation. We had already planned to take our mother home and to report all abuses of this graveyard shift nurse and the graveyard shift aide who had done the "wriststand torture" to the state. This "absolute best nursing home" was in total chaos, with managment not firing anyone for the most flagrant of abuses.

I should mention some other problems we had with this graveyard shift nurse pertaining to feeding tube care. Another reason the tissue of my mother's feeding tube site was inflamed was due to the fact that this nurse was using drain sponges (gauze) around it. The doctor had discontinued the use of drain sponges around the tissue area. The drain sponges were used to soak up residual formula when the stomach gets full and some formula leaks out. Drain sponges are useful for soaking up the formula so it doesn't irritate the skin around the tissue (the stoma). However, the use of drain sponges in nursing homes is counterproductive because the nurses don't remove the drain sponge on a timely basis. Once it gets wet, the drain sponge ends up sticking to the tissue, irritating it more, if it isn't removed for hours. Once "glued on," to remove the drain sponge, causes inflammation and bleeding of the tissue. The graveyard shift nurse had kept using drain sponges despite the doctor's order to discontinue them. Further, my mother's insurance stopped paying for them, so the nursing home billed us.

All that's really needed to keep the tube site clean is to wipe up the residual formula with a warm washcloth dampened with a little soap. Then you remove the soap with a wet washcloth.

However, when my mother left the nursing home, her hospice nurse found a good alternative to drain sponges: Sof-Wik IV ™ sponges. This is a softer gauze.

As for yet other feeding tube problems cause by the graveyard shift nurse, I found out that she'd been shorting my mother on feeding tube formula for many months or even longer. She and her friend, the other graveyard shift nurse, had not been following doctor's orders to give the full amount of formula. Was this euthanasia? Did they want my mother to become more ill and die?

I had previously complained about shabby care by one of the graveyard shift nurses to the director of nursing. I was brushed off by the director of nursing who responded, "You bring problems on yourself." She'd flapped her wrist at me, and began walking out of the room as I replied in a firm monitone, "There is no excuse for patient neglect and abuse." Since it was useless to deal with her, I wrote a letter to the administrator of the extreme neglect and abuse to my mother on graveyard shift, telling her I would contact the state if problems weren't cleared up.

There are nurses who are so unprofessional that they not only harm patients, but they chew out family members for reporting them. The graveyard shift nurse denied having shorted my mother on feeding tube formula and was shouting at me, waking up all the patients, as I left one evening at 11:30 p.m.

The director of nursing, after these incidents and my letter to the administrator, wised up. She was bending over backwards to be nice to me, knowing that I could blast the nursing home to the state when I took my mother out of there, without fear of retaliation. However, she didn't fire the graveyard shift nurse. With a doctor's order, I insisted on giving the graveyard shift tube feeding to my mother at 6 a.m. for the final month my mother was there, because I couldn't trust the nursing home to do it.

Before we left the nursing home, the staff admitted, for example, that the aides were causing my mother's stoma to bleed through their carelessness in moving here around in bed. They finally came up with a solution. Solutions to problems, I might add, are hardly ever found at nursing homes, unless a family member is relentless in pressing them to. They gave my mother a velcro waistband that would keep her feeding tube in place while the aides were changing and turning her in bed. The hospice nurse later recommended a simpler solution. One can buy an elastic cloth at a home health pharmacy. You can cut it into a two-sided waistband and pull the cloth up over the legs to rest on the waist.

Other Feeding Tube Problems and Dangers

I truly believe that any patient on a feeding tube should receive home care. You simply can't trust a nursing home to deliver adequate and safe feeding tube care.

At nursing homes and at the hospital, we saw a particular danger with feeding tubes. There were a few instances when the nurse didn't properly push the medication through the feeding tube with a plastic syringe. I walked in to find some medication spilled on the linen. It was anti-seizure medication which is important not to lose. If a nurse doesn't cap the feeding tube properly after administering medication, it can seep back out. I noticed that aides had a tendancy, being in a hurry, not to question liquids spilled on linens. They come into the room like automatons and change a diaper, not notifying nurses of problems.

The sutured-in peg tube was rubbery and often got clogged, after just six months of use. When it got clogged, the anti-seizure medication would spill back out when the nurse tried to push it in with the syringe. My mother would lose some of her medication, and then the nurse would have to guess at how much she lost and give some medication again. Doing this, you run the risk of underdosing or overdosing the patient with anti-seizure medication, either leaving her prone to seizures or too much sedation, respectively.

Another problem with the feeding tube at the nursing home arose when the nurses didn't properly attach the feeding bag plug to the feeding tube itself. The medication would spill out, or on a few occasions the whole bag of feeding tube formula would spill out and soak my mother's body. Because the nurse leaves the room after she sets up the feeding tube to run, the patient may be lying for a couple of hours in a completely soaked bad. This happened to my mother.

A big problem with nurses running a feeding tube is that they set the gravity bag onto a gravity pole to run at a certain pace, and then they have to leave the room to do other things. It's not uncommon for a bag to have a defective lever, and if so, the formula runs too fast, causing the patient to vomit or to cough too much in discomfort. Even if the bag isn't defective, sometimes the formula flow quickens, so it's hard for the nurse to judge how to set the flow.

Some insurance companies will only pay for a patient to have a tube feeding by hanging a feeding tube bag from a gravity pole. There are calibrated feeding tubes that don't have gravity poles. With a calibrated feeding tube, the formula drops in more uniformly. It doesn't run too fast or too slow. Since the formula drops in slowly, it's harder for the patient to aspirate if she is laid flat by a nurse's aide during the feeding.

Oftentimes, a patient turns red and goes into a coughing fit if the formula drips too fast. The patient could aspirate then, too.

Nurses sometime hang the wrong feeding tube bag on a gravity pole—the kind intended for a calibrated feeding. In this case, the calibrated bag will cause the formula to run through in just about five minutes, rather than 30 to 40 minutes. The patient may vomit. Sometimes, nurses even deliver the wrong feeding tube formula to a patient. Those errors occur when there is more than one tube feeder on the unit.

Often nurses make the mistake of running cold water into a feeding tube. Besides causing discomfort, a patient could get diarrhea. Fluids should always be warm, not hot. Because liquids don't go through the esophagus as when drinking by mouth, the liquids don't get warmed up, but go directly into the stomach. As I've discussed before, juices (without pulp) can go through a feeding tube. I knew a nurse who would administer refrigerated cranberry juice through a feeding tube for a patient who had a bladder infection without warming it up first. She felt she didn't have the time to warm it up. The patient's daughter complained.

Yet another problem at the nursing home with feeding tubes involved the fact that many nurses wanted to save leftover formula in its tin can, if the entire can contained more formula than what was prescribed by the doctor. For one, you don't want opened formula refrigerated in a lead can because that's unhealthy. And number two, cold formula upsets the patient's stomach, especially on an empty stomach in the morning.

Though many nurses do believe it's okay to give liquid medication or crushed pills diluted with water through the feeding bag itself, other nurses feel it isn't good to do this. The drugs might not give the patient the full effect. Liquid medications may stick to the bag unless you shake the bag vigorously and mix a lot of water in. Afterwards, you need to flush the bag with more water. It's best, I've learned, to shoot medication with a plastic syringe directly through the feeding tube itself. First you suck up the diluted medication with the plastic syringe from a paper cup or medicine cup, and then you suck up another 50 cc. of water with the syringe to push it through and flush the tube. Obviously, medication should always be given with water.

One thing that clogged the feeding tube at the nursing home was when nurses would try to save time by mixing my mother's feeding tube formula with her 200 cc. of water for hydration. In their minds, this meant they didn't have to come back a second time after the formula had run, to give the water. However, this causes the fomula to be too thin and drip too fast, and the patient can vomit when the formula runs too quickly. The purpose of giving the water after the formula has run, is to thoroughly flush the tube of formula.

As for troubleshooting with a feeding tube, often the feeding tube gets clogged, even if you're careful about flushing it with 50 cc. of water after medication and 200 cc. of water after the formula has run. If it's not totally clogged, you can shoot water through the tube itself (not through the feeding tube bag.) You shoot the water by using a plastic syringe, just like when you administer medication.

I saw nurses who didn't even wear gloves when working with a feeding tube, plugging the feeding bag into the tube. And, I saw nurses filling the feeding bag with water directly at the sink which was unsanitary. Instead, they should fill a glass of water and pour the water into the feeding bag, without transporting the bag to be filled at the tap.

Sometimes nurses even forget to give a tube feeding on their shift if they get busy. I observed this with my mother at two different facilities. Though it wasn't a common occurrence, it shouldn't happen at all.

If your loved one does have a feeding tube that can easily be replaced, it doesn't do much good if the facility doesn't have a replacement tube on hand if the patient's tube gets clogged. Ask to have a second tube on hand at all times. In one instance, this very thing happened to my mother, and the director of nursing substituted a catheter tube. My mother vomited. Catheter tubes don't work as a substitute. (And, once again, my mother didn't aspirate from vomiting, so this indicated that she had a good swallowing reflex.)

Another feeding tube problem occurs when the rubber lid to the tube gets worn and the feeding bag plug slips out of it while the formula is running. The nursing home should have an extra rubber attachment on hand. If it doesn't, you can tape the plug with non-adhesive (paper) tape.

There are a few points I'd like to make about troubleshooting with a feeding tube. If the feeding tube is dripping too slowly at first, hold up the bag's cord to get it dripping faster.

If the feeding tube won't drip at all, maybe there is residual water in the tube from a previous flushing of the tube, and it has caused air bubbles in the tube. If so, disconnect the plug of the feeding bag which hooks into the tube, drain the excess water, and restart the tube feeding.

I'm giving you these tips because it's often difficult to locate a nurse at the nursing home when you walk in and spot a problem.

With a feeding tube, institution nurses check for any "residual formula" before they start another tube feeding, to make sure the patient digested the previous formula. To do this, you insert the plastic syringe into the feeding tube and pull backwards, (not pushing forwards as you would when delivering medication), to see if you can draw out any residual formula. Once a patient starts recreational eating, if you check for residual formula, you'll pull out regular food, if the food was eaten by mouth after the last tube feeding, and right before the new tube feeding. In this case, maybe it's best not to check for residual. Notify the nurse that your elder has just been fed by mouth.

Recreational Feeding Suggestions

As for recreational feeding, one can keep being fed by a feeding tube, but supplement the formula with real food for enjoyment and to practice swallowing. This isn't for nutritional purposes in such small amounts. If a patient does get pneumonia and die, for some, it would have been worth it, just for the enjoyment of eating real food. This is the way my mother would have seen it, as my brother and I felt. It took one year and seven months for us to get permission to feed our mother— far too long.

For practical purposes, if a doctor doesn't lift the ban on recreational feeding, then how can you call in a nurse to say, "Look, she's swallowing?"

If the patient makes it beyond the recreational feeding stage, have the doctor reduce his formula intake, so he'll be hungrier and eat more food by mouth. Real food is so satisfying, and it provides energy and stimulation (alertness.)

Following is a letter I wrote to my mother's doctor on this issue.

To: John Smith, M.D.

Dear Dr. Smith:

Late each afternoon, I feed my mother about 20 spoonfuls of nutritious foods that I blend. She has gained a great deal of weight from the tube feeding. Currently, she's at 168 pounds. Nursing records show that when she was admitted here 11 months ago, she weighed 145 pounds. Leading an active life at home, she averaged 148 pounds.

Currently, she receives three tube feedings daily, 400 cc. each, at 5 a.m., noon, and 6:30 p.m. These total about 1200 calories. In light of the fact that she is able to eat by mouth without coughing, my brother and I wonder if her 6:30 p.m. tube feeding could be reduced to 250 cc.

Thank you for your attention to this request.

Sincerely ....

How do you feed a patient who hasn't eaten in a long time? What food do you give her?

To awaken a sleeping patient, have her smell something strong, as far as food. Spices, such as oregano, might awaken a patient, helping her to be alert for food by mouth. However, the smell of hot food is much better.

Since my mother loved cooking and eating, and grew up on the smell of basil, garlic, and rosemary, I would stimulate her alertness with those spices in hot tomato sauce.

Speech therapists will tell you to wash a patient's face, swab her mouth with a toothette, and wash her hands to stimulate and prepare her for food by mouth. For my mother, however, the food, if she liked it, was enough to stimulate her. Speech therapists will also tell you that a patient should be sitting upright at 90 degrees to be eating.

The best position is in a wheelchair. Another thing a speech therapist will tell you is that it's helpful to position a patient in front of a mirror so she can watch herself eat.

Don't feed a patient with plastic utensils. She can bite down on them and crack them. Have a fork, spoon, knife, and bowl ready so you don't waste time and the food doesn't get cold. Further, the patient may fall back asleep if you leave the room to hunt for missing things.

Though I'd stimulate my mother with tomato sauce to wake her up, I started her swallowing rehabilitation with simple things. You start with small chips of ice that melt slowly in the patient's mouth. The drops of water usually aren't enough to cause aspiration, since it's like swallowing saliva. Ice cream, sorbet, or fozen yogurt are refreshing as starter foods. Applesauce is often used by speech therapists, in addition to ice cream. It's important to start with tasty soft foods. Even try a popsicle. The latter will taste awfully good to someone whose mouth and throat are dry from not having eaten in a long time. If the patient hasn't eaten by mouth in a long time, his taste buds are shot, so start with sweet things.

Once the patient has gotten used to these foods, branch out. Some families bring in bottled baby foods (pears, peaches, and plums), fruits that aren't chunky. Fruit smoothies through a blender with yogurt mixed in are great. You can even put orange juice and bananas through a blender.

Next try, thick soups, not clear broths, and tomato sauce. (If they contain vegetables, these must be completely pureed, so the patient doesn't choke.)

You can get thickened juices from the nursing home kitchen or from a medical supply store. Start with the thickest consistency. You can also thicken foods and soups by using thickening powder that you can get at the nursing home or at a medical supply store.

Some Other Foods to Consider

1) Pureed corn, carrots, beets, peas
2) Pureed macaroni and cheese
3) Mashed potatoes with gravy
4) JELL-O™ (thoroughly mashed up into small bits with whipped cream)
5) Cottage cheese
6) Clam chowder (take out clams)
7) Campbell's cheese soup
8) Pureed chicken with tomato sauce (through the blender)
9) Pureed ground beef with tomato sauce (through the blender)
10) Custard

If you have a Cuisinart ™, you can puree fruits. Remember that protein helps a patient get stronger. Sometimes a patient can't lift her arms and legs because she's weak. My mother could sometimes repond to lifting her arms and legs, but most of the time she was very weak.

Don't expect too much in the beginning. A nurse told me that when you're bedridden and not expending energy, you don't have much of an appetite.

With pureed foods, I alternated giving my mother one teaspoon of pureed food and one teaspoon of juice to wash it down. What I found with my mother is that it took her a very long time to get her taste buds back and to start liking her favorite foods again. At first, the vegetables she once loved, she didn't like. However, I kept trying until she got used to them again. Early on, I tried bottled vegetables of baby food companies. (At this time, I was in my late 40s, buying baby food at the supermarket. I got a strange look from a man I knew at the checkout stand. He picked up the baby food and looked at me. I just smiled, without explaining. He didn't say anything. He hoped I would explain.)

In the beginning, when you start feeding your elder, if you wish, you can have a nurse check her lungs before and after eating to see if her breathing has changed, and if she's aspirated. (I never did, however.) It might be a good idea, because patients sometimes "silently" aspirate, that is without coughing, or showing other signs.

For my mother, one of my favorite recipes in rehabilitating her was to puree ground beef and tomato sauce and then blend in mashed potatoes.

After pureed food, your elder may be able to work up to mechanical soft food. After that, the next step is solid food. If you work with a speech therapist, she could test at every level. My mother just got to the mechanical soft food stage, that is, food you can mash up with a fork, such as salmon. (Mechanical soft is obviously food that needs to be chewed by the patient.) However, before you go on to mechanical soft, see if your loved one can chew slivers of a banana. Cut a banana into slices, and do not use a fork. Wear a latex glove, and put the banana up to her lips. (Do not mash the banana.) You want to see if the patient can take a small piece of fruit from your fingers and chew. Without a fork, in case she doesn't chew it, it's more likely you can get the piece of fruit out of her mouth quicker. Of course, if the patient doesn't follow instructions well, she may bite your finger. I noted in my mother's case, having her take a piece of banana from my fingers, forced her to dig into it. She practiced chewing.

If the patient who isn't always alert, stops chewing, pat her cheek, and remind her to keep chewing. You don't want her to lose her train of thought.

At the mechanical soft food stage, you can mash up salmon with a fork and pour in some tomato sauce. Try to introduce more spoonfuls of food by mouth at each meal. And, if warranted, have the doctor reduce more and more tube feeding. (At nursing homes, you need a doctor's order for this.) Because my mother was not allowed to eat for such a long time, her swallowing never became proficient enough for her to have the feeding tube removed. For some patients, the goal may be to wean them off the feeding tube completely.

In progressing up the ladder of foods, guard against choking. Follow these rules, and other rules a speech therapist might give you:

- No sticky foods that can get caught in the throat like peanut butter.
- No slippery foods.
- You can steam and mash fruits.
- You can use a strainer to mash vegetables into thick soups. Split pea soup is good.
- You can thicken juice with vanilla ice cream or yogurt, if your elder doesn't like bottled thickened juices from the medical supply store.

It's important after feeding your elder, to swab her mouth with a toothette dipped in a little water, toothpaste, and mouthwash. Make sure she hasn't pocketed any food. Then, use a little water on another toothette to rinse. Or, you can do the same, only with a toothbrush, preceded with using a toothette to check for pocketed food. (I used a few toothettes and a toothbrush to scrub the teeth.)

Postscript

When the speech therapist used the argument that my mother wasn't alert enough to eat, I asked her, "Don't you stimulate a patient to be alert by offering food, and doesn't their desire to be alert and awake increase if they begin receiving more and more food?" She admitted that this was true. Food is often the best stimulant to waking a lethargic patient. Yes, some patients awake with deep massage, family members and friends talking to them, or music.

However, for many, especially for my mother who loved food and was a great cook, food was a stimulant that shouldn't have been denied.

It should be considered that in having a feeding tube, a patient urinates all the time because his intake is strictly liquids. Consequently, his sleep during the night is interrupted to have him changed and turned. How well would you function if you were awakened a few times during the night, not just to have your body repositioned (that you could sleep through), but to be cleaned up? Further, skin breakdown occurs in nursing homes, because patients are often subjected to uncleanliness when they are cleaned up, particularly those who urinate all the time. Therefore, having a feeding tube creates many peripheral problems beyond the quality of life issues and nutrition.

There is the miscellaneous point I raised before: the fact that nursing homes don't cut your elder's base fees that cover room and board, when she's not getting food. Has anyone ever thought of advocating that feeding tube patients who pay extra for a nurse to administer the tube feeding, are not charged for food that they are not allowed to eat?

It's not only unjust to the patient to not allow a family member to carefully feed her by mouth, but it's not right for her to be denied food that she pays for.

Chapter 5

Alternatives to Nursing Homes

Beginning Your Search

There are much better alternatives to a nursing home, but many patients who are placed at nursing homes are misguided by hospital staff into going there. They are quickly dumped out of hospitals, and family members don't have enough time to learn about nursing homes or alternatives to them. In addition, hospital staff, such as social workers, really know nothing about nursing homes other than just through the rumor mill or at best, one visit to particular nursing homes. My brother and I had been repeatedly told by hospital discharge personnel and our mother's doctor that our mother wasn't entitled to substantial free R.N. care if we took her home. What we didn't find out until years later, when we placed our mother in the hospice program, was that from the beginning, just by virtue of the fact that she had a feeding tube (which was "life support"), she had been entitled to up to 27 hours of free R.N. care at home each week, after leaving the hospital. You can imagine the utter disbelief we felt at learning this. Our mother had spent years in unclean nursing homes, paying through the nose for minimal assistance or "care" which led her condition downhill, rather than being at home and getting free, substantial private care. We felt she would have had a chance of recovery at home.

The doctor, his office nurse who was a liaison to my mother's insurance, and the hospital discharge staff shouldn't have made emphatic statements about insurance issues without really knowing. In addition, a family member should never just call Medicare, Medicaid, and private insurance up on the phone and get information from people who might misinform them. The best way of definitively finding out about insurance coverage is to make a personal visit to these offices and ask to speak to someone or even a supervisor.

Further, some family members can be paid by Medicaid to take care of their elder. Medicaid often feels this is cheaper than paying a nursing home for the Medicaid patient.

I remember a few days before my mother was dumped out of the hospital, she was in critical condition, having uncontrolled seizures and the doctor said she might die any day, but the hospital benefits had been used up because it had been a month. What we were to learn years later that besides not knowing about the substantial free R.N. care that she could have gotten at home, she could have been, as an alternative, placed in the hospice program for substantial free care, too.

In my ignorance, I had initially thought that hospice was for terminally ill cancer patients. I didn't know at that time that heart patients, head injury patients, and those with other terminal conditions who were not expected to live beyond six months could be placed in a hospice program by doctor's order. The doctor didn't bother to tell us that this was yet another alternative, at this time, that our mother was eligible for. Her doctor had been practicing for 30 years, so he wasn't just fresh out of medical school.

After a month of nursing home care, my mother was going downhill fast. She had pneumonia and near fatal lung embolisms (clots in her legs spreading up to her lungs), followed by another pneumonia. Her lung problems may not have occurred had she not been totally confined to her bed, without being transferred into a wheelchair twice daily, as per doctor's orders. At any rate, the assistant director of nursing at this bad nursing home suggested we contact the hospice program. We did, but we were concerned that if she was still alive after six months, she would get dumped from the hospice program, and we'd be back to square one as far as needing care for her. We were also very confused at the time, and didn't know what to do. We began looking at other nursing homes. It should be noted that some hospice patients have been kept on hospice for even three years if the hospice nurse and social worker determine that the patient is not getting any better and the family needs the assistance. (We were not told this at the time.)

Whatever condition your loved one is in, this chapter will help you define options for him. You can consult The Eldercare Locator when you decide on some options. This government entity is financed by the Federal Administration on Aging. It can provide information about all services in your area. Its phone number is 1-800-677-1116. Its website is www.aoa.dhhs.gov.

Currently, there are about 23 million caregivers in the U.S. to aged and ailing family members, either who do it part-time or full-time. You may want to join these ranks.

Oftentimes, your local Alzheimer's Association, County Department of Human Services' Aging Division, or State Senior Services Division can recommend a person who is in the business of finding housing options for the elderly such as licensed foster homes. These referrel people often don't charge a fee, but, for example, foster homes pay them for the referrel. It should be noted that they often direct you to some very good options. One woman, we found, a Ph.D., who ran a non-profit referral corporation, gave us some reputable advice on some very good foster homes, both when my mother was ambulatory and memory-impaired, and when she wasn't functional and bedridden, although we didn't end up placing her in a foster home. She also gave us information on residential care facilities. She was paid by the qualifying licensed foster home or facility.

Geriatric Care Managers (GCMs) can also help you decide on care options, for a fee. They will even assist you if you want caregiver referrels for 24-hour home care. They not only do everything from supervising the care of an elderly person and hiring people to do the caregiving, but they arrange for medical, financial, and legal services. They typically charge by the hour from about $60 to $110 as independent consultants. Some work for agencies. They may be a solution, particularly if a family member lives in a different state, or if an elderly person has no family at all.

There are no licensing requirements for GCMs , but some are social workers. Medicare, Medicaid, and private health insurance don't cover the cost. For the names of GCMs in your area, check with the National Association of Professional Geriatric Care Managers, (www.caremanager.org). Its phone number is (520) 881-8008, and its address is 1604 N. Country Club Rd., Tucson, AZ 85716. You can also contact the Area Agency on Aging where your elder lives.

Ask whether a GCM is certified through the National Academy of Certified Care Managers. If you do decide on hiring a GCM, discuss how quickly he responds to calls, how and when he can be reached, and who covers for him when he isn't working. Ask whether it is possible to negotiate a flat rate instead of an hourly rate.

Make sure you have a written agreement with a GCM regarding fees and services provided. Ask him what his patient load is. You should evaluate GCMs in terms of the situation your loved one is in, and their experience with others in that condition. Of course, ask them about their experience and their professional licenses (i.e. social worker, nurse, etc.). Ask if they personally provide any services or how they screen workers they hire. It may be a good idea to check the GCM out with the Better Business Bureau in your area. Of course, when you contact any GCM, ask for client references.

For the extremely wealthy, there are independent health care management firms, sometimes run by nurse entrepreneurs who will coordinate medical and home services; do written assessments and care plans for your elder; train family members and caregivers; and work with healthcare facilities, home health services, or adult day care programs. They have 24-hour on-call availability by phone. Their hourly fees can run a couple hundred dollars an hour. They find and coordinate all kinds of healthcare. If a family member lives far away from his loved one, sometimes this can be an option.

They not only obtain and arrange for services including caregivers and home care services, but even financial and legal services. They work, too, with nursing home administrators, hospital staff, attorneys, and insurance carriers. With 'round the clock aides at home and a care management firm's assistance, the cost of care could even run $15,000 a month. My friend paid this to a healthcare management company for its services including the aide workers.

In this chapter, I'll deal with the basic alternatives to nursing homes. They are adult day care, that would be used as a method of relieving the family member who does home care; Assisted Living; home care through private caregivers; agency home health care; foster homes; residential care facilities; and hospice. Obviously, adult day care wouldn't work for a bedridden person, nor would Assisted Living. It's doubtful, too, that a residential care facility would be able to care for a bedridden person any better than a nursing home would, for reasons I'll discuss later. Therefore, care options obviously depend on the particular condition of your loved one.

For an elder who has extensive physical and mental problems, adult day care is probably not an option. For an elder who needs nursing care, assisted living facilities are not an option, but it may be a good option for someone who suffers from Alzheimer's or a memory-related impairment. For elders who are bedridden and have physical and mental impairments, both home care and foster care are options, as some advanced level foster homes will take bedridden and hospice residents. For the terminally ill, enrolling an elder in the hospice program gives your loved one great healthcare benefits. While a hospice patient can be living at a nursing home, hospice patients are usually at home or in foster care. We placed our mother in the hospice program four months before we were able to move her back home. The hospice program made all necessary arrangements for her transfer from the nursing home, including setting up the home with all equipment she needed. You will discover the great free benefits of hospice in this chapter.

Following is a letter I wrote to my mother's doctor informing him that my mother was leaving nursing home life for good. I decided on home care, after investigating other options as discussed in this chapter.

To: John Smith, M.D.

Dear Dr. Smith:

My brother and I have decided to move our mother back into her home by the end of August. She will be cared for by me, along with private and agency help.

Besides long-standing care problems at this facility, our motivation to move our mother home involves her being able to take full advantage of services offered by the hospice program.

I enclose an emergency medical form for the utilities company with information provided by you that would make it possible for my mother to be a priority customer should a power outage result. Of course, in her condition, heat and electricity need to be restored as quickly as possible. Would you please be kind enough to fill out the back side of the form by August? Please use the enclosed SASE.

Again, thank you for your assistance.

Sincerely......

Prior to my mother's discharge from the nursing home, it should be noted that my brother told the hospice social worker that he was concerned about my taking our mother home. While he wasn't overlooking the fact that she was being abused, not receiving her prescribed amount of tube feeding formula, and was riddled with infections including Strep, due to the staff's uncleanliness, he wondered if I could manage lifting my mother at home. He visited foster homes, and considered other options. He told the hospice social worker that he felt I would lean on him too much if I took her home and that he would get calls waking him up during the night, thereby disturbing his family.

Perhaps he redeemed himself when he saw how well she was doing at home. He pitched in, coming to visit a few times a week, helping with errands and some lifting of my mother, and bringing food.

Moral: expect protests from family members, but hope for the best, and be prepared to give it a try, no matter how much resistance you get from relatives.

Even if hospice and home care aren't options for your elder, you can consider others in reading this chapter.

Adult Day Care

Adult day care is usually offered anywhere from five to seven days a week in a group setting outside the home. This provides a chance for activities, socializing, and it costs about $7 an hour, less than in-home services. It's great for people who are, for example, mildly confused and ambulatory, but not so appropriate for totally confused and wandering elders who are hard to control or even combattive. My mother attended some day care centers years after her brain cancer surgery, when her memory was failing. There were also people in wheelchairs who were brought by relatives. However, adult day care is certainly not an option for people with extensive physical problems and illnesses who should be homebound and receive in-home, one-on-one help. Adult day care is also appropriate for adults who are socially isolated and depressed.

One often finds, as we did for our mother, after her brain cancer, that limited adult day care, one or two days a week at a senior center is available.

You can even check into free bus transportation to and from the center, specifically for the handicapped and elderly, often provided by your local public bus transportation system.

Adult day care usually isn't suitable for someone who is strickly nursing home material with substantial physical and mental impairments. We saw people in nursing homes who didn't need nursing home care and could have benefitted from other options. This is why I'm dealing with adult day care. Adult day care centers tend to improve elders' well-being, even postponing the need for a nursing home, and they allow family caregivers to keep working during the day. Adult day care is in short supply, even in metropolitan areas, and many don't offer the extended hours working caregivers need. If the elder likes being around people, an adult day care center is great. When my mother was still somewhat functional and ambulatory, years after her brain cancer, she enjoyed herself at adult day care. At first, she was resistant to going. They have music, arts and crafts, conversation, visits by dog owners and their dogs, movies, etc.

To find an adult day care center, contact your Area Agency on Aging, or find one in the Yellow Pages of the phonebook. The National Adult Day Services Association, www.nadsa.org, is also helpful with information. The Association's phone number and address are 1-800-558-5301, 722 Grant St., Herndon, VA 20170. There are about 3,500 centers nationwide.

The cost of adult day care, at an average of $56 a day is expensive for most elders. However, it's cheap considering the alternatives of $80 a day or more for a companion home-care aide that you hire privately to do simple tasks. And, it's cheap in compared to about $5,000 a month for an assisted living facility or $7,000 a month for a nursing home. Long-term care insurers may pay for day care. Medicaid funds can be used for adult day care in most states.

You can also check with Volunteers of America that often has adult day care programs.

Adult day care programs are wonderful. Participants sit in a circle reminiscing about childhood and talking about families. They do chair exercises, and play games. Participants are engaged in very simple activities and receive help, so they don't feel as if they aren't capable of enjoying an activity. Some day care centers offer outings, or outside entertainers come in. It's a stimulating environment at many places, not a babysitting service.

At most adult day care places, the activities are simple ones. However, at some day care places my mother was at, after her brain cancer surgery, I saw crafts demonstrated that were too difficult, involving scissor cutting and pasting. At one day care, the leader made peanut brittle and the elders stuffed it in gift bags and tied a ribbon around the bags. This was fun and simple for participants. This leader also told me that with memory-impaired participants, she was careful not to give participants a glass of paint to paint with. She said they might end up spilling the paint, or worse, even drinking it. She was careful not to put them in a situation where they would be harmed or even just embarrassed to have made a mistake.

Sometimes day care places through senior centers have retired nurses leading the program or retired nurse volunteers to assist. Some day care centers offer blood pressure monitoring and medication supervision. Participants are served snacks during the morning and afternoon. And, if they stay the whole day they receive lunch.

It's good to visit day care centers before placing your elder in one. Make sure they are clean, and that the staff greets elders at the door by name and makes them feel at home.

Ask the day care center staff what its policy is about participants arriving with colds and flu. You don't want your loved one to catch germs. Tell the director of any unusual behaviors your loved one has. My mother, after her brain tumor surgery, had squinting eyes. This often concerned people who witnessed it.

Ask the director if your loved one must cancel out on his scheduled day, what the cancellation deadline is to avoid being billed. You should also ask if the day can be made up sometime during the week.

Determine if Medicaid, state, or private funding is available. You can also locate adult day care centers by calling your county office on aging, or perhaps an association of adult day care exists in your state that you could contact. You can also inquire through United Way about adult day care centers in your community.

General things to consider in an adult day care are:

- Is it certified or licensed?
- Can the staff perform CPR?
- What is the staff-to-client ratio? (If your loved one is in a program for dementia or memory impairment, the ratio is usually no less than one staff to five clients. My mother was once in an adult day care program

at a senior center where there was one staff to two
clients. They had some volunteer staff, including a
paid leader who was a retired R.N.)
- Are the policies and procedures for emergencies, complaints, and refunds clear?
- Is half-day attendance possible, or what are the minimum hours a day of attendance?
- Are meals available for special diets?
- Inquire about the activities and consider if they would
be of interest to your loved one. (My mother loved
conversation and music.)
- What about transportation to and from the center? ("Lift
Buses" through the public transportation service in
your community usually offer shuttle bus service for
the handicapped and elderly to special appointments.
You reserve ahead of time. They will even
transport both the elder and caregiver to doctor's
appointments.)

In the San Francisco area, for example, you'll find
"Health For All," a non-profit arts program geared to helping elders suffering from Alzheimer's and related dementia. It's a program whereby participants paint and communicate what they can no longer verbalize. It visits care facilities. To get in touch with the program, you can contact
the Center for Elders and Youth in the Arts, 3330 Geary
Blvd., San Francisco, CA 94118.

In some cities throughout the country, there are adult
day cares that include visits by doctors, nurses, and rehab
therapists. They run 24 hours a day with a medical team
on call at all times. They are for frail older Americans. However, the elders still live at home with their families. For
Medicaid elders, Medicaid picks up the tab.

Although a day care center will have you fill out emergency information for your loved one, make sure your
elder carries an I.D. card in her pocket with, "In case of an

emergency call....." The card should have your name and phone number, plus contact information for her physician and a list of drug allergies. If she has a special medical condition, a medic-alert bracelet should be worn.

It's interesting to note that about eight million Americans care for both their children and their elderly parents in their home. They are called the Sandwich Generation.

Assisted Living Facilities

Unlike nursing homes, assisted living facilities don't provide skilled nursing, but they do offer private living quarters and staff to help residents with basic services, such as providing meals, bathing, dressing, and assisting with medications. They are for seniors who are unable to live alone, but don't require nursing care.

There are about 37,000 assisted living facilities in the U.S. There's little accountability for these facilities. Like nursing homes, they receive complaints about inadequate staffing and patient neglect and abuse. To date, there is really little information about the quality of them for consumers through one's state.

Many people with Alzheimer's and memory-related illnesses who are ambulatory live in assisted living facilities. The key is to determine if the services advertised in their marketing brochures are consistent with those listed in residents' written contracts.

When my mother was ambulatory, after her brain cancer recovery, I'd considered putting her in an assisted living facility and one manager allowed her to test out the idea by permitting her to spend a day or two a week as a day participant in their activities for a nominal charge. At that time, many years ago, the charge was equivalent to that of an adult day care center. My mother didn't feel there were enough activities during the day to keep her busy. They would have a bus ride once a week, ten miles out into the country; they had a library for reading; and some music activities. The facility's main lobby was elegant for receiving visitors. For a facility, the food was very good, according to my mother who was an excellent cook. However, many of the residents were much older than my mother at that time. They were in their 80s and 90s, and she was in her early 70s. They were not as functional or communicative as she was at that time.

Some corporations own, operate, and develop assisted living facilities in states nationwide and do a lot of advertising to hook adult children who'll hopefully place their elderly parents there. They hold open houses with wine and cheese parties for adult children. Since the early 1990s, assisted living facilities have been offered to somewhat functional adults as an alternative to nursing homes. However, in walking through an assisted living facility, you sometimes see ambulatory residents who look about as functional as a nursing home patient. Perhaps given the competitive nature of the business, some accept residents who are actually too frail to be there, or they let them stay on when they aren't functioning well enough.

On the flip side, an assisted living facility can toss a resident out, if she starts failing dramatically. Before you sign on the dotted line, make sure you understand how and why they discharge residents. The Assisted Living Federation of America, the industry trade group, cautions families about this.

The federal government's Long-Term Care Ombudsman Program has volunteers in every state who put consumers in touch with agencies that can help them find assisted living facilities or attempt to resolve complaints against them.

Go directly to your state's Long-Term Care Office to inform yourself of any complaint against the facility and for an inspection report. Again, these reports don't always give you a clear picture of a facility, just as a state's report on a nursing home may not be a clear picture. However, it may be better than nothing.

When my mother was ambulatory and still functional, I even visited an assisted living facility that had a special wing for memory-impaired adults.

Recognize that there are different levels of assisted living. Some offer rental apartments, a communal dining room, and limited personal services and activities. Some offer rental apartments, a dining room for all meals, full assistance with personal needs such as bathing, dressing, and medications, and an on-site nurse for limited help.

"Continuing Care Retiring Communities," allow residents to age in place, by including independent living, then allowing them to graduate to assisted living, and finally to a nursing home, all on the same property. For this, you may have to put up front $200,000 or more for an apartment that you can't pass along to heirs, besides paying monthly charges. Before you enter into any complex agreement, consult an elder law attorney. Some CCRCs make promises they can't keep, so you'll have to weed out the good from the bad. Religious-affiliated CCRCs exist, too. As with all housing arrangements, don't assume that the religious-affiliated ones are the best choice.

To be accepted into a CCRC, an individual must be healthy, but if assisted living and skilled nursing care should become necessary, they are assured for life. (Obviously, if you're reading this book before your elder needs care, you might consider this. But, as with some of the readers of this book, this option comes too late.)

At some assisted living facilities, there may be some surprise fees for services you thought were included. Further, find out when rents are raised and how much advance notice is given. What are staff-to-resident ratios? How often are rooms cleaned? Is the property safe, security-wise? Are residents' call bells answered? (At nursing homes, even hospitals, one can be buzzing for an hour or more!)

You also want to determine if the assisted living facility is financially stable and debt-free. If the company that owns it is public, you can examine the Securities and Exchange Commission statements.

As with all facilities, the staff turnover rate is probably high, every three to six months. I remember that after an initial visit to an assisted living facility to talk to an administrative person, I called back two weeks later and she'd left unexpectedly. They didn't explain where she'd gone. Get used to this. I noticed this, too, not only at nursing homes, but with home health agencies. Often the staff gets frustrated with management policies and leaves.

With assisted living, one can often bring one's own furniture and even bring one's own small dog or cat. Laundry and linens are done by the staff. Some assisted living facilities take Medicaid residents. Limited staff is available 'round the clock.

Assisted living allows people to be more independent by helping them with dressing, for example, rather than doing it for them, as nursing homes want to do for an elder. The latter want to speed up the task.

Assisted living is also a good choice for the individual who is able to transfer himself into a wheelchair. Incontinence aid is also available.

It should be noted that there are now some high-tech assisted living facilities for Alzheimer's residents, allowing them the freedom that they wouldn't have in a locked Alzheimer's ward of a nursing home. These high-tech facilities have a home-like ambiance with plants, pets, and live-in caregivers. They have only a few dozen residents. They allow their residents to "wander" on the grounds, because the facilities have security cameras and high-tech gadgets called "transponders" that the residents wear. These set off an alarm when the resident gets off the premise. These facilities are not short-staffed like nursing homes, so the caregivers can monitor residents' whereabouts at all times. (In the future, with high-tech, family members who live far from their elders will be able to tap into their home computers and track their elder's moves. This will be possible with the elder's transponders and cameras in the elder's home.)

To find out about your best options in facilities for your elder with Alzheimer's and related dementia, contact your local Alzheimer's Association Office.

Assisted living facilites are regulated even less than nursing homes. Further, assisted living bills may be tricky. The base pay may look attractive, as I've said, but the add-on fees such as incontinent care may bump up the price. Ask about add-on fees.

You should also ask the assisted living facility staff how the facility is different from a nursing home. Then ask yourself if you'd like to live there if you were old and frail. Is the facility concerned with a resident's dignity?

A senior center staff member, who ran an afternoon day care for memory-impaired adults, once told me that an elderly woman who occasionally came to her program lived at an assisted living facility closeby. Her daughter would pick her up and bring her there for the activities that were lacking at the assisted living facility. The senior center staff member told me that the elderly woman always arrived with tangled hair. Apparently, she said, the assisted living facility didn't do a good job with personal care, either.

As with anything that you pay for, the bottom line is, "Buyer Beware."

Taking Your Elder Home & Hiring Private Caregivers

If you take your loved one out of a nursing home, even if you do some or most of the care yourself, you'll need either family or friends helping. Or, you'll need to hire some relief help, even just a sitter so you can run out and do errands.

Like most people, you'll ask friends if they can recommend a caregiver. A good friend of mine found a live-in caregiver for her mother at her mother's home. The caregiver has lived with her mother for a year and a half. Her mother is in her 80s, is confused, and walks with a walker. Besides free room and board, the caregiver is paid $1100 each month, and is given weekends off. My friend is fortunate, because it's rare that caregivers stay this long. The caregiver is in her 60s and is foreign. If you find a retired person, of course, the retired person should be in excellent health.

Another friend of mine, (as I did through the years), hired private caregivers through a local hospital's caregiver listing service. Using this method, you pay a few dollars each year to have a monthly list mailed to you of caregivers who run classified ads. They state their experience and what kind of position they seek. For example, they state what kind of elder they are willing to work with, whether or not they are a Certified Nursing Assistant, (CNA) who has experience with bedridden patients, and when they are available to work. You must first interview them by phone, and if you feel you'd like to meet them, schedule a meeting and ask for references.

You can also check with your Area Agency on Aging to see if there are any low cost home health programs in your area or you can check with your State's Department of Human Services that has a Special Aging Division. An alternative is contacting United Way for suggestions.

Hiring home help involves being very specific with prospective caregivers about what your elder's needs are. You must also determine to what extent you are willing to train the caregivers (especially with a bedridden elder), and to what extent they are willing to be trained.

Does your elder need help with:

1) Feeding
2) Bathing
3) Dressing
4) Walking
5) Toileting
6) Constant supervision
7) Incontinence
8) Lifting in bed
9) Medication

You should also describe your loved one for the caregiver. Is she:

1) Visually-impaired
2) Hearing-impaired
3) Able to talk or gesture
4) Confused
5) Wandering
6) Depressed
7) Hostile
8) Totally dependent

Define what activities the caregiver should do:

1) Prepare meals
2) Light housework
3) Read newspapers/books to elder
4) Do laundry
5) Do grocery shopping
6) Offer transporation
7) Give companionship/conversation/sitting
8) Do range of motion exercises
9) Give complete bedridden care

You need to decide specifically when you need to have the caregiver available. Preferences for caregivers should include: their age, sex, smoker/non-smoker. You must decide how much you are willing to pay and whether you want to pay by the hour, by the day,or weekly. Live-in salaries include room and board. Hours of service depend on your needs.

Usually, home health workers want as much as $5 more per hour that the wage that nursing home aides start at.

When caregivers run classifieds through a hospital listing service or in the newspaper, you get a feel for what the going rate is.

One thing you'll quickly find out about home health care workers is that they don't like social security deducted from their paychecks. Actually, most don't even stay long enough for social security to be deducted from their paychecks. Check with your accountant or call the Social Security Administration Office as listed in your phonebook, to find out about how much you can pay home health care workers in a calendar year before you need to withhold and pay their social security. Most calendar years, the cut-off amount has been slightly above $1,000.

You should also check with your insurance agent to find out what coverage you have for an in-home worker, and also check your auto insurance policy for coverage if the worker is to drive your car. With the latter, I would strongly suggest that the caregiver drives her own car for errands or in transporting your elder.

If your parent is bedridden and she requires lifting and turning in bed, recognize that caregivers you hire privately are usually not licensed or bonded. If they can claim they injured their back or even tripped in your home, you could have a lawsuit. They would probably have to prove that they didn't injure themselves taking care of another bedridden person or through some other means, however. This is why some people prefer to hire help through agencies that insure the worker.

If a home health care worker works full-time, you should give him two full days off each week. You must hire a substitute for weekends and you must have an alternate plan in case a worker calls in sick. Can a family member or you substitute? (Oftentimes, you'll get a call in the morning, an hour before he is scheduled, that he is sick.)

When you check references, it's also a good idea to ask the previous employer how often the person called in sick and what kind of advance notice was given.

If you decide to find help on your own, you can also place an ad in a church bulletin, at a college employment office, or at an area nursing school. (These didn't yield any great prospects for me, but sometimes they might work. I hired two nursing students who were unmotivated. I guess they'll be no better as nurses! We couldn't scare up any other nursing students. We were offering them twice the pay that they would have earned doing hospital work as nursing students. I guess between studying and hospital experience, home care wasn't alluring.)

Your ad should include a general description of your needs and preferences. List just your phone number in a newspaper, and run the ad for several days including Sunday.

I believe your best bet will be finding a caregiver through your local hospital listing service, as caregivers are actively looking for work.

One of my friends who had a husband, mother, and father who were ill in the same five-year period, was making care arrangements for all of them. She told me that for every 50 caregivers she called who were advertising, she'd find one suitable caregiver. The process can be grim.

My friend, Julie, kept a list of caregivers whom she would recommend to other friends in her situation, long after her loved ones died. In fact, my best caregiver came from this list. She knew how hard it was to find caregivers. Julie also kept a list of "crazy caregivers to avoid." Especially in a smaller city like ours, they make the rounds, and begin to be well-known to people. One crazy person on her list met her for coffee, and simply got up and walked out of the coffee shop while she was being interviewed without saying a word. Julie's list of good caregivers included detailed notes about who they were and what their situations were.

Yes, private caregivers are hard to find. Caregiving is not seen as being a valuable effort. I contacted nuns at convents I knew, hoping an older, retired nun or a young nun might be interested. No takers. I don't think caregiving is demeaning, and I had professional careers before becoming a caregiver: educator, journalist, and public relations executive.

Ask the pastor of your own church if he'll run a notice in the church bulletin that you're looking for a caregiver. At some churches, they have a group of volunteers who will assist the elderly and homebound. They run errands, drive them to the doctor, take them shopping, and relieve relatives who wish to go out. Unfortunately, they organized this group at my church after my mother died.

Sometimes you run across people who aren't caregivers, but who are willing to help you. You can train them to be caregivers. I ran across a clerk at the laundry service I used. I had been talking to her about why I needed the laundry service with my bedridden mother. She was pleasant, responsible and intelligent. I hired her to do some weekend relief aide work. I trained her. She lasted only a couple of months until she found out she was pregnant, and couldn't do lifting anymore.

You can even call up a senior center and ask if there is an active senior who might want to earn some extra money as a sitter while you're out on errands.

Some caregivers who sounded good in their ads and over the phone already found jobs by the time I contacted them. Some of my friend's referrels were busy working, too.

If caregivers are good, they get enough referrels to other jobs, so they may be busy when you need them. Ask if they know of someone else. Some caregivers have relatives or friends who are caregivers. It doesn't hurt to ask if they know of someone.

Be frank with the caregiver about the duties involved. Don't downplay the difficulty of certain tasks. And, be just as specific about tasks you don't want them to do, such as bandaging sores, giving medications, or giving tube feedings. I wanted to do these tasks myself.

Hire caregivers who have lived in the area for a long time. If someone has moved here from another state, for example, your state won't have any record of their criminal past, if they have one.

I remember that after my mother's brain cancer recovery, I hired a companion aide a few hours a week. Each time she came, she left the house fatter than when she arrived. No, she didn't eat our food. I connected the dots. She was stealing towels from the linen closet.

Sixteen years later, when my mother was a hospice patient at home, some aides were stealing from her. Imagine doing that to a dying woman. Some nice silver utensils and vintage clothing were taken. While you can't lock up everything, it's a good idea to keep jewelry, cash, credit cards, blank checks, and important documents locked up in a safe at home, out of the eyesight of the caregiver. And, make sure your elder's purse doesn't contain any more cash than what she'll need for an outing. Cash and other valuables are too much of a temptation for some caregivers. Oftentimes, you don't notice possessions missing until months later. Whenever someone tells me that his parent's caregiver was honest and never stole from the elder's home, I begin to wonder. How does he know for sure? Especially if the family member doesn't live in the elder's house, he won't notice things missing. One of my friends told me his mother's caregiver tried to extort $3,000 from her. She told the elderly woman that he had not paid her yet for the caregiving, and that she was owed the $3,000. The elderly woman wrote out a check for $3,000. He found out about it just after she deposited the check. He called the police and she was charged with larceny.

Another friend of mine hired a caregiver for her frail grandmother who still had her mental faculties. My friend visited one day and found the caregiver downstairs in the basement smoking dope.

One of my neighbors was an elderly man of 92. His daughter told me that an aide she'd hired actually stole patches, little by little, from an old bed quilt he had, until his quilt could no longer keep him warm.

A nurse once told me that her grandmother went though 32 home health aides in three years. She said many were alcoholics and thieves. Actually, 32 might not be so bad. Most aides last about two weeks, so one could go through 26 in a year.

You can check the caregiver for past criminal convictions and civil suits for theft, for example.

To check for civil suits, call the county court recorders office where the individual to be hired lives or has lived. The search is done by name only and is public record. It costs you nothing.

To check criminal records, call your State's Correction Division. You'll need the date of birth of the prospective caregiver. They can tell you if the person has ever been in the state penitentiary system, booked into a county jail, or has been on probation over the past 20 years and what the crime was. This search is free.

Just because an individual is a licensed caregiver, doesn't mean she doesn't have a criminal record. She may have fallen through the cracks, or the state doesn't check civil records for suits.

If you opt to spend money checking out the background of a caregiver, use www.USSearch.com. You must have the caregiver's written permission to do this, but if he has nothing to hide, he should agree. The site will email you an accurate report of his previous addresses, a check of sex-offender records, driving, bankruptcy, and criminal histories. The search can run from $80 to over a hundred, depending on how detailed you want to get.

After a successful initial visit at a coffee shop, have the caregiver come to your home to meet your loved one. If your elder is bedridden and not very alert, a lot of caregivers might feel uncomfortable being around such a person. They may feel it's lonely and depressing work.

You should ask the caregiver when she left her last position and why. Did she have the same type of situation as the one you're offering her? For live-in help, ask about whether she is willing and able to get up during the night. To be on the safe side, you or a family member may want to take graveyard shift, so you know for sure that your loved one isn't being neglected during this time.

As a live-in, a caregiver will want a private room, bath, and kitchen privileges, of course. Determine specifically when she will be on and off duty. When she isn't on duty, I would allow her to have only one guest visiting at a time. And, I would ask her not to have lengthy phone conversations when she is off duty.

Try to avoid live-in aides, as you lack privacy if you're living in the same house. There is also wear and tear on your home with plumbing, if you live in an old home, besides the added cost of utilities. There is also too much downtime when they are on duty, but have nothing to do. A lot of aides have poor cleanliness skills, and particularly if they live in your home, you might end up being their housekeeper.

If the job applicant tells you about her own personal problems, don't hire her. You don't need a second problem in your life.

Ask for professional references. Hopefully, she'll have three. I would ask the references if the applicant is patient and easygoing, and of course, industrious. You want to know if she is punctual, reliable, and honest. Further, I would ask about cleanliness skills. You don't want your home to be as dirty as a nursing home. Ask the reference person what she liked most about the caregiver, and if there was anything she didn't like about her.

You will find that most caregivers don't last long after the honeymoon period of the first few days.

When I took my mother out of the nursing home, I hired a good aide who had once worked there, but who left the job to work at a hospital. She helped me for two months, after work at her hospital job, and on one of her days off. However, she dropped the job with my mother because she was working too many hours with two jobs. Although I paid her $15 an hour, and she was getting only $10 an hour to work like a Trojan at the hospital, the job with my mother was precarious. If my mother died and she dropped her hospital job, she'd be out of work, or if she went back, she'd have lost her seniority. I also didn't pay her health benefits as the hospital did. At the nursing home, I observed that some family members who got disgusted with it and moved their elder home, offered part-time work to good aides they met there, once their loved one was home.

Although a private care job is a piece of cake for an aide who is inundated with patients at a facility, often these aides feel that private care work is isolating. Yes, the job is easy in comparison, and it pays more, but they feel more comfortable working around other aides and making friends with them in a facility. This is what I found out from talking with aides who worked at the nursing home and had done private work on the side. One even said that she felt scared being left alone with a hospice patient when she took on some private work. Further, when the patient died, she said the family had each other to share their grief. She said she had no one to share her grief with. She prefers nursing home work because she has co-workers to talk to.

Aides who've never worked in a facility or who've left a facility, often take on private care because they don't want a lot of responsibility. They want a simple job, and they only want to work when they feel like it, or need money.

If you need a registered nurse as a caregiver, perhaps you can find a private retired nurse. She'd probably want about $25 to $30 an hour. Chances are, she'd probably only need to come for an hour's visit and not everyday. We hired a retired registered nurse, the wife of a family friend, to check in on our mother at the first nursing home, since the care was terrible. Unless your elder catches a germ or infection, you wouldn't need a registered nurse checking in every day anyway. When my mother was under hospice care (and she got free R.N. care), the nurse would stop in once a week for an hour or so, and instruct me on what to do for her, for practically all of my mother's needs. An R.N. can even teach the private aide you've hired about what needs to be done.

I also paid a retired person to be a sitter for my mother. She used to run the adult day care program at the senior center that my mother attended for a few years, a few hours a week, after her brain cancer recovery. This woman was wonderful, very delightful and upbeat.

You'll find many aides who are just plain lazy. Our next door neighbor was in her late 80s and had emphysema. Her caregiver didn't care that she had emphysema. She wanted to smoke! Further, when she sat down to smoke, she fixed herself a cup of coffee, putting the glass coffee pot on the burner!

Caregivers often show poor judgment. When my mother was ambulatory, after her brain cancer recovery, a relief aide drove her to the bank. She couldn't find a parking spot, so she dropped my mother off. When my mother came out of the bank, she was left for about 15 minutes just standing there, with cash in her purse, until the caregiver showed up again. She probably took a break herself. Another one took my mother for a walk in a park with drug dealers. She later told me that she knew there were drug dealers there, but that they never bothered anyone. The next day, this caregiver locked my mother's purse inside her car in plain view, while they took a walk in the neighborhood.

Many aides are overweight and complain about having to do range of motion exercises with bedridden patients. Further, if you ask them to lift your elder's back a little bit off the already elevated hospital bed to do some light sit-ups, they can't do it. If you want a lot of range of motion exercises done, even physically fit aides will complain. If you're desperate and can't find anyone else, you'll be reduced to giving these aides simple things to do like laundry and folding towels and linen, making the bed, massaging hands, arms, legs, and wiggling fingers and toes for your elder's exercise. You can't expect too much from some of them. You'll often use them as sitters so you can get out of the house.

In hiring aides, recognize that people from Asian countries like China, Vietnam, and people from poor countries like Mexico like to work six or even seven days a week. Although you don't want to burn-out anyone, if you need someone in an emergency, don't hesitate to call them back for more hours.

I've always thought that it was ironic that you can find a competent sitter for children for little money, but you have to sometimes pay three times as much for a sitter for seniors.

Even if you do a lot of the work yourself, you should always try to line up more than one caregiver to take the place of someone who calls in sick—someone who likes relief work on short notice. Tell them you'll pay them more, if they are available at the last minute.

It's interesting about caregivers. The first few times they show up, you may think they are wonderful. After that, you begin to see their idiosyncrasies. As I've said, private aides tend to work only when they need the money. Often, they are the type of people who don't want to commit themselves to full-time work and they want to be free to take time off for vacations, to spend time with their children, etc. They are often unreliable, and will quit at the drop of a hat.

Having your loved one at home requires a lot of commitment on your part. You must be willing to cancel your appointments if the relief aide doesn't show up. Sometimes if your elder gets sick suddenly and requires your special care, you may need to cancel your relief caregiver, though you try not to, especially if the aide needs steady work.

When the going gets rough, and relief help calls in sick, always remember that it's better for you and your loved one to be free of an unclean facility. You don't have control over your loved one's illness, but at home, you do have control over her care.

When my mother lapsed into her coma, the doctor told me that immobile people often get pneumonia and other infections. I always feared taking her home because I wasn't a nurse and wouldn't be able to react in an emergency. However, what I found was what I sometimes suspected. If a patient is away from the germs of an institution, kept clean, and she is moved in and out of bed, she doesn't often fall prey to pneumonia and other infections and doesn't need a nurse. Having my mother at home, despite the hassles of doing 99 percent of the work myself, was well worth it.

When you hire an aide, you may want to start her off once a week on a four-hour shift and try her out. If someone is good and needs more hours, give her more. The going rate for private aides is about $14 an hour in some metro areas. Raise their pay if they are good, after a few months. Don't start out high, but let them earn better pay. Remember, you're not necessarily buying more motivation with higher pay. Some caregivers don't like the job, and won't be more motivated with better pay than what they'd get elsewhere. Some private aides like the idea of home care if they feel no one is around to supervise them. If you get someone who's worked in a nursing home at minimum wage and has had 13 patients to care for with little or no benefits, paying them over double of what they got there, should make them happy. You think? They usually have downtime, and are in a more pleasant environment in your home. However, some people do caregiving because they can't do anything else, and don't fully appreciate a private job with good pay.

You might be thinking that if you hire agency help, there will be less hassle because you don't have to deduct social security from the caregiver's paycheck. This is true to a certain extent. While I inquired of my tax man about deducting social security, he laughed and said that rarely do caregivers stay that long. It's true, often private caregivers quit after a week or two, before they've racked up the $1,000 or so when the government requires social security deducted. Even if they stay longer, they beg you not to deduct social security from their paycheck. If someone is a "long-term" worker, does wonderful work, and you can't bear to lose her, you can offer to pay her social security for her so you're not doing anything illegal. That's what my tax man advised me.

In hiring an aide, don't forget to get her social security number, along with her address and phone. Pay her at the end of each week to keep her motivated.

Don't be afraid to say the obvious when you hire an aide: "If you take dad out in cold weather, he should wear a jacket." Remember that aides often have little common sense.

Although you might be having a bad day, try not to lose your temper in front of a relief caregiver, showing negative attitudes toward your loved one. If you do, the relief caregiver might assume she can treat your elder this way.

Make sure all relief caregivers have an updated list of current medications and immunizations of your elder in case of an emergency and they need to talk to a doctor or call a paramedic. Post the list above the bed, if the patient is bedridden or even above the phone, along with the physcian's phone number and the numbers of other family members.

If you want to fire a worker, don't "fire" her. Just say you won't be needing her anymore because your schedule has changed or that you've run into financial problems and can't afford to pay for help. Wish her good luck at her next job. Some workers are crazy, and may retaliate if you fire them.

If a sibling is willing, make a schedule for him to contribute some caregiving time. This didn't work too well for me in my situation during the first decade plus of my caregiving. My only sibling, my brother, took our mother to the grocery store once a week for an hour or so, while I babysat his daughter! As a substitute for caregiving, perhaps a family member can bring over cooked food, so you don't have to cook. Perhaps a sibling could relieve you for only one week a year, so you can take a vacation. Or, perhaps a sibling could help pay for some in-home relief assistance or housekeeping service.

During my caregiving years, I was single. If an adult child is married with children, and the elderly parent moves in, it usually means that each member of the family must adjust to having grandma or grandpa move in. However, I've known two families who did this, each for about four years until the elderly loved one died. They both said that although they didn't spend as much time as they would have liked with their children, everyone learned a valuable lesson about caring. The two families said they didn't regret the time their elders lived with them.

A caregiver or caregiving family does need relief time, even if they just stay at home while the relief worker is there. When my mother was ambulatory and I cared for her, I was scared to even take time to take a bath. If she fell down, I wouldn't hear her fall.

Besides getting relief help, you should consider making the home a safe place for your elder, and a convenient place for caregiving to take place. Make sure your home has smoke alarms, particularly in the bedrooms and hallways. In case of a fire, it's best for the elder and the caregiver to have bedrooms on the ground floor. Preferably, the caregiver should always sleep in the bedroom closest to the elder's room, so he can hear sounds of distress, or help walk her to her bathroom during the night.

It's important that an elder doesn't have to climb steps to get to a bathroom or a bedroom. And, if your elder is bedridden, you don't want to climb stairs to empty a bed pan or catheter bag in an upstairs bathroom.

As a safety issue, if your elder is ambulatory, you may want to unplug the stove when it's not in use, so he won't inadvertently turn on the burners. Or, you can latch the kitchen door. Keep knives out of his reach in the kitchen. He can cut himself by accident. Make sure pots and pans aren't old and rocky, and that they lay flat on the burner. A fire extinguisher in the kitchen is a good thing to have.

Other Tips:

- Don't wax floors. They can be slippery.
- Don't use extention cords that can be tripped over.
- Avoid heating pads and electric blankets. They can be a fire hazard.
- Avoid cigarette smoking in the home. It's not only unhealthy, particularly for your elder, causing respiratory problems, but it's obviously a fire hazard.
- Get a hand-held hose with showerhead for your elder, along with a shower chair to sit in. Also install grab bars near the shower, so that she can lift herself when getting up from the shower chair.

If an aide is on duty all day long and must cook, tell her not to leave the kitchen while cooking. It's also a good idea not to use an electric coffee pot that is often left on by mistake.

Instead of facility care or foster home care that costs several thousand dollars each month, you might consider adapting your home to your elder's needs. Make his room and hallways handicapped accessible with rails and large door openings for a wheelchair. Remodel the bathroom with a shower with no step that could accomodate a roll-in shower chair, for example.

I knew a woman who turned her garage into an apartment for her aging, ambulatory mother. She thought of raising the roof to put in a second floor so that in the event her mother needed a live-in caregiver, there would be extra space for the caregiver. She said she would put in an electric chair along the steps to the second floor in case her mother could no longer walk. The elderly woman already had a bad memory. I told the daughter that as her mother aged, she probably wouldn't have the good judgment to use the electric chair or maybe she would forget how to turn it on if she wanted to go upstairs to find the caregiver. Or, maybe her eyesight would get bad and she'd misstep as she tried to get into the electric chair. At any rate, building a second floor would have been a mistake, I said. Perhaps the electric chair could have been considered if there was already a second floor there.

One should also consider if your elder's insurance covers medical equipment in the home. If it doesn't, you can contact a medical equipment store that often rents out equipment.

Always sit down with a supervisor at an insurance company, or contact Medicare through the social security office, or Medicaid through the Welfare office to definitively find out what home health care benefits are covered by private insurance or the government, respectively. If your elder is being discharged from the hospital, the doctor and hospital personnel might have misinformed you into believing that your elder has limited equipment benefits. Above all, don't accept verbal statements made over the telephone.

If your loved one's insurance won't cover a hospital bed, rent one with a foam mattress for its comfort, particularly for a frail elder.

If possible, accompany your loved one to the doctor or be present when a nurse comes to the house. Hired caregivers don't always understand what a doctor or nurse is telling them about the patient and her care.

Make a list of medical problems that your loved one complains of, so that the next time you go to the doctor's office or the next time the home health nurse visits, you don't forget to address the issue. Remind them of allergies to drugs and prescription creams. (Doctors don't always consult the chart.)

As a caregiver, always carry the doctor's business card in your wallet.

Keep in mind that physicians are reimbursed by insurance to make house calls to the bedridden, or they can send a nurse practitioner from their office whose visit will be reimbursed. A nurse practitioner has a master's degree, so she is more credentialed than many nurses.

Besides caregiving, doing your elder's bookkeeping is also time-consuming. I knew a family who hired a "Daily Money Manager" at $85 an hour to write checks and organize records for tax returns. Caution: the field is ripe for abuse. There are no federal or state standards for Daily Money Managers. Some have no financial background at all. Ask your CPA if he knows of one. CPAs obviously charge much more than Daily Money Managers do. When you do find a Daily Money Manager, check her references. Make sure she will provide you with a detailed invoice for the hours worked. You can check out the American

Association of Daily Money Managers at www.aadmm.com. Generally, these money managers will provide their services once or twice a month. Most impose a two to three hour-a-month minimum of service.

As for your own business matters, if you provide care to an elderly parent, you may be able to claim a tax credit for it. Ask your CPA.

Hiring Home Help Through An Agency

Home care through an agency for a nurse's aide can run $21 or more an hour in a metropolitan area, again, depending on where you live. Agencies supposedly screen their workers, but with a lot of them, you'd never know it. The good thing is they are licensed and bonded in case of an accident, or if they hurt their back.

Some home health agencies distinguish between caregivers and housekeepers, and won't even allow a caregiver to do light housekeeping even during an eight-hour shift when your elder may be taking a nap and there is downtime. Why should they sit around and get paid, you wonder. Also, beware that some agencies charge during graveyard shift according to whether the caregiver is allowed to sleep through the entire night, get up two times during the night, or be awake working the entire night. The charges get detailed and even nitpicky.

A lot of agencies, though, will allow a caregiver to provide care, run errands, and do housekeeping, too.

Some agencies charge you a finder's fee and then you pay the caregiver directly. In addition, the agency bills you a few dollars for every hour the caregiver puts in. For example, the finder's fee may be $175. You pay the caregiver $17 per hour, plus the agency bills you for another $4 per hour for its take. The agency's rationale is that if the caregiver gets most of the money—unlike most agencies who give the caregiver $10 to $12 an hour—it can attract better caregivers. In reality, one finder's fee agency I worked with had worse caregivers than the other agencies whose caregivers were paid so much less. Paying someone more money doesn't always translate into better skills, more motivation, or more common sense. This finder's fee agency sent me five caregivers, three of which weren't even CNAs and didn't know a thing about care of bedridden patients, despite my detailed description for their supervisors of the qualifications needed by the caregiver to do the work. Of the two caregivers who did know how to do bedridden care, one was morbidly obese. She weighed about 300 pounds, and she was sweating up a storm after five minutes of range of motion exercises. The other complained to me that she wasn't sleeping well at night and was tired because she lived in the ghetto and the police wouldn't answer loud disturbance calls. She emptied my mother's catheter bag down the bathroom sink, instead of in the toilet. She told the agency that she had worked a number of hours she hadn't, which I was billed for. She didn't bring any food to eat during the eight-hour day and was very hungry. When I offered her food, she dug her teeth into the shell of hard-boiled egg because she was in such a hurry to devour it. Further, she called in sick just a half-hour before her scheduled time. No replacement was available, though the agency had previously sworn to me that replacements were available. Lastly, she asked if she could take home cans of my mother's tube feeding formula that were dented and that I was going to throw out. She didn't have enough money to eat, despite the fact that she was making $17 an hour.

The third caregiver that this finder's fee agency sent lasted two days. They bragged that she was a former registered nurse, so that I was actually getting a highly- experienced person for the aide wage that I was paying. In reality, she couldn't ever have possibly been a nurse. She didn't know a thing about bedridden care and didn't even know how to attach the leg rests onto a wheelchair, nor how to operate a hoyer lift. She didn't know about tube feedings, and she arrived an hour late to work the first day. After two days, she told her supervisor that she was "overwhelmed" at seeing my mother in such bad shape with red inner thighs from the Strep infection she had gotten at the nursing home. She said to me that she "highly disapproved" of my not speaking to my mother about death in front of her, and that I should tell her that she was dying, instead of "playing games with her." She complained that my mother's bladder infection meant that she needed to have her diaper changed "101 times a day," a ridiculous exaggeration. In general, she acted imposed upon and repulsed by my mother's condition. If this wasn't enough, she also was afraid to be left alone with my mother and said she didn't want me to leave the house. She refused to wear latex gloves, and was cleaning the toilet with her bare hands, using a thin piece of toilet tissue to scrub the bowl. She wouldn't wash her hands afterwards. She'd emptied out the garbage outside in the garbage bin without wearing latex gloves, and not washing her hands afterwards. And, when she came back inside, she was very offended when she heard me telling my mother to eat so she'd "have more strength." She asked me why I was telling her that. She looked at my mother in disgust like she shouldn't be allowed to live another day.

When I first complained to the agency that all caregivers were unacceptable, the assistant to the supervisor told me that after speaking to the aides about me, she saw "a pattern" with me, that is, that I was the problem. I wouldn't give them "independence" in caring for my mother. I had told her that all were having trouble with the basic skills involved in doing the job, and that I needed to instruct them about basic cleanliness and bedridden care techniques. They had not followed through in sending qualified people as I'd specifically asked for. Worse, I was getting charged at a higher hourly rate for advanced level care, as some agencies charge. (Some agencies charge less for just companion-aides.) Getting nowhere with her, I spoke to the owner of the agency who was apologetic, but said that these were the best aides she had. She refunded practically all of the finder's fee, as I'd requested. I think she was afraid that I'd bad-mouth her business to the hospice social worker who'd recommended her agency.

After I'd dismissed this agency, I noticed that there were some china souvenirs that were missing in the home of value, since they were antiques that belonged to my grandparents. Theft is a problem with a lot of caregivers, since most don't have a lot of material possessions. You often don't notice things missing right away, so it's hard to figure out which caregiver took what.

I've read horror stories of home health agencies not properly screening their workers and even hiring felons to go into homes, some of whom have assaulted or even murdered patients. Two of the aides the "finder's fee" agency sent, had out-of-state license plates. I wondered how this agency could have adequately checked their backgrounds for crime. The answer is, they don't, because it costs money to, and they don't know how long the aides will stay on the job. They may quit after a day.

Some states like Massachusetts have enacted a statute requiring criminal-background checks by all home-care agencies.

It should be noted that this agency originally said, as others do, that they never leave you in the lurch if a worker calls in sick at the last minute. All agencies say this, and all never seem to be able to find a replacement even at any time during that day. Therefore, you're left to fend for yourself. The moral: Never schedule an appointment for yourself on a day when you have "outside" help coming in. Schedule appointments on a day when a family friend or a family member can relieve you.

A placement service that costs just as much as a regular agency isn't a good deal. You're paying for the placement service to find someone—usually a person who is no better than one whom you could find on your own and pay less to. Also, with a placement service, you have none of the benfits of a regular agency. That is, you are responsible for the person they find you, who is your employee and not the agency's. You are in charge of social security matters and liability if she injures her back. With most home insurances, you're limited to about $1,000 medical if a domestic worker is injured. Therefore, if there's a lawsuit, you better have umbrella insurance.

Every once in a while, a great aide may be sent to you from an agency. Most agencies have a rule that you can't hire away their aides privately, because they don't want to lose a good aide. Sometimes an agency will stipulate that you can't hire one of its aides until three or six months after you've terminated your agreement with the agency. Obviously, an aide would love you to pay them directly and get a better wage than what the agency splits with them. While I'm not advocating it, it's a thought that some families consider as an "under the table" agreement. One of my friends did this. She had one aide come privately on weekends when the aide wasn't offered work by the agency. She saved herself a few dollars an hour, by not having to pay the agency's hourly fee. Was it worth it? You decide. Again, I'm not advocating this, because at that time, the aide is strickly your employee and if she's gets injured that day, you are liable.

If you are fortunate enough to find a long-term aide, congratulations! Most grow weary of the job after a short time, or they have crazy personal lives and can't carry on with the job. Aides from other agencies I had, didn't yield much better help with my bedridden mother. For example, I cautioned an aide from another agency to use the toilet to empty my mother's catheter bag. She said she wouldn't think of throwing my mother's urine down the bathroom sink. What did she then do? After she'd emptied my mother catheter bag in the toilet, she put it under the bathroom faucet to get water to rinse it out. As far as I'm concerned, rinsing it out with water does nothing anyway. However, if she wanted to do this, she could have gotten the water from the bathtub faucet.

I can remember back to when my mother was in the nursing home, receiving 100 days of free skilled care benefits. We had an agency aide work with my mother privately to stimulate her. The aide got bored, when my mother fell asleep. She thought my mother's fingernails needed trimming. She clipped them so short that my mother's skin underneath was red and nearly bleeding. To add further injury, she then applied my mother's arm/hand splints. Her fingers were stretched out, with her irritated red skin more pronounced. Incidentally, this aide seemed mentally deficient, and she told me she used to be an R.N., though I didn't believe it.

As for other agency aides, I can remember even further back in years. After my mother's brain cancer recovery, when she was ambulatory, I enlisted the help of agencies. Their aides were just as ineffectual with ambulatory and communicative patients. At that time, I would hire caregivers just to drive my mother around to stores and do errands. They would dump her off, and take off on their own errands, saying that they'd be gone for just a few minutes. Sometimes, they'd come back an hour later. I would always be told by their supervisors, "We'll send you our best person," and when the person was unacceptable, the agency acted as if I was the problem because I'd complained. One agency sent an aide who was such a heavy smoker, that her clothes and her car wreaked of cigarette smoke. Her R.N. supervisor told us she was her best aide. However, being a heavy cigarette smoker, I would imagine families of elders, particularly those who'd had cancer, felt otherwise.

A home health agency—whether you want to hire a nurse or nurse's aide—first sends a nurse to speak to you and evaluate your home. She gives free advice, for example, on putting shower bars on the wall of the shower stall, or she tells you how to arrange furniture and rugs to make your home safe, so your loved one won't trip over something.

If you need a registered nurse from an agency, you'll pay the agency about $70 an hour or more in a metropolitan area. As I explained in the last segment on hiring your own private help, unless a patient takes a turn for the worse, you wouldn't need a nurse for more than an hour a day, or even one hour a week. A registered nurse can train a family member or nurse's aide to do practically any type of care, including giving oxygen, or running a feeding tube, for example, provided one is motivated to learn. (I feel that changing a catheter should be done by a nurse.) In hiring an agency, you should ask how long it takes a nurse to respond in an urgent situation.

A nursing home nurse I knew, who also did private work through an agency on her days off, said that an agency nurse is assigned to a particular patient, and if she is absent she instructs a substitute nurse, updating her on the patient's needs. Therefore, make sure this is the case, if you go through a agency.

It's important to tell the agency that you want a nurse who doesn't have the attitude that the patient is better off dead. Perhaps, you could ask for a nurse who believes in respecting and caring for the patient, and one who doesn't make value judgments on whether a patient should be treated for an illness or infection. To me, it's very sad that you would even have to stipulate this. I always thought it was a given, until I met dozens of nurses and listened to some of their attitudes.

Home health nurses with agencies bring needed supplies with them. They try to send the same nurse each time—that is, the "primary" nurse, unless it's her day off.

If your elder's health declines rapidly, he is near death, and he isn't in a hospice program, make sure that if an agency sends a nurse, she is one with hospice experience. A hospice nurse will know how to adminster pain medication through a pump. Some nurses don't know how.

An alternative to home health through an agency, may be the Visiting Nurse Association, (VNA). If an elder isn't entitled to some R.N. care paid by her insurance, and isn't in the hospice program, if you want a regular visit once-a-week by a nurse, contact the VNA in your area. Having a nurse from the Association visit, may be less costly than having an agency nurse. VNA is not only staffed with R.N.s, but other healthcare professionals including physical therapists.

As for nurse's aides, keep track of the hours they spend at your home. Most of the time, agencies and healthcare associations have a family member sign the aide's time sheet after each visit to confirm hours worked. However, if the agency is essentially a "finder's fee" service, and it takes a cut of each hour worked by the caregiver, it often has the caregiver report hours without checking with you. Even if a caregiver doesn't mistakenly report her hours on purpose, sometimes she gets confused.

In general, in dealing with agencies, be very specific with them about what tasks you need done by their aides, and what tasks you don't want them to do, such as clipping toenails. If not, the aides might feel you don't like how they are performing a task, and that you've chosen to do it yourself.

Tell the aide, for example, that you will bandage a tumor or pressure sore. You can also have a list of Do's and Don'ts.

My list of Don'ts was:

1) Don't wheel mother outside in bad weather.
2) Don't open windows.
3) Don't wash mother's face.
4) Don't clip nails.
5) Don't discuss cancer or death.

I told agencies that I needed an aide to help me lift and turn my mother for sponge baths and changing diapers. I also told agencies that I wanted assistance turning her, to attach the hoyer hammock onto her, and to operate the hoyer lift. With assistance on these tasks, you don't wear out your back with a heavy patient. I told them I needed someone to do range of motion exercises with my mother. However, most of all, I told them I needed a sitter who would relieve me to go out on errands.

Agencies will often tell you that their aides want eight-hour jobs. With a bedridden patient, if a family member does the care, it's not practical for aides to hang around for more than four hours at most. Try to get them to send you someone who will work on their days off for four hours. (At first, I acquiesced and had aides for an eight-hour day, but they got bored not having much to do, while at the same time, complaining about the tasks that they did have to do like range of motion exercises. Most agencies will have at least a four-hour minimum.)

Incidentally, an R.N. supervisor at an agency said I could send away an aide who showed up with a cold. Of course, at nursing homes this can't be done, so you do have some control over caregivers.

Realize that in billing you, agency weekend care is sometimes billed at a higher rate, and holiday care is sometimes billed at double the usual rate. You should also inquire about when the bill is sent every month.

Following is a list of typical agency tasks performed by aides:

1) Preparing meals/feeding patients
2) Housekeeping (depends on the agency)
3) Linen change
4) Laundry
5) Assistance with walking
6) Assistance with transferring patient from bed to wheel-chair
7) Transportation to appointments
8) Grocery shopping
9) Turning/changing diaper of bedridden patient
10) Toileting for ambulatory patient
11) Sponge bath
12) Shower
13) Brushing teeth/cleaning dentures
14) Shaving
15) Shampoo
16) Recording bowel movements
17) Assistance with colostomy
18) Catheter care
19) Assistance with medication (Some won't allow their aides to do this.)
20) Soaking feet
21) Companionship

When contacting an agency, you will not only want to discuss your requirements, but ask questions about their policies.

These were some of my requirements:

1) Don't send anyone with a cold.
2) Send a non-smoker.

3) Don't send anyone with allergies. (They cough and
    sneeze, and often don't know if they have an allergy
    or a cold.)
4) Send a permanent aide. (You don't want to orient and
    train different aides.)
5) Send someone who is fit enough to do range of motion
    exercises with a heavy patient for 15 minutes at a
    time, four times a day.
6) Send an aide who has experience with a bedridden
    patient.
7) No CPR for my mother.
8) Send an aide who can operate a hoyer lift.
9) Send an aide who can read to my mother. (I was told by
    one agency that some of their workers couldn't read.)

These were some of my questions about the agency:

1) Is the agency licensed—are workers bonded and insured?
2) What is the minimum number of hours per day that you'll
    send someone for?
3) If someone works for four hours, should they have a 10
    or 15-minute break, or a break at all?
4) How long a lunch break does an eight-hour shift aide
    get? Does she eat while watching the patient? Does
    she get a snack break, a.m. and p.m.? How long?
5) What is considered overtime work for their aides?
6) Does the agency have any special rates by hour, based
    on the number of hours you hire their aides?
    (Usually, they don't.)
7) Does the agency have alternate people in case someone
    calls in sick? Will they ever leave you in the lurch?
8) Do they have substitute aides who are willing to work
    on the spur of the moment if you need someone on
    a non-scheduled day?

For a live-in agency aide, find out how many hours out of the 24-hour day she is allowed to work, and whether the aide has her own car to drive for errands and appointments for your elder.

Agencies sometimes have a different nurse's aide rate for companionship care and advanced level care, such as for the bedridden. However, as I discussed previously, I found that in paying for advanced level care with one agency, they sent aides who knew nothing about advanced level care and had never worked with the bedridden. Question the agency about the skills of the caregivers they've chosen to send you.

Remember that agencies expect you to supervise and train their employees. Before you plunk down a deposit which they'll ask you to do, ask to meet the person/people they have selected for your elder, or least talk to them on the phone. Most agencies, however, don't even begin selecting someone until they have your deposit, even though they don't like to admit this. It often takes them a while to come up with someone permanent. They'll probably send different people in the beginning or perhaps a "permanent" person who doesn't work out.

The agency that told me that many aides don't know how to read, got me thinking. No wonder this agency didn't allow their aides to give medications. And, how does this help a family member who is at work during the day and can't be home to give medications? What is the point of hiring a caregiver?

In dealing with an agency, it doesn't hurt to ask if any of their aides are nursing students, though I never ran across an agency that did have one. Two nursing home nurses told me that while they were going through school, they worked as nurse's aides through agencies. The average agency aide isn't very competent.

There was one agency aide we had who quit because she couldn't handle looking at and cleaning up diarrhea.

(My mother couldn't have a bowel movement as she'd gotten constipated from some medication, so I had given her a suppository that led to diarrhea.) Further, this aide wanted to wipe up diarrhea with terrycloth towels, rather than first clean it up with tissue paper, and then clean with soap and water using terrycloth towels.

With aides from an agency, keep in touch with their supervisor if the worker starts slacking off. After my mother's brain cancer recovery, a relief aide was driving her around and she would bring her home early. She would short-change her five or ten minutes each time she came. That adds up over multiple visits. She would also run personal errands on my mother's time, stopping at the bank. She would fudge on mileage reimbursement that my mother was paying for. I found that if you didn't speak up the first or the second time, it would continue.

As for cautions in dealing with home health agencies, it might not always be a good idea to allow some aides to do even light housekeeping. Many have trouble even operating dishwashers and washing machines, even after being shown how. They scratch furniture, ramming vacuum cleaners into chairs and tables. They wash dishes with sink cleansers. Maybe it's not so much ignorance, as not caring about the job they're doing.

As for the aide's schedule, you'll often have to give two to four hours' notice if you want to cancel out on a certain day. In case your loved one is too sick and you don't want to leave her, you may need to cancel out on an aide—though you try not to, realizing that the aide needs to earn a living. In this case, if you schedule an aide in the morning, you won't be able to give the agency enough advance notice so they won't bill you for that session.

Further, when scheduling aides, try not to schedule them for early mornings for another reason. You should schedule for afternoons, particularly if you need to leave the house for appointments. The reason is, if they call in sick, you likely won't have a replacement in time to make your morning appointment.

One of the drawbacks of using agencies, is that sometimes if you cancel their services too soon, your deposit money may not be refunded. Sometimes, they'll ask you for advance payment for the first two weeks of service. The reason for cancelling their services is often due to the fact that their workers are unacceptable. They often don't have any that can do the job, particularly if your elder is greatly incapacitated. You should always inquire about the stipulations for getting your deposit money refunded.

Foster Care

Foster homes take in a variety of residents, from those who need minimal care and companionship, all the way up to those who are bedridden and hospice residents. Usually foster homes have no more than five residents, and there usually is no more than one caregiver on duty at a time. If a foster home has five bedridden residents, it should have two caregivers on duty during the day and evening shifts when a lot of care maintenance is done, such as bathing, showers, and feeding. If there's only one caregiver on duty at all times, I would not put an elder there if all five patients are bedridden.

With one caregiver on duty, one usually sees a foster home that has perhaps three ambulatory residents and two bedridden or hospice residents.

I visited many foster homes in my 16 years of caregiving, both when my mother was ambulatory and functional, and afterwards when she was bedridden in a nursing home. What I found was that a foster home that may run as much as $5,000 a month (these days) for a bedridden patient, is much better than a nursing home, especially if the owner is an R.N. and does a lot of the care herself. These are hard to find. Oftentimes, you'll pay about $1500 to $2,000 less for your elder to be in a foster home, than in a nursing home.

Often hospice program patients who don't have family members to care for them and who don't want to be in nursing homes, enter foster homes and receive visits from hospice program staff there. Therefore, there is no need for a registered nurse to be on staff at the foster home, just a responsible caregiver, who much like a family member, is vigilant and contacts the hospice nurse when the patient needs one.

I know of a foster home, run by an emergency medical technician and his wife, that charges $7,000 a month, and has all patients that are bedridden. He has two caregivers on duty on both day and evening shifts, and his wife does all the work on graveyard shift of turning residents and changing diapers. I had learned of him through a hospice nurse, and when I visited his foster home, I was very impressed. It was fully handicapped accessible, having been built for handicapped use. Each resident received a shower three times a week.

I seriously considered foster care when my mother was at the nursing home, as an alternative to taking her home. The reason being, I wondered if my back would hold out in lifting my mother if I took her home. I also wanted to cover my bases. I considered that if I took my mother home, became ill myself, and couldn't be the primary caregiver, she may need a foster home. Once at home, I would never have put my mother back in a nursing home, so if my health broke down or I suffered a back injury, I decided she'd go to a foster home and have the hospice staff visit her there. It should be noted that a hospice program patient can be housed anywhere—a nursing home, a foster home, etc., but the hospice program is mainly set up to give the patient the benefit of care in her own home or in a family member's home.

Foster homes usually have a homey feeling, unlike a nursing home. The positives are that the owners are usually nice people and work hard for their money. Some foster homes have two levels, one for the caregiver to sleep upstairs with her own apartment. I would not put an elderly person who was ambulatory and confused in such a setup. He may try to go upstairs and find the caregiver and fall down the steps. Foster homes with one level, are the most common and have the best environment.

It's my opinion and that of a friend of mine who had three ill, elderly relatives in a five-year period, that foster homes while much better than nursing homes, do have drawbacks. With five residents to care for, a house to keep clean, cooking, laundry, and grocery shopping, a married couple who runs a foster home, or even a single caregiver doing the work, as is often the case, is deep in drudgery. If it's a married couple and the wife does most of the caregiving, she looks exhausted. Further, as you would at home as a caregiver, they also have difficulty finding adequate relief help.

Those foster homes that work the best, are those run by ethnic families who are industrious and share the work with a relative or two, not having to depend on hiring outside help. These ethnic homes also usually feed the residents homemade food.

Since it's a private home, before placing a family member there, you must determine when family members are welcome to visit. (At a nursing home, you are sometimes welcome 24 hours a day because they'd love to have you do all their work for them.) However, at foster homes, particularly during morning hours when they bathe patients and are busy, they often prefer not to have visitors stopping in.

In visiting foster homes, you'll find the rooms are small, and the homes are sometimes drafty with sliding doors in some bedrooms, leading to a patio. If they don't have air conditioning, they'll keep their doors open when it's hot, so it's drafty. There isn't as much privacy as there'd be in your own home.

Often, a foster home owner will own more than one foster home—even two or three, and each one offers a certain
level of resident care. For example, one home might be licensed to give advanced care to the bedridden. Often, an
R.N. will be the owner of mutiple homes. I'm not sure that
these multiple homes do any better a job than your average foster home. It becomes, in a lot of cases, more profit-
oriented for the owner, who is a business owner, rather than
a caregiver.

Often people who run more than one foster home have
relatives who run their other homes for them. I remember
that one nurse who did substitute work at the nursing home
my mother was in, had a foster home, that she, her husband, and their six-month-old baby lived in. She wasn't
around much at her home, but had CNAs from the nursing home, on their days off, help her with morning care of
residents at her home. This nurse owned a second home
that was staffed by her mother and a midwife. Her aunt
owned another foster home. She claims her aunt covered
for her when she was out of town. Obviously, these foster
home owners farmed out most of the work at their homes
to CNAs that they paid very little to, and then charged a
good sum of money to the residents.

As I've said, owners of foster homes who have more
than one home, often offer a different level of care at each
home. Therefore, if a resident is ambulatory, and later becomes bedridden, they can move him to their home with a
more advanced level of care. Often they have homes next
door to each other, so that staff can help each other out in
an emergency.

For Alzheimer's or memory-impaired people, a foster
home should have an aide working, not sleeping, on graveyard shift. When my mother was ambulatory and became
demented, years after her brain cancer recovery, she was
restless during the night and would get up and walk around
the house. Worse, some memory-impaired people can pick

up and leave the premise or wander to the kitchen and turn on the stove. Foster homes that give care to memory-impaired residents in the late stages of their illness or to bedridden patients, should have an aide awake and at work on graveyard shift.

If a foster home has both bedridden patients and wandering demented patients, if only one person is on duty on day and evening shifts, be wary. How, for example, can one adult go in and change a bedridden resident, and at the same time watch the wandering residents? Most likely the bedridden residents will get slighted.

Make sure the foster home you place an elder in is licensed and that there is a vigilant owner. An aide at the last nursing home my mother was in, ran a foster home. I don't know when she was at the latter working, since she put in about four days' work at the nursing home to supplement her income. She was working for minimum wage at the nursing home. You'd think her time would have been better spent at her foster home. She told me that one day, a family member of one of her foster home's residents came to visit. She showed them to the resident's room, and the resident was dead in bed. One would wonder just how much attention she was giving her residents with her double life. Her sister, incidentally, ran the foster home with her, but she also put in a few days' work at the nursing home. Maybe they just couldn't get enough of elder care, or perhaps their foster home residents were behind in rent! I guess it pays to figure out just who will be minding the foster home you put your relative in. One begins to wonder just how many older people die unattended in group situations.

I knew quite a few R.N.s who owned foster homes, but would supplement their income by working a few days a week at nursing homes or doing agency work in private homes. Again, these people spread themselves too thin.

Ask the foster care operators who relieves them. Some look exhausted. Ask for how long they go on vacation. Do other family members relieve them? If outsiders relieve them, they often have the same problems you'd have in hiring caregivers in your home.

Some foster homes were built specifically as foster homes. You see this where the owner owns mutiple homes and has turned them into a real business. These foster homes have wide doorways to accomodate wheelchairs; rails in the hallway at wheelchair height for those who can roll themselves in the chair; light switches placed at wheelchair height; walk-in showers without a step to step over; grab rails in the shower; doorknobs have been replaced with levers; and a rope near the bed to buzz the caregiver in case of an emergency.

It's amazing to me that some foster care operators take in wheelchair-bound residents and bedridden ones, but have, for example, a step to step over in the shower. I saw this in two homes. How can they safely put an immobile person into a shower chair and get that chair into the shower without the person falling off the chair? The answer is simple: safety measure aren't in effect at these foster homes. Just like nursing homes, they don't fear lawsuits. Maybe they feel that if an accident occurs, no one will notice, and the elderly person is too feeble to complain.

I considered placing my mother at one foster home when I knew she could no longer endure nursing home life. The foster home was very professionally run. The owners who did virtually all the work, had a surveillance camera in each of the two hospice patients' rooms and in their bedroom, so that they could monitor their care at all times, even when the couple went to bed. The other three residents were ambulatory.

If at a foster home, the house is not staffed by the owner, it will have a "house manager." Sometimes the house manager is a family member. Ask how long the house manager has been with them, and ask how long the relief aide for the house manager has been with them. If the house manager is married and has small children, you wonder how much attention and energy she has left to give to the elder residents. I saw this situation in two homes I visited.

When I was 23 years old, I ran a foster home for teens. I was employed by a social service agency. At another one of its foster homes, a house manager was fired for theft. She was using money budgeted for meals for the residents for her own personal use. Since the residents were teens and had their mental faculties, they were able to complain to the agency officials that there was little food. My point is, if a house manager is dishonest and works with mentally-impaired and frail adults, will the adults be able to communicate the abuse?

The area or county that the foster home is licensed in, stipulates care requirements, such as, for example, two showers a week for each resident. When my mother was ambulatory after her brain cancer surgery, I considered putting her in a foster home after living with her for ten years. I ended up not doing this, however. I remember asking the operators of the foster homes I visited if they gave more than two showers a week, since many older people need a shower every day, being incontinent. If the foster home offers more than what is required, perhaps that's a sign it may be a good one. However, bear in mind that what is promised isn't always delivered. One house manager told me that each resident got no more than five minutes in the shower.

I ran across foster homes that would accept residents on a temporary basis for a month, either for them to recover after a hospital stay or to give a family caregiver one month's relief. There aren't many of these, though.

Keep in mind that foster care house managers don't have time to stimulate or entertain residents. Between caregiving, cooking, cleaning, laundry, ironing, giving medications, showering, dressing, etc., what time is left? If you're looking for mental stimulation for your loved one, try to find a foster home where other residents can communicate or possibly entertain each other—ones who are in good shape mentally. I ruled out one foster home, after my mother's brain cancer recovery, based on the fact that the other residents were as much as 20 to 25 years older than my mother. She was 75 years old at the time. They sat around staring off into space. My mother at 75 was still very sociable, though her memory was bad.

At a foster home where patients are ambulatory and just need minimal help (sometimes called a "Level 1" home), it often has a live-in house manager for five days and a relief person for two days. The residents are mildly memory-impaired. At a Level 3 foster home, for example, where residents may be bedridden, are on hospice, or have major medical problems, it usually has one aide per eight-hour shift, not a live-in. Sometimes, there will be one aide for each 12-hour shift.

For Level 3 residents, you can expect a variety of services. Some of these would be: range of motion exercises; feeding tube care; catheter care; suppositories or enemas; oxygen; suctioning; medications; and dressing wounds (surface tumors). The worker doesn't need to be a nurse, but should have a nurse to consult with as needed, such as a hospice nurse or a nurse from VNA. For example, I wouldn't allow someone who is not an R.N. to insert a catheter.

Some Level 3 foster homes take residents on respirators. A resident on a respirator must be monitored closely. This type of foster home should be owned by an R.N. or someone in the medical field who has experience with respirators. Further, the resident should be closely supervised.

It seems that with the high cost of nursing homes and poor care they provide, Level 3 foster homes that have access to a registered nurse are a good alternative and will be the wave of the future. If a resident is in the hospice program, she is entitled to the services of a registered nurse who will visit her at the foster home. The hospice-enrolled patient is provided free equipment such as a hospital bed, hoyer lift, wheelchair, oxygen, suction machine, etc. These will be delivered to the foster home. (If the resident isn't on hospice, the cost of equipment may be an extra expense to the resident if her insurance won't cover it.)

One of the greatest advantages of foster care is that since an owner or aide has only five residents, she gets to know each resident's needs, and errors are less likely to occur, especially with "tube feeder" residents. At a facility, aides rotate on a unit, and may have up to 40 patients over a period of a week, so it's hard for them to remember what needs to be done for an individual, such as keeping her elevated for the tube feeding. Again, nursing home care is assembly-line care.

However, foster home owners, if they don't do the work themselves, often have trouble finding or keeping aides. If an aide isn't reliable, she may even leave the house unattended to take a walk.

At any foster home, if the owner doesn't run the home, she should be available by phone to the aide or house manager 24 hours a day for emergency help or questions.

As for locating a foster home, you can look in the Yellow Pages of your phonebook where there are often foster home placement services listed. Some of these are good, and they don't charge any fees to the family. Some foster care placement agencies are bad because the staff hasn't bothered to visit all the places they recommend. Ask the staff when the last time was that they visited a particular home. Of course, you can also contact your Area Agency on Aging for information on finding foster home care. Individual counties usually regulate foster homes.

Foster homes run the gamut of care, from those that take ambulatory and continent residents exclusively, to those that take in Alzheimer's residents, to those that take in bedridden and hospice residents, including tube feeders. Some do respirator care. Most take either sex, but some just prefer women residents. Many foster homes have a weekly menu printed out of the foods they serve, and will show it to you.

If a foster home doesn't have air conditioning, and many don't, make certain they plan on giving enough fluids to your elder in hot weather. Otherwise, your elder can get dehydrated. I once met a nursing home nurse who had her mother in a foster home. Her mother got dehydrated and had to be taken to the hospital's emergency room.

Following is a general checklist of questions to ask foster home owners:

1) What is the room like that is available? (See it.)
2) How many residents share a bathroom?
3) Does the resident have use of the house or is she confined to her room?
4) Are there any staircases that might be a danger to a resident?
5) What about security? Are there adequate locks? Any sliding doors?
6) Is the kitchen area inaccessible by a locked door so that residents can't turn on the stove?
7) Are medications locked up?
8) Are there adequate hallway handrails and bathroom grab bars for the ambulatory?
9) Is there a shower chair in the shower? Is there a handicapped accessible shower?
10) How accessible are various parts of the house if a cane, walker or wheelchair is used?
11) Is there a power generator in case of a power outage?
12) What is the general health of other residents? Do they have any lung problems?
13) Is there air conditioning?
14) Is there any special equipment such as hospital beds or wheelchairs?

15) How often do residents receive showers?
16) What kind of food is served and is there attention to special dietary needs? Is there soft food served? Baked? Fried? Processed food?
17) How is laundry done—with other residents' clothes?
18) Are there men and women residents?
19) Are there pets in the house?
20) What is the monthly rent and what are the extra charges?
21) Who is on duty during the weekdays? Weekends?
22) Does the person on duty ever leave the house at any time?

Above all, don't be afraid to ask obvious questions. Ask the owners how long they've been in business. You should observe if the home is clean and odor free. Observe if the caregiver is cheerful, friendly, and loving. (I've seen some that are strickly business!) Ask if the owner has references from families or professionals such as nurses or social workers who know them. You should carefully read the foster home agreement before signing it. The agreement should clearly state rates, services, and house rules.

It's interesting that some foster care owners are just as lax about safety as nursing homes are. I visited a foster home that was generally an excellent one. However, I noticed one obvious danger. There was a narrow and steep spiral staircase leading from the living room to the lower level. How could anyone have elderly, ambulatory residents in such a setting?

Realize, too that good foster homes often have waiting lists, so perhaps it's a good idea to keep your elder's name on one, in case the present one he's in doesn't pan out. As with any care situation, you should always have other care lined up in case something unforeseen happens, such as the foster home operator becomes ill and has to retire.

Following is a special checklist for foster homes offering bedridden or hospice care:

1) Will the resident's room be large enough for equipment such as a hospital bed and hoyer lift? Where is the fire exit in relation to the room? Do room windows open and have screens?
2) Do you have any special equipment? Hospital bed? Hoyer lift? Wheelchair?
3) Do you have a power generator?
4) Do you take bedridden residents who are heavy? Can all caregivers do lifting?
5) Are all the caregivers experienced in bedridden care?
6) Do you have an aide who works graveyard shift to change and turn patients?
7) How long have the caregivers been taking care of bedridden people?
8) Have you had residents on oxygen?
9) Have you suctioned residents?
10) Do you give tube feedings? Administer medication with a syringe through a feeding tube?
11) Do you know how to operate a hoyer lift?
12) Do you give hospice care?
13) How often do you give sponge baths?
14) Do the residents get a shower? Is the shower handicapped accessible with a shower chair on wheels?
15) Do you do range of motion exercises—how often?
16) How do you handle incontinent care? Do you use diaper wipes or cleanse with soap, water and a terrycloth towel? How often do you change and turn a resident?
17) Do you do catheter care?
18) Are you good at pulling up a resident in bed? Is there a second person to help?
19) Do you do mouth care? How?

20) If a resident needs oxygen, where do you get it from? Do you know a nurse who can deliver it? (One owner told me a resident's doctor dispatched a nurse from the Visiting Nurse Association. She also told me that the Visiting Nurse was sometimes not able to come until hours later.)

21) If x-rays are needed, when you call the doctor, does a mobile x-ray unit come fairly quickly? (One owner admitted that mobile x-ray units weren't always prompt. Sometimes, they aren't prompt in getting to nursing homes, either.)

22) Do you consult a particular nurse with questions, such as in the case of problems with a feeding tube?

23) Will you take a resident back after he's been hospitalized and needs special attention?

24) What residents have you had to have leave?

25) Does your base fee cover all supplies like latex gloves, diapers? What doesn't it cover?

When putting a loved one in foster care, be honest with the owner about the health and personality of your loved one. One foster care owner told me that there had been times when residents didn't work out, and they were frustrated at being there, so after a month, she thought it best for them to leave. I guess the bottom line is that if your loved one doesn't have a nice personality and is too much trouble, no one, for any amount of money, will help them.

Beware that foster care is even less monitored by the government for problems than nursing homes are. They aren't regularly inspected. You are putting your trust in the reputation of the owner and how long they've been in business.

You hear on the news about facilities and foster homes where residents have died in fires. Firemen say their greatest fear is going into a foster home that is on fire and lifting elderly patients out.

The owner of a foster care placement service told me that some foster homes may not want to take a heavy bed-ridden patient because in case of a fire, they'd be afraid of getting her out in time. He said, too, that many foster homes shun heavy, bedridden patients, not wanting to injure their backs. He said that ethnic people who run foster homes and have all their family members working there appreci-ate the money. I found, in talking to ethnic owners of foster homes, that they all seemed to say that they got attached to their residents. (Of course, nursing home staffers sometimes say this too, particularly at religious-affiliated nursing homes. At nursing homes, with the way they sometimes treat patients and family members, this statement is sus-pect.)

Residential Care Facilities

Residential Care Facilities (RCFs) can usually take from 6 to 15 residents. They are usually not set up to give nurs-ing care. Surprisingly enough, I ran across some that claim to. For example, I met an R.N. who owned an RCF, and she said she would take my bedridden mother. She had 12 resi-dents, and one day when I visited, she had one aide on duty babysitting a living room full of residents. There was a cook in the kitchen. However, if I had placed my mother there, who would have been upstairs checking on my mother? There was a fire escape on the second floor, but how would my mother had gotten out alive with so many residents and a narrow hallway?

For ambulatory residents, there were no rails on the stairs going down to the living room. The stairs were steep, too, and there were some brain-damaged residents. These residents often have bad balance. You'd think the R.N. owner would have been concerned about safety.

How could this nurse have thought that she could take a bedridden patient in, given the population of residents she had and the staffing. I should mention that I saw a young resident, mentally disabled, in his room on the second floor. He was all by himself unattended. Would he have harmed my bedridden mother if she had been in her room unattended?

A couple of other RCFs I knew about weren't any better. The services at RCFs are supposed to include meals, special diets, laundry, assistance with medications and personal care.

I found that RCFs were just as expensive as foster homes. After visiting three, I can't imagine that with so many more residents, why a family member would choose one over a foster home. RCFs don't even look homey, because there are too many rooms and too many residents. A hospice physical therapist I knew used to make regular visits to another RCF that I knew of in my neighborhood. She said it was appalling how little attention each resident got. It was just as inadequate as a nursing home, care-wise, she said.

Hospice

Hospice services are fully covered by Medicare/private insurance and Medicaid. Many family members put their loved ones in a nursing home when they become terminally ill, instead of enrolling them in the hospice program. Or, sometimes a family member will enroll a loved one in hospice who is already at a nursing home. The hospice program is great. If your elder is terminally ill, putting him in a nursing home is a bad mistake. I'll give you some examples.

My neighbor's mother was put in a nursing home as a cancer patient with a few months left to live. My neighbor reported to me exactly what I witnessed at nursing homes among terminally ill patients. The terminally ill patient didn't get pain medication as needed. When she approached the nurse to remind her that it was time for her mother's medication, the nurse was busy and postponed giving the medication.

Why does the nurse postpone giving the medication? Usually because the nurse has other patients to care for. Sometimes the nurse doesn't even know how to run the IV for pain medication. Sometimes the nurse is even afraid of overdosing a patient on pain medication and losing her license.

In one's last days of life, if one has cancer, one may need medication every 15 minutes. There is no way a nurse in a nursing home with say, 25 to 40 patients, can be in one patient's room every 15 minutes. The hospice program is set up so that the immediate caregiver is trained to give medication. A hospice nurse cannot live at one's house or station himself at the nursing home giving medication every 15 minutes. Therefore, in the case of one being at a nursing home, it's the nursing home nurse's duty to administer the medication. A family member is not allowed to do this in a nursing home. At nursing homes, as I witnessed, too many patients often died very alert and in a lot of pain, as their relatives watched helplessly. I remember the son of an elderly nursing home patient, who after she died, got very upset at the nurse who had been on graveyard shift. On that shift, the nurse had 80 patients and could not deliver pain medication as required.

If a loved one is in her final days and is at home, a family member is most likely there administering pain medication and will see that she gets her medication on time.

I have known some family members who confided in me that when their loved one was dying, they didn't want to keep them suffering an extra few days, so they gave them more than the prescribed dose of medication. I'm not condoning this, but they did it. I wouldn't.

A hospice nurse can address all of the family member's questions and concerns about medication. Hospice nurses don't advocate illegal acts.

I watched many terminally ill patients die at nursing homes and each time, the nurse would struggle to set up the IV for pain medication. Sometimes, the nurse would call in another nurse from another unit to help out, and they would scratch their heads about what to do while the patient was moaning in pain.

One nurse confided in me that she was glad she wasn't on duty when Mr. So and So died, because she wouldn't have known how to run the IV with pain medication.

Further, there is another factor to consider. Nursing home employees often don't like outsiders giving them instructions about care issues. When the hospice nurse makes a visit and gives instructions about bandaging a patient's tumors on a regular basis, the recommendations are sometimes ignored. This isn't in the best interests of the patient. However, as with a family member's wishes, the nursing home nurse sometimes doesn't follow through on instructions.

The solution is to either put a hospice patient at home, at a foster home, or at a hospice house.

The patient's physician makes the recommendation for the patient to be placed in the hopsice program, if she feels the patient has six months or less to live. The medical director of the hospice house and hospice staff determine admittance of a patient to a hospice house, if home care isn't feasible.

Although hospice nurses at your home usually make one visit a week, if more visits are necessary, they will come. For example, my mother's hospice nurse said he had been at a hospice patient's house every day for one week. She wasn't in her final days, but she was having some medical difficulties.

A hospice nurse is just a phone call away, 24 hours a day, on holidays, too. He can give instructions by phone or help in a real crisis that the family member can't handle on his own. But, what you'll find, is that the hospice nurse can train you to do practically any task, except catheterize a patient, for example. All care equipment needed, from wheelchairs to oxygen and suction machines to feeding tube supplies, are delivered by hospice.

Hospice even gave me miniature pillows that their volunteers had made to place between my mother's ankles when she was resting on her side. This prevented ankle sores. More importantly, they gave me a drawsheet with handle straps to allow me to more easily slide my mother up in bed. The drawsheet is a thick pad placed under the body of a patient.

If your loved one needs medication , and it's a late hour when the hospice nurse can't deliver it, hospice will call ahead to a nearby pharmacy where the drug will be waiting for you to pick up and hospice will be billed. If only this kind of care were available to everyone!

Hospice is a team approach among a number of support people for the patient. While a patient is in the hospice program, he is entitled to physical therapy, occupational therapy, and speech therapy visits as ordered by the doctor. Massage therapy is sometimes available for hospice patients. A hospice nurse's aide will give a bed bath and a shampoo, and foot and back rubs, once a week, (or more if the hospice nurse deems necessary). A hospice volunteer will spend four hours a week, either reading or helping with some care. You should ask for a retired hospice volunteer. My mother had two hospice volunteers during eight months . They weren't always diligent about coming as they had demanding jobs. This left me in the lurch on about six different occasions, when I couldn't leave the house as scheduled. Neither hospice volunteer made up the time. Perhaps the hospice volunteer program needs a volunteer floater who can fill in when your volunteer can't make it.

If a patient in the hospice program is in a nursing home, certain benefits won't kick in, such as visits by the nurse's aide to do a bath or shampoo. The hospice program doesn't want to duplicate the nursing home duty, even though the nursing home doesn't do this task well.

I remember the frustration of having to question pharmacy bills and laboratory bills when these services were contracted out by the nursing home. However, when my mother moved home, and was enrolled in the hospice program, we never had to question bills, since hospice received these bills directly and paid them. The hospice nurse arranged for lab tests through the doctor.

While in the hospice program, if one can't be cared for privately at home or in a foster home, there are hospice houses. Each nurse there has about four patients. Here, hospice nurses will see that a patient gets his pain medication on time. However, had we put our mother in the hospice house we visited, there would have been certain restrictions. For a hospice house, there is such a waiting list that one often can't stay there as a long-term patient. Usually, the patient is accepted for the last two months or so of her life. Years ago, when funds were more plentiful, patients could stay several months or a year at hospice house. Further, at hospice house, tube feedings are not permitted, though one can continue getting chemotherapy medication and antibiotics to prolong one's life. The idea is not to treat the cancer so much, as to make the patient more comfortable.

While some healthcare professionals consider chemotherapy and antibiotics to be measures to prolong life for the terminally ill, other professionals say that you allow a patient to die on his own terms. Obviously, when a patient becomes very ill, antibiotics will no longer work. There are many gray areas in hospice care, as far as treating the patient, or not continuing to treat the patient.

Hospice houses lack space, so we were told that if we wanted to continue our mother's tube feedings, a hospice facility would not accept her. Perhaps in another area where a hospice facility isn't in demand, this rule could be negotiated. The medical director of the hospice facility and your loved one's doctor might be able to negotiate something.

At a hospice house, they tend not to treat pneumonia, because they consider it to be a natural process of the terminally ill. However, they do treat bladder infections as a comfort measure. (A bladder infection, that is untreated, can lead to kidney problems.)

However, if one is in the hospice program and is at home or in a foster home, a family member can request that the patient be treated for pneumonia. My mother's hospice nurse said that they often treated pneumonia for ambulatory patients, but usually not for bedridden patients, unless desired.

When my mother was on hospice at home, she was also entitled to 30 hours of free care from an agency aide that hospice would foot the bill for. These 30 hours were available during the first six-month period. Beyond that, the free agency aide care was dependent upon hospice funds available. (Don't confuse this with the weekly visit by the hospice program aide employed by hospice. This was an added benefit.)

In the hospice program, one is assigned to a regular hospice nurse and a regular hospice social worker. The latter makes visits every six weeks, or more frequently as needed. She's also available by phone.

When I expressed to the hospice social worker that my mother's doctor never even suggested the hospice program, she said this wasn't unusual. She said often doctors know very little about hospice. I found that even hospital and nursing home nurses don't know too much about hospice and its benefits.

If you're so inclined, a hospice program chaplain is available for counseling for the patient and family members—both emotional and spiritual counseling. Further, the hospice social worker is available for up to a year after your loved one has died for counseling by phone. You also receive grief counseling literature after the death of your loved one.

I should mention another hospice benefit that involves respite care for the caregiver. For every two months of caregiving, a hospice house will relieve a family caregiver by offering a five-day respite when the patient can go live there and be cared for. I didn't take advantage of this, because I didn't want to shuffle my mother around in her bedridden condition.

A hospice nurse told me that when a family member is taken home to die, the hospital bed is often put in the living room or dining room, because they are often the larger rooms. We put our mother in a small room, but it was still big enough for the hoyer lift and her wheelchair. It was the warmest room in the house, right directly above the basement where the furnace was.

As I will discuss in Chapter 6, "You Can Care For The Bedridden," in setting up the home for my mother's return, I had a power generator installed, so we would always have heat and light. It was the simplest portable natural gas generator that I could buy, with limited features from an electrical panel. In other words, the stove and other heavy appliances such as the washing machine couldn't be used while the power generator was on. Further, I contacted our local utilities company to make our mother a priority customer, with her doctor's authorization, so that when power was restored, we'd be back in service sooner.

I should mention that the hospice program isn't all peaches and cream, although it's excellent. One weekend, when my mother's nurse wasn't on duty, a substitute nurse came in an emergency when my mother had a bladder infection and high fever. Although it's usually hospice policy to treat bladder infections, as a comfort measure, this substitute nurse took the attitude "Why bother?" Yes, even in hospice there are "independent-minded" nurses who don't follow procedure. When I told her that we wanted the infection treated, she did go ahead and call the doctor for a prescription. When I later reported this to my mother's regular hospice nurse, he said I should report her to a supervisor at hospice. I didn't do this, because knowing the healthcare system as I did, I didn't want to complain and perhaps later cross paths with this nurse in another emergency. I felt she might hold it against us.

Hospice first came to be in the U.S. in 1974. Hospice knows no age limits. Even babies can be in the hospice program. My mother's hospice nurse once told me that he'd just come from the hospital and comforted the parents of a dying baby.

Hospice is a philosophy. While hospice workers like to talk openly about death with the patient, I asked that they not do this with my mother because being Italian, it was a cultural matter of her generation not to talk about death, even though I'm sure she knew she was dying. Not all hospice workers felt comfortable doing this, however, and I had to keep reminding them.

Clearly, hospice isn't the answer for everyone. Some people may refuse pain relief for religious or philosophical reasons. Some may prefer quantity of life over quality of life, not being prepared to embrace death, but to keep being aggressively treated.

The main appeal of hospice is that it treats the patient, not the disease. Hospice neither hastens nor prolongs dying. It doesn't use heroic measures, such as resuscitation. If there is an emergency, the family member usually doesn't call 9-1-1, but lets the patient die naturally.

With all the help from hospice, my mother's weeks were full. For example, on Monday, a hospice aide would come to give a bed bath and shampoo in the morning. And, I had hired a private aide to come for four hours in the afternoon. On Tuesday, the hospice physical therapist would come for an hour. On Wednesday, the hospice volunteer would come for two hours. On Thursday, our family friend would come for four hours. On Friday, the hospice nurse would come for one to one and one-half hours. On Saturday, the hospice volunteer would come for two hours. And, on Sunday, we had a private caregiver we'd hired. (We could have used up the 30 hours of free agency aide help that hospice would pay for, but I found private caregivers that I preferred to pay for myself.)

I had feared it would be lonely at home with no one coming, but to the contrary, people were coming in and out regularly. With a private caregiver, a hospice volunteer, and the family friend that we paid (as she was retired and needed the money), I had plenty of time to get out of the house and do errands.

In caring for my mother at home, after the first month of bad agency aides, I decided to go it practically alone, since these aides weren't very functional and weren't helping too much with care. I had used these aides primarily as sitters to read to my mother and to keep her company while I did errands. They'd come in the afternoon, after I did her morning care.

I did have a private R.N. come who had helped my friend's father. She asked for only "aide wages," because she was not doing nursing care. However, in my mother's final days she came in the evenings, and helped give medication every 15 minutes and oxygen, so I paid her R.N. wages then. It should be noted that in one's final hours, if it's in the evening, a hospice nurse doesn't come. They instruct you on what to do, and you're on your own. This is the only disappointing thing about hospice. However, if you need moral support, after your loved one has taken her final breath, if you call hospice, they will notify your social worker to come and comfort you.

My mother died in the morning, just before 10:30 a.m. We had known she was in her final days, and the hospice nurse had instructed me days before on what to do. We had known that my mother's death was approaching, as many of her organs had started to fail. That morning of her death, the social worker had arrived just for a half-hour visit, since I hadn't seen her in six weeks. During the half-hour she was visiting, my mother died. My mother's friend was also with us. It was a humbling experience, and I can say nothing more.

Besides having access to pain medication, when a patient is in the hospice program, you don't run into resistance about discontinuing tube feedings in a patient's final days. At the Catholic facility my mother was at, the last facility, the nun administrator, as a policy, wouldn't allow a doctor's order to discontinue tube feedings when the patient was dying and in pain. At home or at a hospice house, no one stands in your way of doing this. One nurse at the Catholic facility told me in confidence that you could ask a doctor to reduce the tube feeding to such a minimal level, so the patient's life wouldn't be prolonged. However, the point is, an administrator shouldn't be allowed to dictate how someone dies. And, if your loved one is at a nursing home in her final days, you shouldn't be burdened with thinking about how to circumvent the system in his final days.

(As I've said, the bureaucracy at nursing homes makes little sense, and is often contradictory. At a Catholic facility, the administrator will allow the patient or patient's family to refuse antibiotics for infections, so the patient's life is not prolonged and she will die. However, they see withholding artificial feeding as wrong. And, if a patient can't swallow and wants her feeding tube taken out, the Catholic nursing home will ask the patient to leave the facility and die at home.) However, as I've said before, if a patient stops swallowing while at the nursing home, a Catholic facility will allow him to die without requiring a feeding tube. Of course, Catholic facilities won't allow physician-assisted suicide in a state where it's legal. Again, in the latter case, the patient must leave a Catholic facility and go home to die.

As an added note: if your loved one is at a nursing home and is enrolled in hospice, you will especially need its assistance. For example, if your loved one has a tumor on the surface of her body, the tumor will likely ulcerate (break open and bleed) at a nursing home. Aides will carelessly turn the patient, and touch or rub the affected area without noticing. Once it ulcerates, the odor of the tumor is very unpleasant. As doctors will warn you, nursing home staff will often shun the patient's room, and even poorer care of the patient will result. The nursing home simply adds insult to injury in these cases.

At a nursing home, you will need the hospice nurse to visit to lend his expertise in bandaging the tumor that often gets infected with poor nursing care. The patient will often die from the infection of an ulcerated tumor. (At home, as I did, you can often prevent ulceration of a surface tumor, just by being careful not to break it open and keeping it freshly bandaged.) As doctors warned me, nursing home nurses don't often take the two minutes required to bandage tumors. We found this out firsthand, before we took our mother out of the nursing home.

In Chapter 6, "You Can Care For The Bedridden," you will see that it is feasible to give your bedridden loved one care at home. Yes, it requires strength, and it's a full-time job, but you needn't be a nurse.

Chapter 6

You Can Care For The Bedridden

Getting Started

You may choose to take your loved one home, when he leaves the hospital, or from out of the nursing home at some point, perhaps for the final months of his life. Or, maybe you'll decide that you never want to put your loved one in a nursing home under any circumstances. You may decide that you'll care for him yourself, taking an early retirement from your profession. Unless you have a very high income, it may work out better to pay yourself to care for a family member than to pay a nursing home. While I'm not advocating that someone spends years of caring for a family member, it might be a cheaper alternative than placing someone in a nursing home. What if both your father and mother needed care? You could pay yourself a handsome salary to take care of them, but it would be cheaper than what it would cost them to pay a nursing home. Personally, I didn't pay myself a salary to take care of my mother at any time. I figured that if something should happen to me, she'd need as much money as possible to seek outside care.

You may not want to be a full-time caregiver to your bedridden family member. Maybe you just want to know some basics to supplement nursing home care, if your elder is in a nursing home.

Whatever your motivation, this chapter will help you understand basic care issues, especially for the bedridden person, but not limited to the bedridden.

During the last eight months of her life, I took care of my bedridden mother practically single-handedly, using relief caregivers mainly as sitters. My mother became very heavy as a bedridden person—weighing as much as 25 pounds heavier than she normally weighed. She had big bones, and weighed at times as much as 170 pounds in her inactive condition. I have a small frame and weigh 117 pounds. My point is, if I could take care of a heavy patient, with no one else in the home, anyone can. And, many single people do.

You don't need to be a Certified Nurse's Aide (CNA) to take care of your elder. Once you read this chapter and get some actual hands-on practice with your elder, you'll find it's mechanical work that anyone can master.

Being a caregiver, especially to a bedridden person, means getting used to doing everything slow motion. You can't hurry tasks along, like "hoyering" (operating the hoyer lift), feeding by mouth, and giving sponge baths. Don't be afraid of getting behind on tasks. Slow and steady is the way to go.

As a caregiver, you don't have control over someone's illness, but in doing the care at home, you do have control over the elder's care, unlike at the nursing home where you have to follow their rules. There, you need to get permission to do things. You are prohibited from doing things without good reason. You wait for the staff to react to administering needed care, by calling the doctor for even a simple order, thereby wasting valuable time. At home, for example, you wouldn't waste time in letting a cold get worse. You'd give a cold remedy. Further, you wouldn't need a doctor's order for cough syrup or even nasal spray, as a nurse would need to get at a nursing home.

If your elder has just gotten released from the hospital, you may have observed the way nurses and nurse's aides handled your bedridden elder. (Hopefully, you didn't pick up any bad habits from the nurse's aides, and that they were lifting your elder properly.)

If you don't know a nurse and you need basic immediate training in caring for your bedridden elder, you may wish to hire a nurse from a home health agency when you first take your elder home. She can show you the ropes of caring for him. If you can afford it, you could even pay a health management company to assess your loved one's needs as far as care, equipment and supplies, and to train you, so you don't ruin your back in lifting your elder. You'll need to know, among other things, how to operate a hoyer lift, for example, to transfer your elder from his bed to a wheelchair.

One may not need to privately pay for a nurse for training, as your elder may be entitled to some good home health care benefits for a limited amount of time, as far as skilled care. Or, he may even be entitled to some home care benefits long-term, depending on whether your elder needs, for example, life support such as a feeding tube.

If you decide to care for your elder yourself, the important thing is not to feel like it will be hard for you to master the tasks. All it takes is observing the right way to do it, and practice. Further, don't feel insignificant as a caregiver. Remember that you are a valuable person giving care to a loved one that no one else would give the same care to. Providing home care for an elder does require a lot of commitment on your part, but ultimately, it is rewarding to do so.

Before you move your loved one home, make certain you've selected a good room in the home for him. If possible, the elder's room should be on the first floor in case of a fire. Make sure the windows open, not only for fresh air, but for evacuation purposes. The windows should have a screen for fresh air. If possible, your elder's room should be next to the bathroom. Make sure that you will have a working sink and toilet. They will get a lot of use. Even though my mother was bedridden and didn't use the bathroom, I was always washing my hands and emptying the catheter pan into the toilet. (I'd first empty the catheter bag into a pan.)

I picked the warmest room in the house for her. Our house was very damp with no insulation. However, I picked a room right over the basement where the furnace was. It was a room with a lot of bright light, with a high ceiling. The room was also next to the kitchen, on the other side.

Pick a room that is big enough for all the equipment, including a hoyer lift. In my mother's room, there was space for:

•The hospital bed. (Bedridden people need to keep their backs elevated for easier breathing and healthier lungs, and they need to keep their backs elevated for eating food.)

• A dresser chest to hold medical supplies.

• A tray table. (This isn't only useful for eating, but you can position the hospital bed so that you can wheel the tray table around to either side of it to do a sponge bath, cleaning each side of the body. If your elder's insurance won't cover the tray table, one is available through a medical supply store or through the Harriet Carter Catalog in North Wales, Pennsylvania.)

• The wheelchair.

• The hoyer lift. (Also, two hoyer slings. An extra sling is helpful in case your elder urinates on one through her diaper. The sling can be washed with mild soap and then rinsed with water. Then hang it up to dry. It takes a day to dry.)

• A comfortable chair for the caregiver to sit in.

• An end table with a television.

•The gravity pole, feeding tube pole, provided by private insurance and Medicare.

• A suction machine. (This is helpful to have on hand at all times, because lung problems often come on quickly.)

If your elder is in the hospice program, it will provide for all of the above, except the chest of drawers, the chair and the end table, of course.

Make sure you have a second electrical outlet in the room of your loved one to operate all machines, such as oxygen, etc., and even the hospital bed which is plugged in.

Undoubtedly, in caring for a bedridden elder, your home will look like a mini-hospital with equipment, medication and supplies. It's filled with Milk of Magnesia™; cough and cold remedies, (Sudafed™, Dimetapp™, and cough syrup), that can prevent a worsening condition such as pneumonia; Ocean Spray™ (nasal spray); Vicks Vaporub™; and suppositories, etc.

Our house was very old, built in the 1920s, and I constantly worried about, "What if such and such breaks down?" Don't worry about things like the water heater breaking down. Just consider that at nursing homes, for example, it's not uncommon for them to not have hot water or their washing machine breaks down and there's no fresh linen. This happened at two nursing homes my mother was at. You won't do any worse. Just heat water and let it cool for a warm sponge bath. At nursing homes when there's no hot water, it gives them an excuse not to do a sponge bath or give a shower, according to what one aide told me. Care problem solved!

(Incidentally, I remember at the nursing home when there was no hot water on the unit, I went to the kitchen to get hot water from the sink. They put my mother's sponge bath tub right into the sink where they washed pots and pans and rinsed vegetables!)

I was also worried about power outages that we had every winter at home. I therefore had a portable natural gas power generator installed in the patio before my mother came home. If you can afford one, it makes sense if you do have power outages. A portable power generator can run $5,500 including installation for minimal electrical service. You'll always need heat and lights. Big appliances such as using a stove and washing machine while the power generator is on—when you have minimal electrical supply—can shut down the whole system. You have to plan with an electrician just what usage is absolutely necessary in case of a power outage, so he can rig up the electrical system accordingly.

Whether or not you have a power generator at home, you'll want to make sure your local power company makes your elder a priority customer for restoring power in a power outage. The power company, when you first notify it, will send you a form that your elder's doctor can sign stating that your loved one, for medical purposes, should be a priority customer.

The power company will recommend that you get a power generator, to be safe. It's not hard to operate a power generator. It was my fear that I wouldn't be able to start it up. This didn't turn out to be true. You keep the power generator outside, under a patio roof or awning. You always keep a flashlight handy so that as soon as the power goes out—often after dark— you can make your way down to the basement to your electrical panel to pull the switches, and then back upstairs and out the back door to start up the generator. (As a substitute for a power generator for heat, don't use a propane heater. It is a fire hazard if it's tipped over.)

If you have a bedridden elder at home, have a list of electricians, furnace people, and plumbers who are available 24/7, and who are members of the Better Business Bureau. Although you may live in an old house, as a caregiver you make do. There will be some unexpected events, so you can expect the unexpected. For instance, there was a water main malfunction in our neighborhood, and we were out of water for five hours. Fortunately, it wasn't longer. I needed water for medication and for a sponge bath, and to wash my hands. I frantically called the City Water Bureau, and explained my mother was a hospice patient, and that I couldn't leave the house to get bottled water. They sent an employee who delivered five bottles of water from the grocery store, and they didn't even want to be reimbursed.

Keeping Your Elder Clean: Sponge Baths

Giving an adequate sponge bath, morning and evening, does a lot not only in keeping your elder clean, but in keeping him refreshed. My sponge baths were pretty comprehensive. They are what nursing homes call a "bed bath," that is, something in lieu of a shower or bathtub bath, (head to toe). Incidentally, sponge baths can be given to an elder for years if she is too frail to enter a bathtub or be given a shower. Good sponge baths can maintain an elder's skin indefinitely.

I wouldn't attempt giving a shower to a bedridden/paralyzed person in your home unless you had a walk-in shower (without a step), that a shower chair could slide right into. (You would hoyer-lift your elder into the shower chair.) You don't want to try to push a shower chair over a step to get the paralyzed person into the shower. If you do, even with a seat belt on the shower chair, your elder could fall off.

You give a sponge bath when one wakes up in the morning, (after range of motion exercises), and another one just before bedtime. Be organized. If you have a hospital tray table to place a sponge bath plastic tub on, that's great. (If you've never been hospitalized, the sponge bath tub looks like a plastic tub that people wash dishes in, in their kitchen sink.) Have everything out on the tray table for the sponge bath, ready to go, so that you don't run in and out of the room getting things you forgot. Your elder can get cold being uncovered. Have your soap in a soap dish, warm water in the plastic tub, and enough washcloths, (face size, not hand size), so that you can grasp them and wring out water. Use a bath towel for drying.

You go head to toe. Start with the forehead and work your way down the body. Don't be stingy with face towels. If you don't use enough, then you're just transferring perspiration, etc. from one part of the body to another part. Follow these steps, after lowering the back of the bed. (Raise the back of the bed a little if your elder coughs.)

1) Wet a face towel, wring it, rub soap on it, and start washing. (i.e forehead, face, neck, shoulders and chest.)

2) Dunk a fresh washcloth into the tub of water to rinse the above parts of the body.

3) Dry these parts of the body.

4) Take another face towel, rub soap on it, and do the arms, hands, in between the fingers, and armpits. Rinse with another washcloth. Dry these parts.

5)Take another damp washcloth, rub it with soap and do the stomach and sides of the body. Then, rinse with another washcloth. Dry.

6) Roll your elder over and do her back, using the same procedure.

7) Proceed down the body, first doing the urinary area, then the rear end, using different washcloths for each area.

8) Then do the legs, feet, and in between the toes. Don't forget the back of the legs, too.

It's important to keep a sheet over the rest of the body as you're washing so your elder doesn't get cold. For cleanliness, remove the dirty diaper, of course, before you give the sponge bath, and place a fresh one under the body. This fresh one will obviously get wet with the washing, and you'll change it again. Or, perhaps your elder will urinate while you're washing, so you must keep a diaper on the body, so as not to wet the bed. Another way of not wetting the bed while washing your elder, is to keep a fresh bath towel underneath the body. Remember to wring out the face cloth well, so you don't make a wet mess out of the bed.

It's very important not to dunk dirty washcloths into the plastic tub. Further, always soap the fresh towel after you've dunked it into the tub, but once the towel is soapy, don't dunk it back into the tub. You want fresh water for rinsing.

After the sponge bath, you can powder the body, particularly under the armpits, in between the thighs, and on the rear end. Or, you can use bath gel that contains aloe vera and Vitamin E on the legs. As an alternative, simply use some body lotion sparingly on legs, arms, and hands.

At night, your sponge bath needn't be a bed bath. Perhaps you can wash under the armpits, do the urinary area, and the rear end.

As for a shampoo, it's nice to give one once a week. There are two ways to give a shampoo to a bedridden person. The easiest is to have your elder up in a wheelchair. Fill the sponge bath tub with warm water. Put it on the tray table. Apply some shampoo to a damp washcloth and soap the hair. After you've soaped the hair, rinse with a few wet washcloths, and blow the hair dry. It's good to keep a towel around the neck of your elder to catch any dripping water.

You can actually do a shampoo in bed if you have a plastic tray that you can get at a medical supply store, or that hospice will bring you, if your elder is in the hospice program, and you prefer to do a shampoo without the help of the hospice aide. My mother's hospice aide would get a pitcher of water, place my mother's head over the tray, pour water over her head, and then soap her head. The soapy water from the tray would drain out of it into a bucket on the floor that was placed at the side of the bed. To empty the water from the tray, you'd press on the edge of the tray, without having to lift the elder's head. You would simply drain out the soapy water and pour in a fresh pitcher of water over the elder's head to keep rinsing the hair until it was no longer soapy.

If your elder has a cold, and you don't want to give a shampoo, then you can give a "rinseless shampoo" with just a terrycloth towel—no water needed. You can get this at a home health pharmacy.

Incontinent Care & Repositioning Your Elder

Probably the hardest part of taking care of a bedridden person is dealing with incontinence, turning her body in bed, and repositioning her.

If your elder uses diapers, she should be checked every two hours. (If your elder is bedridden, but alert and can communicate well, a bed pan could be used, or a male patient could use a urinal.) Catheters may work well for patients who aren't prone to bladder infections.

If your elder is heavy, as my mother was, or heavier than you, it's strenuous to turn her, pull her body up in bed, and reposition her body.

To change a diaper, just as with giving a sponge bath, you lay the bed flat. If your elder begins to cough a lot, raise the back of the bed until the coughing stops. When you change a diaper, you turn the body to one side and start rolling up the dirty diaper. After removing the dirty diaper, you can put a disposable blue pad — a cotton-lined sheet that you buy at medical supply stores in quantity— underneath the body while cleaning up your elder. This is done just in case she urinates while changing her diaper.

You wipe in between the thighs and urinary area with a soapy washcloth, then rinse with a wet washcloth, and dry with a hand towel. (At nursing homes, rather than take the time to use terrycloth towels and use up towels that must go to the laundry, they usually would clean a patient using diaper wipes. This sometimes irritates the skin, especially if the wipes are alcohol-based instead of aloe-based.)

I would also clean the buttocks with terrycloth towels, instead of using diaper wipes. It should be noted that when you clean a person who's had a bowel movement, you wipe the feces away from the front part of the body. (The elder is turned on her side.) If you don't wipe the feces away from the body, you can infect the urinary area. If your elder has had a bowel movement, don't use your wet terrycloth towels, until you've wiped away the feces with tissue paper. Toilet paper doesn't wipe the feces away as well, I think.

After you've cleaned and dried the urinary and buttocks area, you slide in a fresh diaper while your elder is turned on her side. As added protection, you can also slip a disposable cotton brief up over her legs as you would a pair of underpants. This would give added protection when she urinates so as not to soil the bed.

Because urine can easily seep through a diaper and even the cotton brief, you should also place a blue pad underneath her body.

Finally, the drawsheet, a cloth pad goes between the blue pad and fitted bedsheet. The drawsheet allows you to draw or pull the body up in bed. The drawsheet is placed slightly above the buttocks, and runs under the thighs. (Hospice gave me a homemade drawsheet with handles for extra leverage in pulling.)

In nursing homes, they often use flimsy drawsheets that resemble miniature tablecloths to pull a patient up in bed. These are often useless because they don't give you much leverage in pulling up the body. At the medical supply store, you can get quilted cotton drawsheets that give you a lot of leverage for pulling. After you've positioned the draw-sheet slightly above the elder's rear end, first you pull up one side of the drawsheet, then you go to the other side of the bed, and pull up the other side of the drawsheet. I'm assuming you may be alone in caring for your elder, as I was, for the most part, when I took my mother out of the nursing home.

If you had a nurse's aide with you, the two of you could simultaneously pull up each side of the drawsheet.

It should be noted that when my mother was in the nurs-ing home, oftentimes I did the changing of her diaper and pulling her up in bed without assistance. It was either that, or leave my mother soaking wet, and wait for an hour or more for an aide to come and help.

After you've pulled your elder's body up in bed, you position a pillow underneath the body. If you position the body on one side, you position a pillow under the lower back and rear end to prevent rear end bedsores. Two hours later, you turn the body to the other side, and position the pillow under that side of the body. In addition, when the body is turned to one side, you don't want one leg resting on top of the other, because the elder can get sores on the legs, ankles, and inner knees. Therefore, you place a pillow in between the knees, a little above the knee caps. Be care-ful not to position the pillow so it's right next to the uri-nary area, since urine can spill out of the diaper and brief and onto the pillow. You can also use mini-pillows—the kind little girls use for their dolls—to place in between the ankles. (Mini-pillows are also used under the armpits to prevent sores there.)

Sometimes my mother's body, as many stroke patients' bodies do, would lean to one side, if she was laying on her back, with the back of the bed elevated. In this case, I would prop a pillow underneath her shoulder, to block her from leaning off to the side. (This works well, too, if one is lean-ing off to the side while seated in a wheelchair.) When she was receiving her tube feeding, often I would lay her on her back, with the back of the bed elevated. She appeared to look more comfortable this way during her tube feeding. If your elder is laying on her back with the bed elevated, you can't elevate the bed too high, otherwise a paralyzed person will slide down in the bed. You pull your elder up in bed, elevated at about 30 degrees, and place a pillow under her rear end to prevent bedsores. You should also place a pillow under her ankles.

One of the worst instances of positioning my mother was done by an aide at the nursing home. My mother was on her back and the back of the bed was elevated at 90 degrees. She was tilted very far forward, and one of her legs was bent inwardly at the knee so badly, that the leg pointed out to the side. Apparently, the aide must have thought she was doing my mother a favor by keeping her so elevated while her feeding tube was running. Yes, it's important to keep the patient's back and head elevated while the feeding tube is running so the patient doesn't aspirate. However, this grossly exaggerated position was foolish in causing such pain to the leg,and pain around the feeding tube site with the circular plastic button piece of the tube pinching against her skin.

(When I complained to the nurse, I called her in to witness it, and she told the aide that this was uncomfortable. The aide retaliated by saying that if I complained, she didn't want to work with my mother. Instead of the staff going to bat for my mother, they didn't even reprimand the aide.)

In positioning an elder in bed who is immobile, consider that being kept on one's side facing a wall, isn't stimulating. While it's healthy for a bedridden person's lungs to be positioned on his side, perhaps he can be positioned facing the window on more occasions. Of course, you don't want to keep him on that side all the time, for fear of him getting bedsores.

As for catheters, since tube feeders, in particular, urinate often with all their liquid intake, the at-home caregiver often prefers a catheter, rather than changing diapers. With my mother, because of the Strep infection in her urine—caught at the nursing home—that caused a chronic skin infection in between her legs, we had no choice but to catheterize her five weeks after she got home. The prescription creams needed to be chronically used, and urinating into the diaper with leakage aggravated the skin and even washed away the creams.

With a catheter at home, germs aren't as likely to occur as they are with catheter use at a nursing home or hospital where they don't practice the same cleanliness procedures as a family member would. Many patients in institutions develop infections with catheters because they aren't sterilized well after patients use them.

Catheters are acceptable for home use. You'll need an R.N. to catheterize your elder, and probably also a nurse to irrigate it periodically so it doesn't get clogged. I remember in the middle of one night, my mother's catheter clogged, and her urine was seeping out onto the bed. I quickly put a diaper on her to catch the urine. I had to keep changing diapers until a hospice nurse was able to come at noon the next day.

Another caution with a catheter is that you should always make sure the catheter tubing isn't kinked. Coil the tube for better flow. Keep it from hanging beneath the bladder, otherwise it may not drain properly and the bladder will get backed up with urine. This may cause a bladder infection. Further, when in bed, make sure your elder's legs aren't trapping the catheter's tubing, otherwise the tubing won't drain and the urine will spill out onto the bed when he urinates.

In addition, sometimes when transferring a person with a catheter from the hoyer lift into the wheelchair, the catheter gets yanked a bit and you see bloody urine. Don't be alarmed, because the bleeding will stop. You can get a catheter leg band that will keep the catheter tubing from moving when you transfer your elder. The leg band fits comfortably around the leg.

When you empty a catheter bag, wipe the tip of the hose with a rubbing alcohol wipe. The bag should be emptied of urine every 200 cc. (Also empty the bag before transferring your elder by hoyer lift.)

With a heavy patient, a catheter is easier for the caregiver. You're obviously not changing a diaper every two hours, but you're still turning the patient from side to side. Your elder's skin doesn't get irritated from urine spilling onto it. However, with a catheter, some people develop bladder infections, even though cleanliness is being practiced. Sometimes those with catheters for a few months or more develop infections. Giving a glass or two of cranberry juice each day may help prevent them. A nurse once told me that some catheter patients receive a low dose of antibiotics to ward off bladder infections due to catheters.

Cranberry juice helps to prevent some bladder infections, though not always. Some people who have catheters get them anyway, and people who aren't kept clean who don't have catheters, can get them despite drinking cranberry juice.

When my mother got bladder infections, her fever tended to be high, more than 102 degrees. If someone has a history of seizures, be vigilant if she gets a bladder infection and has a high fever. Seizures may occur. My mother died from a recurring Strep infection in her urine, that she first got before she left the nursing home. Her fever was 104 when she began having seizures.

If a person with a catheter has urine that is dark and cloudy, that doesn't necessarily mean she has a bladder infection. Catheters often cause this.

Without a catheter, dark urine can mean a bladder infection. If a person's urine is cloudy, it may be due to hot weather, for example. Have your elder drink more water or cranberry juice.

Bowel Care

You can stimulate a bowel movement a number of ways, often without an enema as nursing homes use.

People who are immobile have trouble with bowel movements. That's why it's best to do a lot of range of motion exercises with the legs. Bend the knee to the chest to see if a "BM" will occur. Another method is to pull the person to the edge of the bed, and in sitting position let his feet dangle.

Drinking more water helps. Prune juice often works, as does split pea soup. You can thicken the juice and soup with thickening powder if your loved one has trouble swallowing. Oatmeal, fiber food, and wheat germ might be a solution, too. Include these in an elder's diet on a regular basis. Apple juice, incidentally, constipates a person.

Your elder should have a bowel movement every three days. If he hasn't had a bowel movement, the night before the third day, give prune juice. The juice takes about eight hours or more to take effect.

You can stimulate a bowel movement digitally by sticking your index finger gently, but not too far up the rear end. Of course, wear a latex glove. Be careful, as you don't want bleeding to result. At one nursing home, an aide with long fingernails tried to do this, and the patient bled very badly and needed to go to the hospital. She punctured the skin. Stimulating a bowel movement is often done for quadriplegics.

Don't be afraid of giving suppositories, if none of the above works. However, a hospice nurse told me that you don't need to worry about an impacted bowel if someone has at least small bowel movements, passes gas, and the abdomen isn't hard. Those three things. If you're worried anyway, give a suppository. It's easy to do. Wear a latex glove, put some K-Y Lubricating Jelly™ on your index fingertip and apply it to the suppository so it slides in. After a few hours, if your elder hasn't had a bowel movement, do leg exercises. This often works.

Respiratory Problems

With a bedridden elder, don't, as nursing homes do, wait for a cold to turn into pneumonia. At the first sign of a cold, give Sudafed™. Dimetapp™ is good for colds and coughs.

Mucous travels down the throat and then to the lungs. Unlike what many nursing home nurses will tell you, don't let a cold run its course with a person who's weak and can't blow her nose. If your elder has a feeding tube, instead of crushing a Sudafed™ tablet and dissolving it in water, get Dimetapp™ liquid, as a pharmacist suggested to me.

It's obviously important to give plenty of liquids such as water and juice. If your elder has a feeding tube, give these through the feeding tube. However, in the latter case, orange juice that may have pulp can clog a feeding tube. Cranberrry juice is better in that it is acidic with no pulp so it doesn't clog a feeding tube. Further, when my mother had a cold and cough, I would cup my hand when pounding her back.

If your elder's fever reaches 100, give Tylenol™. Respiratory problems are signaled by shortness of breath, pale skin color, cough, loss of appetite, and fever.

The pneumonia vaccine only prevents bacterial pneumonia, not viral pneumonia nor pneumonia from aspiration. The latter involves swallowing difficulties. Futher, flu shots don't prevent all flu.

If your elder has a cough, try to determine if he is coming down with a lung problem. Listen to his cough. If his cough sounds like it's coming from the throat, that's not bad. If his cough sounds like it's coming from the lungs, I would contact the doctor.

A nurse told me that sometimes bladder infections cause coughing. Or, if someone's bowels are full, he may begin coughing.

If someone lacks oxygen, their lips and hands can turn bluish. If you press below their fingernails, the skin color won't come back. However, my mother's lips turned bluish on a number of occasions while bedridden. Her breathing was normal and her oxygen level was fine. Sometimes if an elder is slumped in bed with her head down or at a strange angle for a long time, lips turn bluish.

When my mother had pneumonia at the nursing home, she had shortness of breath and she was pale. The nursing home nurse kept her oxygenated at 90 or above. Therefore, she needed the oxygen tube if her oxygen level dropped below 90. The nursing home nurse checked her oxygen level with an oxygenator.

If your elder has pneumonia, arm exercises are good for the lungs. You can also turn your elder over on his back or side, rubbing or massaging the back to loosen congestion or phlegm.

If your elder is coughing a lot, resposition him. Movement is good for him. Coughing can also be a good exercise for the lungs, as nurses often told me.

Remember that the hardness of the wheelchair's back— rather than the back of a mattress which is softer— is much better for the lungs and breathing. If an elder has pneumonia, it's good to transfer him to a wheelchair for a few hours, twice a day.

If your elder needs x-rays because you fear pneumonia or some other condition, a mobile x-ray service can be sent to your home, if ordered by the doctor. Respirators, even electrocardiography and kidney dialysis can be set up and covered by insurance. Lab technicians' visits, authorized by a doctor, for blood tests and urine samples, for example, are also possible at home. They are covered by private insurance and Medicare.

Bandaging Sores/Tumors

Bandaging sores and tumors is something a nurse will have to show you how to do. How you bandage depends on the type of the wound. I know I was intimidated by the task, thinking that I wouldn't have enough dexterity in my hands to wrap bandages. The hospice nurse, however, demonstrated and I knew I had to do it.

In my mother's final months, my mother's circulation was poor. When my mother developed a foot sore on the heel of her foot, the hospice nurse had me spray wound cleaner on a gauze pad, then hold the pad to the foot sore. I then attached Optifoam™ dressing. I rolled gauze around the Optifoam ™ and taped the gauze. Finally, I rolled a brown adhesive bandage over the gauze. The brown bandage looked somewhat like an Ace™ bandage, only it was sticky in order to hold the gauze in place.

As the nurse described, the wound was black in the center, and had an open pink area in the outer circle. The wound was oozing, but there was no odor to the discharge, so it wasn't infected. The wound needed dressing each day. Of course, you keep the part of the body elevated that has the sore. Therefore, with a foot sore, you put a pillow underneath the ankle, so the foot overlaps the pillow.

If you bandage a sore that is on the rear end, you lift the side of the body that the sore is on, and stick a pillow underneath that side, but not touching the sore. Incidentally, just because a person develops a rear end sore doesn't necessarily mean she can't sit in a wheelchair. Normally, you have a foam cushion on your elder's wheelchair to prevent getting a rear end sore from the hardness of the seat. However, if your elder gets a sore on her buttocks, anyway, depending on the location of the sore, sometimes a "donut-hole" type of cushion can be placed on the wheelchair. This way, the sore is not touching the cushion, but it sinks into the hole of it. In addition, the back of the wheelchair can be tilted so pressure is lessened on the rear end.

The month before my mother died, she developed a sore on her bottom. We used the Optifoam™ bandage. It's very strenuous to try to lift a heavy person onto her side to bandage a rear end sore. Because I was alone, I had to hold my mother on her side with my left hand, leaving me with one hand to cleanse the wound with spray and bandage it. The sore needed to be dressed three times a day. When the hospice volunteer came, she would tilt my mother's body onto her side, so I could work with two hands.

Bandaging my mother's breast tumor on the surface of her skin wasn't hard to do. It was emotionally, but I focused on the nursing duty itself. It had to be done, and I was the only one to do it. I'd spray saline on the tumor to cleanse it. Then, with a Q-Tip Single Tipped Applicator™, (that is, a Q-Tip™ with a long wooden stem and a swab only on one end), I would wipe off the old skin. I would then apply potent Vitamin E cream (with 10,000 i.u. potency) that the home health pharmacy special-ordered for my mother. I would generously apply the cream with the Q-Tips™ over the tumor. I would bandage the tumor with a Telfa™ bandage and cover it with a piece of Tegaderm™, a clear bandage that seals the Telfa™ in place. I would dress the tumor every two or three days, when the bandage looked bloody.

At the nursing home, incidentally, the nurses never changed the bandage, leaving the tumor prey to infection with dried blood. Further, at the nursing home, the aides would actually rub the tumor, a horrible looking raised sore, and try to dry it after a sponge bath, despite instructions that it shouldn't be touched. Rubbing the tumor could cause it to ulcerate, and the patient would then need to be sent to the hospital.

At home, after two days, I would remove the bandage from the tumor, spray the tumor with saline, and take Q-Tip ™ applicators to carefully remove the old cream. Then, I would apply new cream and bandage it again.

At home, I would keep gauze, bandages, and paper tape (non-adhesive white tape) stored in a large plastic storage box. It was see-through, so I could easily see when my bandage supply was getting depleted. In addition, I would wrap batches of bandages and gauze in zippered sandwich bags inside the box.

Beware: a nurse once told me that if a patient is frail, bedsores can also come about if the drawsheets underneath the patient are wrinkled.

Physical Maintenance

A) Using The Hoyer Lift

Maintaining the body physically means "hoyering" your elder into a wheelchair twice a day to encourage good circulation, breathing, and sustaining back muscles.

Before I took my mother home, I was scared about operating a hoyer lift on my own. It's actually quite simple, after some practice. In fact, my major motivation in hiring aides once we got home was to receive help with the hoyer, besides to have sitters to relieve me so that I could get out of the house. I later found that hoyering was an easy task, and that I didn't need to have aides come regularly just to help with this task, as I could do it on my own. Once you "air-lift" a person, you can leave the "pumping lever" of the lift behind, position the wheelchair under the lift, and the go back to the pump side to turn the knob to lower the person into the wheelchair. No doubt, it's easier to have a second person helping so that he can slide the wheelchair more easily under the lift, and so that you can focus your attention on turning the knob of the lift in order to lower the elder in. However, a hoyer lift was actually built so that one person could operate it. In the beginning you may want to enlist the help of a neighbor, if you're feeling insecure.

It's actually easier for your elder to land softly in the wheelchair if you have a foam cushion on the seat. A thick, high foam cushion is not only necessary so an immobile elder doesn't get sores from sitting on the hardness of the wheelchair seat, but the elder seems to land more smoothly into the wheelchair with it, without the body tilting sideways in the chair. The pillow must be foam, otherwise your elder can slide out of the chair. For good circulation, after the elder has been sitting with legs outstretched in bed, it's good to let the legs hang from a wheelchair without the support of the chair's leg rests. (However, if you put your elder's splints on, while she's in her wheelchair, you'll need the leg rests to support the splints. The leg rests support the heaviness of the splints, thereby allowing the feet to lay hard and flat against the splints. This helps delay foot drop, that is, dropping of the anterior portion of the foot.)

If your bedridden elder can stand and pivot, instead of using the hoyer lift, it's better exercise for him to get into the wheelchair with your assistance. When pulling your elder to the edge of the bed, you're actually swinging his torso upwards. You get as close to the bed as possible. You slide your elder's legs over the edge of the bed. You place one of your arms under his shoulder and the other arm under his lower legs. You draw him to sitting position.

I once watched an aide at the nursing home transfer a weak patient from his hospital bed to his wheelchair. The aide lowered the bed to its lowest level possible and positioned the wheelchair at an angle to the bed. The aide applied an elastic wasteband (transfer belt) to the patient. She then supported the patient's knees by placing her knees in front of his knees. She placed her arms under the patient's armpits, pivoted him, and lowered him into the wheelchair. You must always remember to keep your back straight and bend your knees slightly so you don't hurt your back. Before you attempt this, try to have your elder's doctor authorize an insurance-paid visit from a physical therapist to your home and he will demonstrate this technique.

(For elders who aren't totally bedridden but who have some ambulating skills, you can keep them walking to the bathroom, if you stand on their weak side. You'll need to apply a transfer belt to the elder. With one of your hands grasping his transfer belt and with your other hand on his shoulder, you can walk him. You are beside him, though slightly behind him. You keep him close to your body.)

If your elder should somehow fall trying to get out of bed, despite your efforts to keep the bedrails raised, or if your hoyer lift malfunctions and you can't get your elder back to bed, you can call your local Fire Department. One evening, my mother was sitting in her wheelchair. I had transferred her there by hoyer lift. When I tried to transfer her back to bed, I suspected that something might be wrong with the hoyer lift. It didn't seem to be lifting my mother as well as usual. I lowered her back into her wheelchair. I first called the 24-hour emergency number of the hospital home care equipment department that contracted with hospice for the hoyer lift. They said that rather than dispatch a man after hours to fix the lift, I should call the Fire Department. Four firemen came to lift her back to bed.

You can reduce the risk of a bad hoyer lift accident. For example, before you hoyer your elder out of bed, lower the hospital bed in its flat position to its lowest level. You can then raise your elder up in the hoyer at a lower level to transfer her into the wheelchair. A hospice nurse once advised me to do this, so that if my mother fell to the floor in a lift malfunction, it would be less of a fall to the floor.

B) Range of Motion Exercise

It's best to do range of motion exercises first thing in the morning for about 15 minutes to one-half hour. Your elder has been in bed during the night without the benefit of too much movement. After the morning workout, do it at different times during the day. It would be great if your elder gets one or one and one-half hour's total range of motion exercise each day or even more.

It's also wise to do range of motion before the sponge bath, so if your elder has a bowel movement with the exercise, the sponge bath will clean her up. Further, if you limber up the arms and legs with exercise first, the sponge bath will be easier for you to give, lifting your elder's limbered up extremities.

When you do range of motion, keep your elder's body flat, unless her swallowing difficulties won't allow it. Do range of motion exercises on arms, wrists, fingers, legs, ankles, and toes. Try to get your elder to initiate movement. Repeat "bend" and "stretch", when you work on these extremities. Maybe your elder will start bending and stretching on her own, depending on her physical strength and mental acuity.

It's best to loosen your elder's arms up first by rotating the arm at the shoulder. Then you bend at the elbow and stretch the arm out repeatedly. As for range of motion on the legs, when you bend the leg at the knee, you can also move each leg from side to side.

If your elder is bedridden and can't move, the legs begin to contract at the knee. One nurse told me that when one bedridden patient died, her legs were so contracted that her coffin couldn't be shut. Her ankles overlapped on the side of the coffin. In fact, I witnessed a patient at a nursing home who had lived there for 12 years. Her legs were so contracted at the knee, that her ankles weren't hanging from the wheelchair. Rather, they rested sideways on top of the wheelchair's seat, pointing toward the armrests, one leg on top of the other. She had obviously not received enough range of motion exercises on her legs.

At the nursing home, despite the range of motion exercises I did with my mother's legs and arms—three half-hour sessions a day—her legs became contracted because of the way her paralyzed legs were positioned in bed by the nurse's aides. Oftentimes, I felt those exercises I did were negated by the aides, who constantly socked her legs sideways at the knees. They did turn her body on its side and stick a pillow in between her kneecaps to avoid pressure sores so the knees wouldn't rest of top of each other. However, there are ways of doing this comfortably with the person fully pulled up in bed, so the back of the bed isn't tilted too far forward and the person's full body weight isn't resting on the knees.

It's important when positioning an elder to consider the fact that bending her legs too much will force more contractures. If you religiously do range of motion exercises to stretch out the legs, and then keep them bent when you're not giving exercises, the range of motion is in vain. In positioning an elder immediately after range of motion, you could perhaps keep her laying flat or nearly flat on her back for 15 minutes while observing her to make sure she doesn't cough. You could put a pillow underneath each calf of the legs to stretch out each leg.

If you don't want to do a lot of range of motion yourself, if you hire a private aide to help with caregiving, have him do range of motion exercises. You can train him. (I remember at the nursing home, we were willing to pay a few nurse's aides we trusted, more money than what the nursing home paid them per hour, to do just a half-hour range of motion session with my mother, before or after their shift. We got no takers. Motivation and financial rewards aren't high on the list of priorities with many aides.)

C) Massage

While licensed massage therapists make house calls, and many charge $100 or more, it's hard to find someone who'll travel even a few miles for an elderly bedridden person. After about five phone calls to traveling massage therapists, I gave up, and did the massage myself. I knew a hospital physical therapist who was also a licensed massage therapist. She took a few minutes to demonstrate how to give an adequate massage. Basically, to massage an elderly person's back, you don't want her on her stomach. She may have trouble breathing. You place her on her side, using your fingers to make upward movements. To massage even the wrist, for example, massage upward toward the arm, so the elder's hands don't contract more.

Leg massage is particuarly soothing, too. However, if an elder has had blood clots in the legs, deep massage may be harmful. It may burst the blood vessels in the legs.

If you don't want to do massage yourself, you can buy a back massager, one with a long handle and a vibrating square piece. I used one of these while my mother was up in her wheelchair, and it worked well for below her neck and her shoulders. Beside the massage itself, the massager serves to stimulate the alertness of lethargic people. While it's obviously not a doctor-ordered medical nerve stimulator with electrodes that sends electrical impulses to the brain stem, (used for some coma patients), it non-medically serves a purpose.

When my mother was bedridden, she would sometimes get swelling (edema) in her hands, arms, or legs. In my ignorance, I wondered if range of motion or massage might help. The answer is no. To reduce the swelling, you must elevate the swollen part of the body with a pillow. Too much liquid intake sometimes causes swelling. Water pills, taken for this condition, sometimes make people feel uncomfortable. My mother vomited after taking them. You can test for edema by poking your finger into your elder's swollen body part, and if the skin doesn't pop back out, you obviously know it's edema. You can also poke someone's abdomen as a test.

D) Physical Therapy

Although I've dealt sufficiently with physical therapy issues throughout this book, I have one more point to discuss before dealing with the issue of splints.

When I had my mother at home, I called up a physical therapist's agency that sent therapists to facilities. I asked the agency staff if they knew a physical therapist who could make home visits for range of motion and other exercises because my mother's hospice benefits were limited in this area. My mother received about 10 visits, one each week, from hospice physical therapists to do range of motion and sit her up in bed. We wanted to hire a physical therapist who would work privately with her. The agency referred us to someone who used to work with them, but had started her own business. This therapist's office happened to be in our neighborhood, and she made home visits. However, after two visits at $80 an hour, we found that she really didn't want to strain herself by doing any range of motion with a heavy patient, as she'd initially agreed to. She was into alternative methods of stimulation for semi-alert patients. (She didn't tell us this before.) She would apply pressure to each of my mother's inner wrists along the veins for 15 minutes. I asked her if I could do this myself or be trained to. She said I couldn't, and that only she could do it properly. Since she didn't do range of motion as she'd originally agreed to, and I couldn't see any value to applying pressure to my mother's inner wrists, after two visits, I'd figured she'd had a chance to do something for my mother. (The hospice nurse said she'd never heard of this technique she used.) I didn't have the physical therapist return. In two visits, she merely evaluated my mother and squeezed her wrists which apparently didn't seem to have any visible effect on my mother. Beware of advice or service these days, even from people who are professionally licensed. The botton line is, are they following your wishes, and do you see any benefits for your elder?

E) Splints

I've discussed splints throughout this book. However, I'd like to add a few points. Contractures occur in the legs, ankles, arms, wrists, hands, and fingers of paralyzed people and brain-injured people. If you are going to apply splints, apply them after you've done range of motion exercises, when the arms and legs are loosened up and aren't stiff. If applied before range of motion, splints can be painful for your elder.

Leg splints, that are positioned below the knee, can help retard foot drop. They also help retard the curving of the feet inwardly at the ankles. Arm splints are used to help retard contractures at the elbows, wrists, hands, and fingers. Wrist splints can also keep the fingers from digging into the palms of hands. If you don't have arm splints or wrist splints for your elder, what nurses do is they often roll a face washcloth into the palm of each patient's hand to protect the fingers from contracting, and therefore, the fingernails won't dig into the palm. One should beware, however, that by not using arms or wrist splints, and just rolling washcloths into the palms, the person's wrists and fingers are more prone to contracting in gripping the towels. Therefore, many physical therapists fault nurses for doing this.

It's cumbersome for a caregiver to move a person around in bed with the extra weight of splints. I, therefore, applied splints when my mother was in her wheelchair, and removed them when I put her back to bed. She was always in her wheelchair for a few hours at a time, twice daily.

Nutrition

When you have your elder at home, with all the caregiving tasks, it's nice to know that Meals On Wheels can deliver hot food to your elder for lunch. To be put in touch with the program, contact either a senior center close to where you live or your local Area on Aging. Meals On Wheels is administered through the Meals On Wheels Association of America, and it is funded through donations. There is no cost to seniors who can't afford to pay, but a suggested contribution for those who can. Volunteers deliver the meals. The program is largely volunteer-operated.

As people get into their 80s, they may lose their taste buds, or if they take a lot of medications, food doesn't taste good to them. This is what I was told by a nurse. It's a good idea to have fresh fruit in the house at all times for your elder. You should also have a variety of fruit juices.

Although I've dealt extensively with the feeding tube issues in Chapter 4, and also focused on foods that can be eaten by an elder if a family member chooses to begin recreational feeding, I'd still like to make a few points.

If you are operating a feeding tube for your elder, you will likely need to troubleshoot if the tube doesn't function as needed.

Following are points that will help you if you have difficulties with the feeding tube formula not flowing:

1) Squeeze the feeding tube bag, and this may get the formula flowing.
2) Is your elder's arm resting on top of the feeding tube? If so, remove the arm from it.
3) Could it be that the tube is clogged? With a plastic syringe, squirt a teaspoon of a carbonated beverage into the tube. This won't upset your elder's stomach.

Always wrap a terrycloth towel around the lid-opening of the feeding tube in case a little formula drops out either while the tube is running or afterwards. This way, your elder's gown doesn't get soiled. This is also a good idea to do after you've inserted medication through the tube with a syringe. You can then tell if any medication has dropped out.

It's best, too, not to unhook the feeding tube right after the formula has finished. Some formula will probably spill out. Wait about 20 minutes. Or, if you haven't waited 20 minutes, be prepared to bend the rubber around the lid-opening of the tube in case some formula starts seeping out. This will contain it.

If your elder coughs after the feeding tube formula has run or near the end of its flow, this might mean the stomach is full.

When your elder is not being tube fed, always make sure her arm isn't pulling on the tube when you change her diaper or lift her in the hoyer lift. This will cause the tissue (stoma) to bleed.

At home, your elder's private insurance and Medicare will pay for a gravity pole feeding, rather than a tube feeding with a calibrated pump. A calibrated pump often needs to be regulated by a nurse. You see calibrated pumps in hospitals.

Medications

In my years of caregiving, I learned about a variety of drugs and problems that can occur with certain medications. My mother often had allergic reactions to medication, even when she was younger and ambulatory. When she was bedridden, she had an allergic reaction to an antibiotic. She had trouble breathing and her face turned puffy and red. I soon learned that introducing new drugs was usually a problem with my mother. Consequently, when she had infections as a bedridden patient, I always reiterated to her doctor or the on-call doctor what drugs were okay, and what drugs she'd had problems with.

On more than one occasion, I found that doctors prescribed drugs that contained elements that my mother was allergic to. Moral: Don't expect a doctor to always check the patient's chart. Question him and ask, "Does this drug contain (such and such) that she's allergic to?" Sadly, some doctors may not remember all the elements a drug contains.

Always pay attention to medication usage, and have the doctor reorder for your elder before she runs out. This is obviously vital when it's a life-sustaining drug or a narcotic for seizures. Incidentally, if your elder is taking a narcotic, such as an anti-seizure drug, for example, keep the old empty medicine bottle on hand to store some medication in it. In case you spill one bottle, you've got an emergency reserve. It's really easy to tip over a medicine bottle.

If your elder is on a feeding tube, remember that any medication is probably hard on her stomach because she's not taking solid food. If an elder is taking too many medications, it saps her appetite to eat some food by mouth if you're trying to rehabilitate her to swallow.

As I previously discussed in this book, my mother was taking a potassium supplement because a blood test revealed she was low in potassium. In retrospect, this potassium supplement could have been substituted for prune juice, taken via her feeding tube, or it could have been thickened with powder for her to take by mouth. An eight-ounce glass daily of prune juice is very high in potassium. Potassium supplements are hard on one's stomach. You must question the doctor about whether a vitamin supplement is necessary or if it can be substituted with real food. If it is necessary, then ask him how long it needs to be taken. With supplements, doctors may have an elder take them for too long. (Six months after my mother began taking the potassium supplement at the nursing home, the staff nurses still hadn't called the doctor to question its continuation. An agency nurse told me that I should call the doctor. When I did, he discontinued it.)

Miscellaneous Care and Troubleshooting

I want to say a few words about mouth care and ear care. Further, hair care, that is haircuts, are especially necessary for a bedridden person who is always being pulled up in bed, and suffers the discomfort of hair being tugged at around the neck.

As for mouth care, if your elder can open his mouth, you might want to get him an electric toothbrush—one with regular power, not a high-speed 3-D. Use a little tartar control toothpaste and mouthwash, (even a non-alcohol based mouthwash like Biotene™ .) You can take out the residual toothpaste with a toothette, and even use toothettes dipped in water to rinse the mouth. An electric toothbrush obviously massages the gums. You can tell when a person't gums are improving. Instead of being red and soft, they'll turn salmon pink and harden. According to one nurse, she advised me not to stop brushing my mother's teeth if the gums bled. If the gums bled, she said they needed work, and I needed to keep up the hygiene. Further, brush in between the teeth. Flossing is hard to do, especially if the plaque is thick. Some people use a wire brush and pull a flossing string through the teeth, though I found it hard to do this. (If your elder has swallowing difficulties, you may not want to use an electric toothbrush, nor do flossing. Use a child's toothbrush or a soft toothbrush as discussed in Chapter 4.)

As for ear care, in nursing homes, the nurses often don't want to take the time to clean ears. Then, when wax accumulates, they don't want to take the time to irrigate an ear with a syringe and water. If the family member requests cleaning of the ears, the nurses get a doctor's order for special wax softener to loosen wax for three days. Then they shoot water in the ear with a syringe, and swab out the wax. At home, I'd used Q-Tips™ and baby oil every few weeks. I'd put a few drops of baby oil in each ear each day for three days to soften the wax. The baby oil doesn't drip out of the ear when you put it in, if you turn the elder on her side when in bed. You can also clean the ears after you've given a shampoo in bed using a shampoo tray. Having poured pitchers of water to rinse the hair, with water making its way into the ear, you may have softened up your elder's ear wax.

As for haircuts, there are some traveling hairdressers, if you don't want to cut hair yourself. Usually if you ask your own hairdresser, she may know of one, or she may make a house call just for your elder. Your best bet is to ask someone connected with hospice. Even if your elder isn't a hospice patient, you could call a hospice program up on the phone. If worse comes to worst, you can clip your elder's hair yourself. Especially in summer months, hair along the neck is especially uncomfortable in bed. A haircut is obviously best scheduled when your elder is sitting up in her wheelchair.

Following are some tips on care for the bedridden and for the elderly, in general. There are also some points about symptoms of illness:

- Bedridden people who don't get a lot of fresh air can get face rashes. Use Cortaid™ for this. (If one has a face rash, don't wash the face or apply face cream.)
- If a bedridden patient has crusty/mucous-like eyelids that "glue" them shut, place a large wet cottonball over each eye for a few minutes. Gently brush over the eyes and this will unseal them. (Don't, as I've seen nursing home aides do, scrub the eyelids harshly with a dry washcloth.)
- For a crusty nose, use a Q-Tip™ with some lanolin on it.
- Bedridden and immobile people feel cold. Cover their arms with blankets.
- With fevers, use cold washrags on the forehead and use a little rubbing alcohol on arms and legs to cool your elder off.
- Use baby powder with corn starch for diaper rash.
- Some people believe that wearing a copper chain bracelet helps prevent arthritis. They are sold at pharmacies. Truthfully, this didn't seem to help my mother, but it's worth a try since they are inexpensive.
- Some older people suffer falls, and later think they've tripped over something, when in fact, they fell

because they had a stroke. If your bedridden elder somehow hits her head in trying to get out of bed, for example, head injury symptoms include lethargy and a reduced level of talking or (walking).

• Signs of heat stroke can involve: dizziness, rapid heartbeat, breathing problems, diarrhea, nausea or vomiting, throbbing headache, weakness or confusion.

Laundry and Linens

I enlisted the help of a laundry service when I took my mother home. If your loved one is bedridden, this may be a good idea. Since I used a lot of linen and washcloths for sponge baths and for incontinent care, this made sense to me. You can sometimes find a laundry service that will pick up and deliver that isn't expensive, if done by the pound. My first attempt at finding a laundry service didn't work out well. For towels and linen, I was averaging $39.50 a week plus another $10 to pick up and deliver. They'd only pick up and deliver once a week, so I'd have to pay a sitter to relieve me, to make it over there to drop off more laundry. After a couple of months, I did even more checking, and found a wonderful laundry service. It would pick up and deliver free twice a week, and the total bill was $40 a week. I had three full "lawn" garbage bags each pickup. It pays to make about 15 phone calls. With this second laundry, because my mother was a senior citizen, the kind manager said he'd pick up and deliver for free.

The first commercial laundry charged $12 for the first eight pounds and $1.25 for each pound over eight pounds. As for the second laundry I found, it was a family-owned drycleaner that did laundry for a $1 per pound, including free delivery. They gave me a special rate because I gave them a lot of business.

Don't go to a laundry charging by the piece. Some charge as much as $1.25 per piece. Find a laundry that charges by the pound, anywhere from $1.25 to $1.50.

Remember that heavy bath towels add to your laundry bill, and they aren't necessary for a sponge bath.

Make sure the laundry service weighs your laundry not when it's wet, but after it's done and dry. Some will have a nominal delivery charge, if they don't give seniors free delivery. Make sure they wash your laundry separately and not with the laundry of other parties. Make absolutely sure, too, that's it's a commercial laundry and that they don't use coin-operated washers that the public comes in and uses.

Incidentally, look under "Drycleaners" in the Yellow Pages of the phonebook, and you'll find more laundries because they are connected to drycleaning businesses. (Don't just look under "Laundry.")

If you don't enlist a laundry service, be sure to keep up with doing laundry every day, instead of letting it pile up. In this case, you'll need a good washer and dryer that aren't about to break down.

It's a good idea to keep dirty, wet towels in a large plastic storage bin with a lid in the bathroom until they are hauled off or washed by you. This is what I did, so I could disinfect the bin every once in a while.

As for other laundry, my mother, being bedridden, wore hospital gown "substitutes," that were actually very pretty. Real hospital gowns with the open back, suitable for changing diapers, etc., are really expensive at medical supply stores. The solution is to buy inexpensive cotton smocks at stores such as K-Mart, and cut the back side of them from the neck downward, sewing in ribbons that can be tied like hospital gowns. These smocks obviously make changing diapers simple. They also have another useful purpose. If one's arms are bent at the elbow, because the elder has contractures, the smocks allow the arms to slip in easily. That is, you don't have to push the bent arms backwards to fit into the sleeves, as you would with a garment that opens in front.

As for changing dirty linen, you'll often have to change the linen while your elder is in bed. To change soiled bed linen while she's in bed, you first remove the old linen by starting at the top of one side of the bed and turning your elder on her side to roll the dirty linen under the body.

Once the linen reaches your elder's body, you turn the body to the other side, and continue rolling the linen off the bed. It should be noted that as you go, you're also fitting the new bedsheet onto the bed as you're removing the old one. That is, after you remove the fitted sheet at the top of one side of the bed, you quickly insert a new sheet there, and as you're scooting out the old sheet, you're inserting the new sheet under your elder's body before she urinates onto the mattress. This technique also saves the elder the trouble of being rolled back and forth too many times to take off the old sheet and put on the new sheet.

The following is a schedule of care that I made up for my mother. Some of these tasks won't apply to your elder, particularly if he doesn't have a feeding tube.

Sample Schedule of Care For The Bedridden

8 a.m.—Changed diaper/swabbed mouth with wet toothettes.

8:15 a.m.— Range of motion exercises. Arms, wrists, hands, fingers, legs, ankles, toes. Bending and stretching, plus circular motions. (i.e. Gently bent fingers back and forth at the knuckles. Then did circular motions with them. Gently turned ankles in circular motion. Gently moved toes in circular motion.)

8:30 a.m.—Sponge bath—head to toe.
—Cleaned eyelids, if needed, with cottonballs dipped in warm water.
—Cleaned feeding tube site with washcloth dabbed with soap and dampened with water. Then rinsed

with damp cloth, dried and applied Vitamin E cream around the tube site.

9 a.m.—Changed diaper.

9:15 a.m.—Ate by mouth.

9:45 a.m.—Brushed teeth. Filled a styrofoam cup with a half-glass of water. Put a dab of toothpaste on the inside edge of the cup. Wet the toothette and added a dab of toothpaste. Wrung out the toothette against the inside edge of the cup so my mother with her swallowing problems didn't get too much water in her mouth. Brushed teeth with toothette. Then took another styrofoam cup, filled it with water and some mouthwash, and rinsed with a new toothette.

10 a.m.— Medication (liquid given through the feeding tube) with a plastic syringe, along with 50 cc. of water to wash down the medication. Then, flushed the tube of any residual medication with another 20 cc. of water.

10:05 a.m.—Feeding tube formula ran for one-half hour. Flushed the tube with 200 cc. of water (a small glass), so the residual formula didn't clog the tube. Note: The feeding tube bag and syringe should be changed each day.

10:35 a.m.—More medication through feeding tube. (Note: if medication doesn't come in liquid form, you can get a small, inexpensive pill masher at the pharmacy, rather than try to crush the pill into granules yourself. If you mash a tablet, dissolve it with water in a cup before pushing it through the feeding tube. Then flush the tube again with 20 cc. of water to make sure all medication flowed through the tube.)

11:30 a.m.—Changed diaper. (Changed an hour late to allow mother to digest feeding tube formula and medication.)

11:45 a.m.—Hoyer-lifted to wheelchair.

12:45 p.m.—Ate by mouth.

1:15 p.m.—Brushed teeth.

2:30 p.m. —Hoyer-lifted back to bed. (Changed diaper one hour late due to wheelchair sitting.)

3 p.m.—Dressed foot sore and put "moon boot" (cloth foot boot) on. Kept foot elevated with a pillow, so the sore would heal.(Note: You can dress the foot sore each day.)

3:30 p.m.—Dressed tumor. (Dressed it every two days according to hospice specifications.)

4 p.m.—Range of motion exercises (one-half hour).

4:30 p.m.—Changed diaper. (Note: It's good to change a diaper after range of motion (ROM) with the legs, as it stimulates urination.)

4:35 p.m.—Hoyer-lifted to wheelchair.

4:45 p.m.—Ate by mouth.

5:20 p.m.— Brushed teeth. (Note: At night use a toothbrush, instead of a toothette to massage the teeth. Use same method as outlined before with the toothette.)

5:30 p.m.—Feeding tube formula.

7:35 p.m.—Hoyer-lifted back to bed. (Changed diaper one hour late due to wheelchair sitting.)

9:35 p.m.—Changed diaper.

10 p.m. —Medication (liquid pushed through feeding tube, with syringe.) And, flushed tube with 20 cc. of water.

10:05 p.m.—Feeding tube formula followed by 200 cc. of water to flush tube.

11:05—More liquid medication followed by 20cc. of water through feeding tube.

12:05 a.m.— Changed diaper one-half hour late to allow digestion of formula and medication.

12:15 a.m.—Sponge bath.

12:45— Range of motion exercises (10 minutes).

1 a.m.—Changed diaper again before bedtime.

6 a.m.—Changed diaper (after five hours, since I needed to sleep).

8 a.m.—Changed diaper. Another day begins.

During the day, I would read to my mother; play music tapes and Italian language tapes (of her native language); and show family photos and picture books, among a variety of activities.

As a caregiver of a bedridden person, I was scrupulous in charting daily in a notebook. I would chart the amount of each medication given; the amount of the feeding tube formula given; estimated calories of food eaten by mouth; and liquids given. I would also, of course, chart the time. I would keep track of bowel movements as small, medium, or large. When I bandaged sores or the tumor, I would also note those times. Further, I would record daily activities such as reading, listening to music, showing family photos, using flash cards for math skills, etc., noting the time of day of each activity. Not only is a record good for you, but it is essential for outside caregivers who relieve you. Never rely on your memory, especially for medications. A lot of medications are given 12 hours apart. When you're under stress and tired, you can't often remember what medications you gave in the morning. When my mother had a bladder infection, she would take more medications than usual, so I highlighted all medications with a felt pen.

Supplies

You should use a pharmacy for supplies that specializes in home health care products or get them through a medical supply store.

If you buy a lot of home health care supplies, often home health pharmacies and medical supply stores will work out discounts for you, particularly if you buy a product in bulk. For example, I'd go through a lot of toothettes for my mother. If I bought two large boxes, instead of one, which would last her a few months, I'd get a good discount.

To simplify your life, the medical supply store will have supplies shipped for free if you spend over a certain dollar amount (about $75). This is cheaper than having to pay a sitter to come while you're out to pick up supplies.

For general household products, latex gloves and adult diapers, you could get a membership at a discount store for big savings.

   While the following is an extensive list of supplies, you can pick and choose which ones you'll need and make your own list.

A)Regular Healthcare Products

1) Bandaids
2) Baby oil (for ears)
3) Large cottonballs
4) Box of tissues
5) Ear swabs
6) Vaseline™ —(To soothe and heal little sores and dry
      skin. Good for chapped lips, too.)
7) Baby powder with corn starch
8) Baby shampoo
9) Body lotion
10) Nail clipper (Don't use if your elder has diabetes or
      other foot problems. In this case, get help from a
      nurse.)
11) Depends ™ (Pads for incontinence)
12) Toothbrush
13) Diaper wipes (without alcohol). Can be used in between
      sponge baths, if you don't want to use up a lot of
      terrycloth towels.
14) Disposable cotton briefs.(To fit over a diaper for added
      protection. Available at a supermarket pharmacy.)
15) Poise Pads™ —(Insert these pads inside a diaper, espe-
      cially during the night. They will help absorb urine.)

B)More Specialized Healthcare Products

1) Suppositories
2) K-Y Lubricating Jelly ™ (to apply a suppository)
3) Cough syrup

4) Extra Strength Tylenol™ (for fever)—Liquid Tylenol for tube feeders.

5) Sudafed™ (for colds—dries up drainage quickly)

6) Dimetapp™ (for colds and coughs)

7) Digital thermometer (to put under armpit)

8) Q-Tip ™ Single Tipped Applicators (For cleaning under the feeding tube site where residual formula accumulates or for cleaning a surface tumor).

9) Toothettes (Available at home health pharmacy or medical supply store).

10) Paper tape for gauze (Ask a nurse about particular gauze and creams for special conditions.)

11) Surgical masks (In case you have a cold, to protect your elder from it. Available at pharmacies).

12) Blue pads (Disposable cotton liners which absorb the overflow of diaper leaks. Available through a medical supply store).

13) Latex gloves—Can be bought in bulk at a discount store rather than paying much more at a pharmacy or medical supply store.

14) Rubbing alcohol wipes (To disinfect a patch of skin, or to clean an oxygen tube or the insertion plug of a feeding tube bag, in case the latter brushes the floor).

15) Bottle of rubbing alcohol (To clean pan that you drain urine from catheter into, before dumping urine into the toilet.)

16) Bed pan

17) Medicine cups (30 milligram cups, to measure out liquid medication.)

18) Milk of Magnesia™

19) Pill crusher

20) Ocean Spray™ —saline spray for nasal dryness

21) Vicks Vaporub™ —(You can even put a dab on the patient's nose to clear up nasal passages, as a nurse suggested to me.)

22) Saline—(Sterile water that you can use to cleanse skin around the feeding tube site. Apply saline

with a Q-Tip Single Tipped Applicator™.)
23) Lanolin—(Comes in a tube. Works well for removing crust around the nose nostrils.)
24) Shampoo tray (For shampoo in bed, available at a medcal supply store).

C) Special Clothing/Linen

1) Twelve smocks (Instead of hospital gowns. Should be cotton as it is easier on the skin than polyester).
2) Two washable bedspreads (cotton).
3) Four pillows (for side/head/under legs). Pillows should be "springy," that is fiber-fill. These prevent bedsores with immobile people. More pillows are often good to have on hand, in case the hospital bed malfunctions and the back of the bed can't be raised.
4) Terrycloth washcloths/hand towels (Buy in bulk at a discount store.)
5) Three bath towels
6) Extra pillow cases
7) A terrycloth bathrobe (for wearing in a wheelchair)
8) Laprobe for wheelchair
9) Two fitted sheets for hospital beds (Can buy them at a home health pharmacy).
10) Four drawsheets (Available at a medical supply store).
11) Miniature pillows (For in between the ankles, when an elder is resting on her side, to prevent bedsores. Also good to prevent sores under the armpits).
12) Cloth boots to prevent foot sores.
13) Old towels/old clothing—(To be used under the chin, in case your elder vomits).
14) Two flannel shirts (These can be worn over smocks when an elder is in a wheelchair. These shirts will help keep them warm.)

D) Regular Household Products

1) Toilet paper
2) Paper towels
3) Garbage bags—for dirty diapers
4) Air freshener
5) Mild bar soap
6) Pine Sol™ or Lysol™
7) Large plastic storage bin (for dirty laundry)
8) Plastic storage box (to store gauze and bandages)
9) Zippered sandwich bags—(to wrap up gauze and bandages)
10) Paper cups (to stir medications dissolved with water)
11) Plastic dishpans (For sponge bath use and to place on floor to drain a catheter).
12) Extra plastic wastebasket (for dirty diapers)
13) Extra outside garbage can (For dirty diapers, etc. You'll have a lot more garbage than usual).
14) Nine-volt batteries (for smoke alarms)
15) Batteries (for flashlight and transistor radio)

E) Useful Products/Appliances

1) Fire extinguisher
2) Space heater—(In case furnace conks out. Must not be left unattended).
3) Fan—(In case you don't have air conditioning).
4) Hair blower
5) Flashlight
6) Television
7) Radio
8) Two alarm clocks

F) Foods

1) Prune juice
2) Cranberry juice
3) Carbonated beverages (for upset stomach)
4) Fresh fruits
5) Peppermint tea (For cancer patients to soothe their stomach).
6) Thickened juice and thickening powder (for foods/ soups). For elders with swallowing problems, these are available through a medical supply store.

For a tube feeder, formula, bags, and plastic syringes will not only be covered by private insurance and Medicare, and Medicaid, but they will be delivered for free from a special supply department through a hospital.

Keeping Yourself in Good Health as a Caregiver

If you should burn out on caregiving, and your loved one isn't in the hospice program, sometimes foster homes offer respite care for a couple of weeks or a month to elders.

As a caregiver to an elder, the stress is substantial. A nurse can go home at the end of the day—you can't. Don't bite off more than you can chew, otherwise you may become an abuser, just like some of the aides at nursing homes who handle patients wrecklessly, while turning them in bed.

If you decide to truly devote yourself to your loved one's care, then don't try to achieve a whole lot in other parts of your life. Take the attitude that you've made this your priority and you can't burn yourself out by trying to do a lot of other things, too. Just do small things for yourself until such time as you feel you no longer want to make caregiving such a large part of your life.

As for the physical demands of being a caregiver to a bedridden person, consider ways to prevent ill-health and injury to yourself.

As for my getting sleep, the last month of my mother's life was truly taxing on me. My mother was never frail and had beautiful skin until her nursing home days when she had bouts of skin breakdown. At home, I was worried about my mother being able to get enough care during my bedtime hours. Throughout my life, all I've needed is five hours of sleep.

I tried to give my mother all of her liquids and feeding tube formula well in advance of my bedtime, so that she wouldn't be urinating as much during the night and I could get four hours, sometimes five, of uninterrupted sleep. Yes, a patient is supposed to be turned and changed every two hours, but this rarely happens at nursing homes—it's more like every five hours at a nursing home. Therefore, at home, during the night, my mother wasn't any worse off, than she would have been at a nursing home. I don't think that having had a graveyard shift nurse's aide at the house, would have helped much. You see, some who work graveyard shift do their sleeping while you're not watching. And, many work dayshift, so they look for a graveyard shift position so they can doze off at that time and still earn money. Two of my friends experienced this when they hired graveyard shift aides.

In fact, agencies will sometimes send you someone who's already worked 8, 10, 12, or even 16 hours that day, to work graveyard shift. A day aide from an agency once bragged to me that she once worked 24 hours straight, going to three different homes.

Therefore, no matter what you do at home when you're caring for your elder alone, it's often much more than what several hired people will do, or a nursing home could ever do.

slippers. When you wear slippers all day long, and don't get the type of exercise you should from walking, that stationary position often leads to circulatory problems in your legs—swollen legs, feet, and ankles. I began having to wear support stockings, prescribed by the doctor. When you go to bed at night, you remove the support hose, and elevate your legs with a pillow. After my mother died, after a couple of months of normal activity, my leg, feet, and ankle problems disappeared.

Arm soreness and swollen rib cartilage problems aren't uncommon among caregivers of bedridden family members. My problems started at the nursing home.

In pulling my mother up in bed and turning her, and in doing range of motion exercises with her arms and legs, my doctor told me to do strengthening exercises for myself, since I obviously had no time to go to the gym and work-out. For my arms, I had some hand weights at home, lifting my elbows up and down, while holding the weights. I'd also bend over at my waist, doing circular motions with my arms pointing downward. In lifting my mother, although I'd try to keep my back as straight as possible, my neck would give me problems. Therefore, I did neck exercises, tilting my head back slowly, looking up at the ceiling, then lowering my head downward.

Pulling an elder up in bed, and lifting her legs to place pillows in between them is also extremely physical work. If the elder is paralyzed and dead weight, doing range of motion is physically demanding, too. I weigh 117 pounds. My mother, when she was ambulatory and active after recovering from her brain cancer, weighed 145 pounds. However, after being bedridden and receiving feeding tube formula, she ballooned up to 170 pounds. I was able to do this very physical work by wearing an elastic back support, the kind you can get at either a medical supply store or even at a discount store. People who work in factories who do a lot of lifting use these back supports that have straps fitting of lifting use these back supports that have straps fitting over the shoulder, and two bands that run from across the back to meet at the waist. In addition, you should always wear tennis shoes or rubber-soled shoes in lifting and turning your elder.

To preserve your back, you should roll your elder over in bed by placing the hospital bed at your thigh level. Make sure your elder's arms are at her sides. Use the drawsheet to turn your elder toward you. Keep your knees bent and chin up.

Another problem that caregivers face is severely chapped hands. You wear latex gloves when you give sponge baths and clean your elder. However, you constantly wash your hands, too. At bedtime you should slather on hand lotion so that your hands get a few hours of good treatment.

Chapter 7

Stimulation For The Elderly Person

Whether your elder is institutionalized or not, try to keep her as functional as possible. One way is to exercise her memory by talking about family members. Does it really matter if an elder has her sister confused with her daughter? At least some of the time, perhaps she has some concept that someone is a family member.

Structure is important. If you have an elder in a nursing home, go visit her on a regular schedule, so that the staff will tell her to expect your visit. If she's at home, take her out on a regular errand each day, if she's capable of leaving the house. Take her into a grocery store and walk her through the aisles. Keep reminding her where you're at and what you're shopping for.

It's hard to take an elder shopping for her clothes. With my mother, when she was ambulatory, she would complain about being hungry or tired, and I'd be under so much stress I'd end up hurrying and buying the wrong size shirt for her. You're better off just going on your own, and taking your chances that the garment will fit.

In nice weather, you can wheel your elder outside for a walk, if she's not ambulatory, whether or not she is institutionalized. The smell of fresh air, a fresh mown lawn, flowers, or the sound of traffic is stimulating.

Stimulating Your Elder's Communication

With an elder, you can try stimulating her alertness and language skills with a number of exercises. These exercises were told to me by a speech therapist.

At one nursing home, when I wanted a speech therapist to evaluate my mother for speech so that she could progress in her communication abilities, I stated in a letter to the doctor that she was talking in complete sentences at times, and at other times she would communicate by laughing, making sounds, smiling, opening her mouth ahead of time to signal that she wanted another spoonful of food. Because there were no liability issues with speech therapy, I found that speech therapists in this field were often more willing to work with lethargic patients, than those who specialized in swallowing problems. A speech therapist can always give you a set of exercises to do so you can stimulate your elder's speech. Further, if your elder doesn't respond verbally when a speech therapist evaluates her for language, and your elder's insurance says it won't pay for any future visits until she shows improvements, then document the alternative communication skills she uses. Document the sounds she makes and if she nods, and what they were in response to. Call the speech therapist to get recommendations on how you can elicit more responses, either verbally or otherwise.

For my mother, I would take an object that made noise like a bell, and I would ring it in front of her to get her to look at it. I'd repeat this exercise a few times, trying to get her to focus on the bell a little longer each time. Next, I'd move the bell to her right side, and then to her left side to try to get her to track the object.

The next step was to get an object that didn't make noise, going through the same routine as above.

Another exercise involved using strickly my voice as a stimulus. I would stand in front of my mother, and say her name, trying to get her to focus on me. Next, I would stand on her right side, and repeat her name, seeing if she would turn her head my way. Then, I'd go to her left side and do the same. I would also just sit in front of her wheelchair and talk to her, trying to increase the amount of time she would pay attention to me. This works well for those who suffer from Alzheimer's, too.

As for language stimulation, I would play tapes of Italian songs (in her native language) that she used to like, and I'd sing along with the tapes, holding her hand and rhythmically beating out each syllable of the piece. I'd encourage her to hum along. I'd repeat the song a few more times. When I sang the words, I'd see if she could produce one or two words of it. She didn't seem to be able to do this.

Using a family photo is important, too. I would talk about a family photo and try to get my mother to focus on it. I would point at a person in the photo and ask if she remembered that person. Then I'd ask, "Yes?" I was trying to see if she would respond "yes" or nod her head. Then I'd say, "That's Omero, your brother, isn't it?" I'd see if she would respond yes or show some expression of recognizing him. If she was responding, I'd ask another question that involved a "yes" answer. "Did you live in Italy with Omero?" If she was really alert, I'd give her a multiple choice question such as, "Did you live in Italy or America at that time?" If I got no response, I'd have her repeat the right answer to stimulate her speech.

In performing these exercises, I'd close the door to the room, making sure there were no outside distractions or sounds of a television or radio. I always explained to my mother what speech activities I was going to do with her, and why I was performing them.

Mumbling and slurring words is normal after a stroke if an elder hasn't talked in a long time or exercised her vocal chords.

If your elder is having a good day, the exercises could be performed twice a day, once in the morning and once in the evening. If your elder is not paying attention, she could be approached later in the day. Each day, give your elder choices. Ask, "Would you like to watch television or listen to the radio?"

With comatose or semi-comatose people, there might every once in a while be a burst of speech. It's like electricity coming on without warning. I noticed that sometimes my mother would say, "Hi" or "Thank you," or say a sentence in her native language of Italian or speak in English. Other semi-comatose people at the nursing home did this, too. If my mother was in discomfort, she would sometimes say a few words.

Sensory Stimulation

My mother really responded to sound such as music. Tapes of music are great, particularly if there are words sung in someone's native language that she hasn't spoken in a long time. They may awaken her from sleep. You can do simple things to stimulate your loved one's senses. To have her utilize the sense of sight, show her pictures on calendars, and read the description underneath. Show her flash cards with pictures of animals. You can find these flash cards at educational stores for preschool and kindergarten kids. Addition and subtraction flash cards are good, too, for those who've had a stroke.

As for the sense of smell, when I'd put a bottle of perfume up to my mother's nose, she would lean forward to smell it. You can also stimulate response by having elders smell the spices in the kitchen. If an elder can verbally communicate, have him guess what a particular spice is.

Touch is therapeutic. Give massages to comatose people. A nerve stimulator has been used for coma patients injured in car accidents. We read about this in our local newspaper, two years after my mother's head injury accident, but we were never told of this option by her doctor. Electrodes are taped to the wrist at the median nerve. They send electrical impulses from the wrist up to the arm to the brain stem. Some comatose patients begin to awaken and gradually show interaction with others and cognitive function. Some begin responding to commands, such as holding up a finger, taking food by mouth, standing with assistance, or they start talking within a few months. Some continue to miraculous recoveries. As for my mother, too bad we didn't hear of this before. Our mother could perhaps have awakened from her coma much earlier and made better progress.

Another method of stimulating your elder, if he isn't too heavy, is to have two people each put one of their arms underneath his armpits and lift him to standing position. Incidentally, my brother and I didn't want to attempt to lift our mother to standing position. She was too heavy. However, movement is such a powerful stimulant. If my mother slid down in her wheelchair, I'd lower the wheelchair's back until it was flat, and I'd be able to pull her up in her wheelchair by placing my arms under her armpits.

With a bedridden stroke patient and even an Alzheimer's sufferer, you can sometimes intiate movement, even walking, by standing them up. You place your arms under their armpits and balance them against your knees. On their own, these same people won't move, stand up, nor even be able to lift their torso if they slump over.

For a bedridden person, being up in a wheelchair— even the motion of getting her up into the wheelchair by hoyer lift— is stimulating. Little by little, you can increase the time your elder spends in her wheelchair. This also builds physical endurance.

As I've said, wheelchair rides outdoors are great. When my mother came home, the hospice physical therapist set up a ramp going out the back door of the house so I could get my mother to the patio.

Too much activity for a bedridden person in one day isn't good as he'll probably just tune out at some point and fall asleep. Spread out special activities over a period of a few days. For example, after you've worked on stimulation through speech exercises, let your elder rest. Try not to have a visitor drop in. Have the visitor come the next day.

If your loved one is ambulatory, encourage walking, even if it's just a few steps from one side of the room to another, or to the bathroom. She should wear rubber-soled shoes or slippers that have back support and provide traction. If dementia is a problem and she's at home, then block off steps with one of those wooden toddler fences. Make sure halls are well-lit, and be sure to remove miniature throw rugs that can be tripped over. Don't polish floors.

Instead of sponge baths, the stimulation of a shower is great for ambulatory elders. Put a bath seat in the shower, install a grab rail, and help your elder to use it to lift herself up from the chair after the shower. You should also encourage using the toilet, if possible. Install a grab rail that fastens onto the back of the toilet seat. If she is able to get to the bathroom, keep a hall light on during the night outside her bedroom, so she may be able to get to the bathroom on her own.

Encourage some independence if she is ambulatory. Have a sitting chair with armrests that are suitable for your elder to lift herself up out of the chair with.

If your loved one is semi-functional, try to keep her using her mind for as long as you can. When my mother's memory began to deteriorate years after her brain cancer surgery, I'd tell her exactly what we were doing when we went out on an important errand to the bank to involve her. At the bank, I'd explain to her how we were depositing her social security check.

If you have your elder at home, and you have relief caregivers coming in, you need to instruct them on how to keep your elder stimulated and entertained. Even alert and responsive elders have trouble entertaining themselves. Relief caregivers don't know anything about how your elder used to occupy himself before he became old, so they'll look to you to give them suggestions. Again, if you can, try to space out visitors and activities so that your elder isn't super busy one day, and has nothing to do the next day.

My goal, when my mother was ambulatory, was to get her out of the house twice daily, if only to accompany me on errands. She wouldn't get restless if she could get out and about.

Both for elders who are ambulatory and for those who are bedridden, dehydration is a concern. It causes mental confusion, besides physical problems. Giving an elder enough liquids, about five or six glasses daily, is good. Particularly if one is ambulatory, give him water before exiting the house. On a hot day, carry a water bottle for him in the car.

Elders sometimes have blood sugar problems. I often thought my mother had blood sugar problems, but it was never revealed on tests. When she was ambulatory, one minute she might not be making any sense. She would be speaking of stolen or missing items. (Many elders with dementia fixate on theft and "missing" money.) Then, five minutes later, after eating and drinking water, she would be a completely different person, appearing normal and making sense again. She seemed 20 years younger. To a caregiver, it's confusing, exhausting emotionally, and even frightening to see an elder go through changes like these during the day. With my mother, I wondered if I could leave her alone in the house for a half-hour, worrying that her confusion might be the onset to a seizure, for example.

In extreme summer heat, a lot of elders become confused. They can even become ill if they are on certain types of medication. Check with your elder's doctor about medication she takes, and whether it's harmful in the heat.

Chapter 8

Long-Term Care Insurance

To Have Or Not To Have

Long-term care insurance doesn't just cover nursing homes, but all kinds of care including home care. You may not only want to check into it for your elder, but for yourself.

Do you need it? Are you even eligible for it, given your medical history or present condition? These are questions to consider. Financial planners usually don't recommend this coverage for those under 45. Insurers start talking to you about it when you're turning 50. My homeowners' insurance agent cornered me at the age of 49.

My mother had enough assets for care, and even if she hadn't had them, she wouldn't have been eligible for long-term care insurance at the age of 65. Due to medical misdiagnosis, her breast cancer— that she had surgery for at 57 that was also misdiagnosed—had spread to her brain. Would she even have been eligible for the insurance at age 57?

Most people consider a long-term care policy at age 60. If you do get long-term care insurance, make sure your policy will pay for the widest choice of care options.

Private health insurance companies sell long-term care insurance. Life insurance companies do, too, along with financial services companies. You can even ask your insurance agent who insures your home and car.

When you're younger, you often have more pressing financial obligations than long-term care insurance. With Baby Boomers often becoming parents in their 40s, some at age 60 are still saving for their children's college education. Besides, they often feel they have little chance of collecting on their long-term care insurance any time soon.

Younger buyers pay lower premiums, but face more years of payments, and a greater chance they'll get stuck with an obsolete plan.

If you have few assets and little money, the premiums are out of sight for you. A retired person could pay $3,000 a year in premiums, depending on when he initiated the coverage. Conversely, the wealthy can afford to pay for their own care. It probably would make little sense for a single person with $2 million in assets, who's in her twilight years, to pay premiums for long-term care insurance, because if she gets to the point of needing care, she'll be able to afford it.

Start by asking yourself if there's longevity in your family, or if your family has a history of debilitating disease. With some nursing home costs running about $7,000 a month, people with less than $125,000 would soon exhaust their assets and savings and qualify for Medicaid, the government's insurance for the poor. Private insurance and Medicare, the federal healthcare program for seniors, will usually only provide for a few months of skilled nursing home care to help one recover from a short illness or injury.

Types of Coverage

Have a knowledgeable friend or financial adviser figure out the break-even point of a long-term care policy. That is, how long you would have to be in a nursing home to get back all the premiums you paid. What I have learned myself from my insurance agent is to avoid policies that require a hospital stay before benefits start. An important question to ask, is how long you must pay for care before the policy takes over?

You'll have to take a physical and pass a cognitive test to get most individual policies. The insurance agent who offered to sell me a plan warned, "Don't get cute with your answers during the cognitive test. If they ask you who the President of the United States is, don't say Abraham Lincoln."

You should also buy only a guaranteed-renewable policy with premiums that remain constant.

Further, find a policy that covers cognitive impairment, as well as medical necessity. As my mother's memory began to fail, years after radiation to her brain from her brain cancer, she could perform daily living tasks, such as brushing her teeth, etc., but she had to be reminded to do so. Does the coverage kick in when assistance with tasks such as eating and bathing are needed? Diseases such as Alzheimer's and Parkinson's should be stated as being covered.

You can get unlimited long-term care insurance for any situation, including home, assisted living, and nursing home for an indefinite period.

As a caution, make sure there isn't a cap on benefits. I read the policy of a friend's mother who had Alzheimer's and the policy has a five-year limit on benefits. The Alzheimer's sufferers I've known have gone on for ten years or more.

If you do decide to get long-term care coverage, buy the coverage from a company that is financially stable. If a company fails, or a new company takes over the claims process, this could get really complicated. Ratings for companies can be found in Standard and Poor's Directories at your library. You want a company with at least $1 billion in assets and years of experience in long-term care. It's necessary to compare benefits among companies. Make sure the policy pays for skilled care once you leave the hospital, intermediate care at a nursing home after you leave skilled care, assisted living care and custodial care. Ask if the coverage is valid in other states. What if you move to a different state to be close to your adult children? You want to know, too, if adult day care and homemaker services, such as cooking and cleaning, are covered besides home health care.

What is the daily benefit for each type of care? Is there a fixed daily amount, no matter what your expenses? Your daily costs will depend on where you plan to retire. You won't need, for example, to cover the full cost of a nursing home if you have a good pension. Another question: What is the maximum payment amount over the life of the policy?

A tricky point in the coverage is who determines when you're eligible for the benefits to kick in. Your doctor or one appointed by the insurer?

In addition, look at the options that can reduce premiums. What is the benefit period? Do you want only one year of coverage, three, five years, or unlimited lifetime payments?

Finally, what sort of inflation protection is available? With costs rising so quickly, look for a generous inflation rider.

Group Plans

If you work for a corporation, you may have the chance to sign up for long-term care insurance through it. About 20 percent of U.S. companies with 500 or more employees offer this coverage, usually at the worker's expense. However, with a group plan, you'll be limited to the options your employer chooses. Beware that since the insurance contract is with your employer, not you, your employer might one day change the terms or allow a premium increase. Conversely, an individual policy's terms can't be changed, and the insurer normally has to petition the state insurance department for a rate hike.

When weighing an employer policy, make sure you can take it with you if you leave the company and the state. Next, ask if it is "tax-qualified," meaning that it meets federal guidelines for coverage and therefore pays tax-free benefits and could entitle you to a tax deduction for the premiums.

If you go with a group plan, ask for a copy of the policy from your employer, not just the company's description of it.

The National Association of Insurance Commissioners in Kansas City, MO puts out a guide called "A Shopper's Guide to Long-Term Care Insurance." The NAIC is an association of state government officials. Its members consist of the chief insurance regulators in all states. It protects the interests of insurance consumers. Have the Association send you its free guide by calling (816) 842-3600.

The American Association of Retired Persons puts out numerous publications including one on long-term care insurance. Contact the Association toll-free at 1-888-687-2277. Its address is 601 "E" St., NW, Washington, DC 20049.

Above all, have an attorney look over any long-term care insurance policy before you get it.

What To Do Without Long-Term Care Insurance

Without long-term care insurance, when an elder becomes ill and needs care, if an adult child has the means to help, an elder could sell his home to her over time. This would allow raising cash and remaining in one's home. Then the adult child could sell the home at the time of the elder's death, and recoup her investment or even come away with a profit.

To raise money for your parent's care, you could buy his car from him or his personal possessions. I had a friend who bought her mother's jewelry.

Inquire of your CPA, too, under what circumstances you can claim your parent or other elder family member, such as an aunt, as a dependent if you contribute financially to her care.

You can explore subsidy options by starting with the website of the National Council on the Aging, (www.ncoa.org). Also look for local agencies and regional resources.

Chapter 9

How Family Members Can Cope With Illness and Death

Ways for Caregivers to Find Strength

Many people will spend at least some time caring for an elderly family member, either before he reaches a nursing home, or even in his final months of life.

Caregivers often live in isolation, and isolation breeds phobias. Oftentimes, counselors, psychologists,and medical people are quick to give advice, many of whom have never spent a day of their lives caregiving. I remember watching on television as a counselor talked about working with family caregivers. She said she decided not to care for her own mother. She didn't get along with her. Her mother was in a foster home. I wondered if she could truly understand the emotions of caregivers who deal, for example, with the frustrating memory problems of elders, their repetitive statements, and the repetitive tasks that elderly people with dementia perform?

The elder you care for becomes like a mate. When my mother was ambulatory, she went on errands with me—actually, practically everywhere with me.

As a caregiver, I tried to focus on the positives, that is, turning lemons into lemonade, as the cliche goes. I wrote books, something I'd always wanted to do, and being homebound with her made it possible. I also did public relations consulting. (I'd been a teacher, a journalist, and public relations executive before my mother's 16 years of illness.) Now I teach again full-time.

I've always believed that career caregivers should take care of their own, if possible. I met a foster home manager who had a mother in a nursing home. She said she didn't need nursing care. Why was she at a nursing home? Why not a foster home like hers? The caregiver said she couldn't take care of her own mother. She said it would be harder to do that, than caring for a stranger. Perhaps this caregiver didn't get along with her mother. I don't know. Caregiving is demanding, so if an adult child feels her parent was neglectful of her when she was growing up, for example, perhaps she should not take on the burden of caring for her. There's too much resentment from the get-go. I met so many caregivers in 16 years, who were caregivers to others, but who left the caregiving of their own parents to someone else. Many worked at minimum wage at caregiving jobs, while their parents paid for expensive foster home care.

At the other end of the spectrum, I once considered an unusual woman for a relief caregiving position for my mother after she got out of the hospital from her brain cancer surgery. She said she cared for her own mother single-handedly for eight years until she died. Her mother had Alzheimer's and her three brothers never helped. When her mother died, she began caring for other people. (While I was impressed with this woman, I wouldn't recommend someone carrying on as a caregiver after that many years, unless you, as a caregiver of your parent, can't find any other work, having been out of the job market for a long period of time. When a parent dies, it's time to get out of the illness mode, and start living again. Personally, I feel a tremendous sense of independence now, besides a deep feeling of loss.)

This woman-caregiver, unlike the other woman, became a professional caregiver after caring for her mother.

As a caregiver, if you only have time for one thing a day that you can do just for yourself, do it. For example, set aside a half- hour for a favorite television show or read a book of poetry. Force yourself to take the time, so you don't lose interest in life. Just remember that for most of us, a loved one's health problems are harder to cope with than if we had our own.

For many caregivers, a deep faith sustains them. They read passages from the Bible, such as psalms. They listen to religious-affiliated radio stations and religious televison programs. Oftentimes, if you're not religious, you beome religious and start searching for help beyond this earth as a caregiver.

Though I wasn't religious before my mother's first bout with illness, after her brain cancer I tried very hard to be. I'd take the Bible in my hands, and highlight in yellow every verse that I thought I'd need to keep me and my mother going. Perhaps it would help others to do the same. Commit each verse to memory. Try to believe in God's peace and presence. Attend a church service and expect something positive to come about as a result of it. Faith alone usually won't help your loved one. Faith and your caregiving work will help your loved one. Maybe as a result of prayer, you'll at least gain some insight. Though I've never been a religious person, per se, prayer has helped at times in my life. It really helps, too, to believe your prayers will be answered. My mother recovered from brain cancer, and I knew that this was the work of a Higher Form. Sometimes, not always, our prayers are answered to our liking. My mother never really came out of her coma to a great extent, except to say a few words or sentences in five years. They were the longest years of her illness.

Perhaps you can believe in intercessory prayer to heal your elder. I believe that my mother recovered from her brain cancer because of all the people who continually prayed for her from across the country. My mother wasn't really religious, but studies have shown that even those who weren't religious recovered, believing that intercessory prayer was helping them.

Often, you fluctuate in your religious beliefs. Sometimes you try to believe in God. Other times, it seems impossible to.

If you're not inclined toward religion, sometimes reading poetry helps or looking at the beautiful scenery in books of famous painters.

I had a friend, a recovering alcoholic, who had been sober for 30 years, who gave me the AA Credo Book, "One Day At A Time." Although I'm not an alcoholic, he gave me the book because it has a lot of good principles to help all people going through a stressful time. Its principles, of course, teach you to live each day without fearing the future.

My Italian upbringing taught me that adversity is part of life, but that you should keep plugging away no matter what. Taking illness one step at a time works. Listen to restful tapes, write a poem, or do a crossword puzzle while your loved one sleeps. Don't lose sight of planning your life. As a caregiver for 16 years, I started my self-employed writing career, and planned for my long-term goals in writing and teaching for when I would cease being a caregiver.

Besides the AA book, books with affirmations through adversity, such as Norman Vincent Peale's timeless classics will help you. His book, "The Power of Positive Thinking," is still on my bookshelf after 16 years. Being a caregiver involves adversity that often erodes one's self-confidence in all areas of life. Peale's books restore one's self-confidence and give ideas on planning one's day-to-day activities and even the rest of one's life, no matter what their situation.

While contemplative activities are good, it's important to invite visitors and neighbors in. You can bake something and have coffee in the house to offer them. I did this in my mother's final months when she was at home under hospice care. Visitors make it less lonely and more cheerful.

If as a caregiver, you don't have time to have friends over to your house, at the very least, talk on the phone with them each day.

As a caregiver, even letters from friends from far away mean so much to you. After my mother's brain cancer surgery, I awaited mail eagerly each day. Now, years later, in the era of email, it takes a friend only a minute to connect with you.

If a neighbor is willing to sit with your loved one for an hour, consider it a blessing. Don't be bashful about accepting.

Some people are wonderful. I had a friend who, for my birthday, besides giving me flowers, enclosed a handwritten coupon in my birthday card. Her homemade coupon entitled me to three hours of relief caregiving. Years after my mother's brain cancer surgery, when her memory was failing, I was afraid to leave her alone for a few hours, so this gesture from my friend meant so much to me. During these three hours, she talked to my mother the whole time. Perhaps a priest at your church might have some ideas on a parishioner who would volunteer her time or of one you could pay to relieve you from time to time.

In coping with caregiving, try physical activities such as walking or working in the garden. Sometimes it's even tough to do this, if your elder is badly confused.

I remember the stressful years after my mother's brain cancer surgery when my mother was ambulatory, but her memory started to fail. Sometimes I couldn't even leave the house to take a brief walk. You end up doing what the situation calls for in order to keep your loved one safe. For example, instead of sleeping upstairs, I moved a mattress downstairs to sleep in a bedroom next to hers. She would get up during the night because she couldn't sleep. She'd start cooking and then leave food on an open burner while she'd go down to the basement to do laundry. She would have caused a fire, if I hadn't have been sleeping downstairs and was awakened by the smoke alarm.

Throughout the discouragements along the path of caregiving, I met other caregivers who did beautiful things for their loved ones. One caregiver took in her elderly grandparents for a year and a half. Her husband used to carry her grandfather to the dinner table by lifting him in his chair up steps so he could eat with them. Her grandfather had a stroke and couldn't walk.

Adult children seem to be able to tell you how long, right down to the month, their elders lived with them. It's not that it was so dreadful that they counted the days, hours and minutes. However, it's a long haul. You know, if you asked them if they'd do it all over again, I'm certain they'd say yes.

Sometimes, it's the things others say to you that will keep you going as a caregiver. On one occasion, a clerk in a store said,"I often see you with your mother in here. She tries so hard." I thought it was compassionate for her to notice that my mother, who was recovering from brain cancer, inched along as she walked, looking as though she was 85 rather than 65. The clerk also said that I had a lot of patience with my mother. That felt especially good.

Six months after my mother's brain cancer recovery, another store clerk said, "Your mother is a real trooper who's been through so much." Then, the miracle of survival hit me. I focused not so much on the trials of caregiving, as on being grateful for her survival.

You have to savor these moments of people saying nice things to you. More often, however, you'll be bogged down by people's insensitive remarks.

Coping With The Negative Attitudes of Others

Caregivers need to be praised—not meant to feel like they are insignificant and do caregiving because they can't do anything else. Some family members who refuse to help will make you feel that way. I know my brother did during the first decade of my caregiving, before my mother entered a nursing home.

If a sibling belittles your efforts as a caregiver, remind him how much nursing homes cost, or even how much it would cost to hire someone to run errands, do caregiving, housekeeping, and bookkeeping for your loved one. It's certainly not insignificant work when you consider that complete care for an elderly person—that isn't even executed well— can run $100,000 or more each year. Most people don't even earn that much a year. When you consider the costs, a family member who works for free, caring for an elder, is indeed doing very significant work.

I think that a lot of siblings cause more stress for the caregiver than give support. When my mother's memory began to fail, my brother often didn't know how hard it was to care for her because he didn't see her in her worst moments during the day. He would even criticize my caregiving skills, though he never spent a minute doing any care himself. When my mother was ambulatory but confused, after her brain cancer, my brother never offered me a day off. I felt resentment toward him. He never took my mother even for an overnight visit in the first ten years when she was ambulatory, after her brain cancer recovery. However, you come to the conclusion that you can't make someone care enough to be a caregiver. As a caregiver accept this, and stop fighting it. The best you can do is try to set up a schedule of caregiving with your sibling.

If a sibling doesn't want to share in caregiving, at least ask him to invest time in interviewing and hiring suitable relief caregivers. This is time-consuming, too, and an ongoing task since caregivers don't stay too long. I rarely opted for relief caregivers when my mother was ambulatory, since the few I tried didn't have the patience to deal with her memory problems.

When my mother reached the nursing home stage, my brother and I did agree on one thing. Some adult siblings go to court, battling over whether to "pull the plug." My brother and I agreed on letting her live, despite our many differences regarding her care in 16 years.

Too often, you read in newspaper articles about how adult children are more concerned about who gets guardianship of the elder's pursestrings than about caring for the frail and failing parent.

The insensitivity of family, people you know, and strangers alike, often drags you down as a caregiver. A lot of people in the American culture have no respect for caregivers of their parents and what we do. Often, they tell us how badly our elders function and how we should put them in a nursing home. This makes it so hard for the caregiver to focus on the positive—that is, that your elder is still talking or walking, and that his memory isn't completely gone. The latter is what I considered when my mother was ambulatory after her brain cancer. At this time, I fully learned how difficult it was as a caregiver with my mother in the home. She needed so much attention, just like a child. However, it gets worse in a nursing home where the staff often consists of "adult kids" who need to be monitored for doing caregiving.

You'll often get unsolicited advice. As a caregiver, many people such as neighbors, will tell you that you shouldn't be a caregiver, and that you should have your own life. This isn't helpful. If they truly cared, they'd support you in your efforts and even offer to run an errand for you.

Conversely, the mentality of others when an elderly person becomes old and frail is often well-meaning toward a caregiver. A friend of my mother's told me, "When your mother dies, you'll have a clear conscience because you helped her so much." However, people should focus on the real issue—focusing not on death, but on the fact that caregivers strive to think about giving quality of life. They don't dwell on death. They don't have the time.

During the course of someone's illness, insensitive comments are often made by people and this not only drags down the ill person, but the caregiver, too. None of us know how long we are going to live, so it makes no sense for outsiders to ask questions like, "How long has she got?" Or, "Is she going to hospice?" Amazingly, they even ask this in front of the ill person.

After my mother's brain cancer surgery, a woman my mother met at a church social group, came to the hospital to visit and asked me if she was going to hospice, right in front of her. I politely said my mother's surgery was successful and that the whole tumor was removed, followed up by five weeks of radiation. Incidentally, I could tell this woman wasn't very sharp. When she first walked into my mother's room, she didn't recognize my mother with a bald head, so she walked right back out. She came back in when she put two and two together and realized that people who have brain surgery have bald heads.

A friend of my mother's, when she learned my mother's brain tumor was malignant, broke down over the phone. She then said, "Maybe she can live another two years." I told her not to have that attitude, and certainly not to display that attitude in front of my mother, because we were hoping for total recovery, even if it was just a dream. Ironically, the woman got cancer shortly after that, and died two years later. My mother recovered from brain cancer and lived ten and one-half good years before her damaging head injury accident that put her in a coma. Even when things seem hopeless, there are always people who recover from diseases that are considered fatal such as brain cancer.

Another church woman wanted to visit my mother after she returned home from her brain cancer surgery. She told me she wanted to tell her that she was "going to a better place." I told her not to do this—that it wasn't helpful to someone like my mother who was determined to recover. Many people were acting as if we shouldn't be hoping for her recovery and that we were just deluding ourselves.

Again, if your loved one isn't dead, the focus should be on caring for her and improving her quality of life, even if her quality of life is minimal.

There was a friend of a friend who told my mother, after her brain tumor surgery, about her aunt who was a vegetable in a nursing home with incurable brain cancer. We badly needed to hear stories of people who had recovered, not those who didn't make it.

A relief caregiver from an agency that I'd hired to drive my mother on errands, years after my mother's brain cancer recovery, was always conjuring up ideas about how my mother must be having a seizure. She was scared to be around her. In reality, my mother wasn't having seizures. This caregiver didn't help us.

As a caregiver, I found I needed to divorce myself from negative people and activities. I tuned out the television if there were programs about tragic illnesses and events. I've heard other caregivers say this, too. These serve to increase your dark thoughts.

The best thing that a family caregiver can do is to not allow negative people to visit or be relief caregivers. Don't listen to other people when they offer you a horror story about a relative who had your loved one's illness and died a painful death.

In most cases, I don't think people try to be insensitive and cruel, but they aren't thinking about what they are saying.

We need sensitivity in dealing with ill people. Over 25 years ago, one of my mother's friends asked her if her radical mastectomy had "damaged" her psychologically. Was this tactless?

My mother, due to her brain tumor, had a chronic eye muscle condition called blepharospasm. Even after her successful brain cancer surgery, she continued to squint and blink her eyes. Sometimes the pain was so bad, that she'd bob her neck. Clerks in stores would ask me, "What's wrong with her?" You wonder what the point of asking is. Certainly, if they've noticed it, the family member has, too, so there's no point in calling attention to it.

Seven years after her brain cancer recovery, my mother's memory was very bad. It was as if she had Alzheimer's. Even some rude store clerks would ask, "Does she have Alzheimer's?" You'd wish people would mind their own business. I simply said "no." It was the truth, after all, as she had brain damage from radiation treatment after her tumor was removed.

Get used to strangers and outside caregivers making comments like, "What does she want?" They never ask the person directly, when the person may be perfectly capable of communicating. Or, they ask, "Is she okay?" They don't have the courtesy to ask the individual first.

A funny thing was asked to me in the years after my mother's brain cancer. Someone who knew us, asked in front of my mother, "How's her mind?" I laughed and asked, "Fine, how's yours?"

You learn to take every comment as it comes. Even people who work with the elderly say silly or patronizing things. I know elder care workers who call elders "young lady" or "young man."

The caregiver is often burdened with stress and fear. Often you feel that life is a bad dream—"Stop the world, I want to get off." You fear doctor's visits and tests that might reveal health problems with your elder.

As a caregiver, after a while, you learn to live in the moment. You try to avoid as much as possible, fearing the future. Personally, I wrote haiku poetry as therapy. Haiku is, at its core, poetry of the moment.

Dealing With Fears and Stresses

In your worst moments, you feel really old. One day I was really burned out from caregiving. It was after my mother had come home from the hospital after her brain cancer surgery and radiation. I remember driving her to the store. I saw 60 and 70- year-old people in the street. I marvelled at their energy, and felt sorry for my mother. I wondered how they ever got to be "that old." Further, you know you're really burned out when you feel you can't enjoy anything anymore, not even a movie. You always are preoccupied with illness.

The fears and stress of illness are incredible and hard for anyone to imagine unless they've experienced them firsthand. When I took my mother home after her brain cancer surgery, I worried each minute, fearing a seizure. If she fell down because of bad balance, I'd worry that she had had a seizure or a spell of some kind. If she felt dizzy, I didn't have any way of knowing if this was caused by the radiation to her brain or whether her tumor had come back. Day after day, I'd worry about the brain cancer returning, because the doctor said, "Any day cancer could return."

Years later, when my mother's memory problems were evident, people used to point them out, as if I didn't know. They'd say, "Maybe she's sick again." This only made it worse.

What adds to your stress and fear is the response of professionals in the healthcare fields, and in the counseling or guidance fields.

You listen to doctors quoting death statistics from a particular disease matter-of-factly. Doctors and nurses even raise their voices when you question their statistics. If you suggest your loved one can defy the odds, they speak to you in a tone that suggests,"Are you so naive that you're not listening to the statistics?" They seem offended, like they feel like shaking you so you'll understand.

You listen to all people in healthcare quoting statistics who don't consider that each patient is an individual who may defy the odds with proper attention and care. I remember that after my mother's brain cancer surgery, a speech therapist told me that my mother would not be able to remember how to even sweep the floor. I responded, "Did you see her make her bed this morning?" Incidentally, this speech therapist had only worked with my mother once, and she job-shared patients with another therapist. Further, a statement such as this was out of her expertise.

Not only at nursing homes, but at hospitals—in all healthcare situations— nurses, doctors, therapists, and social workers often make emphatic statements that a patient will "never" be able to do this or that. It's simply unprofessional because ultimately some patients do defy the odds.

In caregiving for an ill loved one, I'll tell you what got me though my 16 years of home and nursing home caregiving. I always remembered to focus on what my mother could do, rather than what she couldn't do. The healthcare professionals seem to talk to you about and focus on the "can't dos." Try not to give into the negativity of healthcare professionals.

After my mother's brain cancer, my mother and I were both fearful of the future. Her doctor suggested we go to a psychologist for family counseling. The young psychologist in his early 30s knew nothing about people with chronic illness, though he rented space out of a physician's office. When we told him we were fearful that my mother would get brain cancer again, he said, "We all worry about illness." He missed the point. My mother's illness wasn't a problem of the future, it was a present and real problem.

It's amazing the ignorance that caregivers meet up with. If your loved one has a chronic illness, and you feel you need counseling, ask for experienced counselors in the area of illness your parent has. Private insurance and Medicare will pay for physician-referred joint visits for elder and family caregiver counseling, but it does no good to waste time with a neophyte.

I should also mention that when you talk to clergy members about a loved one's illness, sometimes they are no more helpful than others. The parish priest, who came to visit my mother in the hospital after her head injury, said that being in a coma and dying wasn't a horrible death, but dying of cancer and being reduced to 80 pounds was. There are problems with comparisons. First of all, comatose patients who don't get proper care, fall prey to pneumonia, blood clots, infections, and contractures, and those can be horrible.

A priest I went to for counseling when my mother was in a coma didn't even read to me from the Bible. He didn't pray with me. He merely concluded that "Life will be hell for you for the next year," and that if the doctors didn't expect my mother to recover, she wouldn't. As I later walked out the door he said, "Did my talking to you help?"

When the going gets rough as a caregiver, try to keep focused on keeping yourself in good physical and mental health. You can't do anything to change the condition of your elder outside of giving the necessary care or helping him obtain it.

My fear of getting sick myself was real, too. I wondered who would help my mother if I had a sudden emergency, since there was no other family member in the home to relieve me when she lived with me. Further, when she was at the nursing home, there was no one to monitor her and give all the required care. At the nursing home, lifting my mother who had ballooned up to 170 pounds had caused me some physical problems such as swollen rib cartilage. To remedy this, I did circular motion exercises with my arms, bending over at the waist. I lifted three-pound hand weights, and I used hot pads. I took over-the-counter muscle pain relievers or I took anti-inflammatory prescription drugs for muscle pain. (Anti-inflammatory drugs aren't safe over a long period. They can be taken for a week or so, not a month. Kidney problems or stomach bleeding is a danger with these drugs.)

Caregivers often neglect their own health, being so preoccupied with their loved one's health.

If you're the sole caregiver of an elder, you must realize when you've reached your burnout point. Sometimes it comes when you begin to age yourself. Or, as I've seen in other caregivers, it's when you begin overeating or undereating, or abusing drugs or alcohol.

Don't engage in the self-destruction of drugs and alcohol. This never happened to me. However, it happened to a friend of mine who was caring for his disabled daughter. He became dependent on anti-depressants and couldn't even gradually withdraw from them.

I also knew a mother who took care of her autistic daughter who was totally dependent on her for 35 years. The mother died at age 75. It was a long haul. The mother was widowed when the daughter was six years old. Her other children didn't help with caregiving when they became adults, nor did the woman's siblings who lived far away. There is always a caregiver who has just as difficult a time as you, or even worse. Try to live through each day, adjusting to the situation as it is.

Caregiving takes strength you never knew you had, besides compassion and love. There are many sorrows and frustrations. I found I had an enduring capacity to find meaning in my caregiving situation. You make a choice not to emphasize the part of the experience that is terrible. Yes, some caregivers do snap and even abuse their loved ones.

A nurse in a nursing home once told me, "I understand how elder abuse at home can happen when elders with dementia ask to go to the bathroom every five minutes, not remembering they already went. That's why you don't do caregiving 24 hours a day." She had one thing right. That is, that adult children of caregivers run the risk of losing it and abusing their elders. I took only eight days off from caregiving in 16 years. I never abused my mother. However, if this nurse didn't realize that it's more dangerous in nursing homes for an elder as far as abuse, she was naive. The aides, with all the patients they are given, are often exhausted and lose their cool, and are rough with the patients to the point of bruising them or worse. The crazy aide who did the wriststands with my mother, had bruised other patients, according to other aides on my mother's unit.

Incidentally, The National Center on Elder Abuse not only keeps track of statistics on elders who are abused physically, but elders who are abused financially by relatives and outsiders, such as relief caregivers.

The stress of worrying about your loved one can bring about changes in yourself.

If your elder is at home, chances are, you're going to end up doing some of the care yourself, if only as a substitute when a worker doesn't show up. If you get in too deep as a caregiver, caregiver counseling and support groups are often available through your local hospital, county mental health office, or Alzheimer's Association chapter. If physician-referred, your insurance may cover your counseling if you can't find free help. You can also contact your County Department of Human Services for suggestions.

After my mother's brain cancer recovery, when her memory started to fail, repetitions in her speech occurred frequently. Rather than lose my temper, I would walk into the bathroom and remove myself from her. Sometimes, this separation would relieve her of her jag. I also found that it added to my stress to correct my mother if she got her facts wrong. With an elder who has dementia, perhaps correct her only once. If she still doesn't get it, drop the issue.

With my mother, when she was able to speak, I often felt frustrated when she repeated herself. Sometimes I coped by keeping the radio on low to mitigate the repetitions. Or, sometimes if the same questions were repeatedly asked, instead of excusing myself and saying I was going to the bathroom, I'd say I had an important phone call to make. In later years, when she couldn't speak, I felt such guilt about how I used to feel when she repeated herself. Life is ironic.

Stress, anger management, and depression are common with caregivers. However, the worst part is allowing yourself to feel guilty for those feelings.

Caring for an elder isn't really like caring for a little kid. Yes, a little kid needs a lot done for her. However, if you reprimand an elder, she doesn't get scared as a little kid would. Elders are often stubborn. Further, it's so difficult watching your elder fail in physical and mental health.

I'd often think that if I'd had a kid, I could send him to spend the weekend with another family. Then the following weekend, I'd take the other family's kid. However, with an elderly parent, there's no family friend to trade off with. Perhaps in the future, families with elders will start doing this, as more adult children take in their elders.

I became a caregiver at age 33—rather young, but as Baby Boomers have children well into their 40s, their children will become young caregivers, too. More options such as day care for elders will have to be available.

As a caregiver, it's normal to feel resentment and feel like you're in a no-win situation, and then feel guilty for having these feelings. However, if your work life and social life is non-existent, and you feel you've had enough, then don't do caregiving anymore or scale back.

It's normal as a caregiver to feel sadness over the things you've given up in order to be a caregiver. It's only human to have sadness and regret that you're no longer in the world of professionals. You sometimes feel envious of others who don't have your situation. Guilt for feeling sad, burnout, anger at your loved one's illness, and criticism from other family members who don't do their fair share of caregiving can wear you down. These things can even do a caregiver in. Further, sometimes you feel anger toward your loved one for not realizing the sacrifices you're making in caring for him. Elders with dementia can't put the situation into perspective. They don't know how lucky they are to be living at home instead of in a nursing home or other facility. They don't realize their adult children need time off from caregiving. I once told my mother, after her brain cancer, that she didn't appreciate me. I remember shouting at her. Then I felt guilty. I thought, "What if she gets upset and has a seizure or heart attack? As a caregiver, you feel so totally responsible for your elder and every-thing that happens to her.

Sometimes you really feel hopeless when your loved one has dementia and he rants and raves. In nursing homes, a patient is given drugs for this. However, drugs often don't help.

When times get hard as a caregiver at home with a memory-impaired elder, just be glad she's not in a nursing home spaced out on drugs, confined to a wheelchair or bed, and that you're not visiting her in a stench-filled environ-ment. There's always a worse situation. Live in the present. Hope for a better future.

I must admit there were times of black humor. When my mother ranted and raved, I'd sometimes say, "Oh, you're crazy." You deal with it any way you can. As a prac-tical matter, I found that getting my mother to drink water during a spell of confusion or some jag often calmed her. Dehydration often causes confusion.

I know friends of mine are always afraid that their par-ents will become mentally-impaired to the point where they can't live independently. If the elder's memory isn't as sharp as it used to be, adult children begin to fear Alzheimer's.

After a person develops Alzheimer's, he could live up to 20 years. In the final stages of the disease, weakness causes susceptibility to infections such as pneumonia, a common cause of death in the Alzheimer's sufferer.

However, an Alzheimer's victim isn't someone who oc-casionally forgets a name or can't think of a word. She is someone who gets lost in familar places or fails to recog-nize people she knows. She has trouble balancing her check-book. She may forget to eat a meal she prepared, or put things in the wrong places, such as a personal possession in the refrigerator. Although my mother didn't have Alzheimer's, years after her brain cancer recovery, the effects of radiation to her brain caused these typical Alzheimer's symptoms.

As a caregiver, don't anticipate the future of an illness, such as Alzheimer's or cancer. For example, if an elder has cancer, don't fear he'll get it again. Don't anticipate what an elder will die from. Try not to look too far ahead. Deal with each episode as it comes, without wringing your hands about the next hurdle. However, do look ahead to future care options.

In addition, do look for respite options for yourself. For example, the National Easter Seal Society sponsors respite weekends for caregivers.

Be grateful for what you do have, such as your own good health. Try not to worry about what others think of your caregiving efforts. Many will think you're wasting your time or have nothing better to do.

An interesting thing about caregivers is that when they are through caregiving, no matter how much they've done, they feel guilty at not having done enough.

What really kept me going as a caregiver was my belief that elders deserve care. Certainly my mother's will to live kept me going, too. Particularly after her brain cancer, I was touched at her courage and attitude to keep plugging away. I felt that if she was so determined, the least I could do was to help.

My mother was courageous, much more so than I would have been. She never expected life to be perfect or to have everything like we Baby Boomers often do. After her brain cancer and radiation, at 65, she looked like a victim of war. She'd had a radical mastectomy with a long scar and no lymph glands, a bald head with scars and indentations, she looked gaunt, and she had squinting eyes. She never had the benefit that women have these days of having special counseling for breast cancer survivors and support groups. There weren't any brain tumor support groups, either, as there now are in our area.

I really admire my mother. She never complained about her breast cancer, nor her brain cancer, but was happy to have recovered despite her diminishments. She used to have unusually thick silver hair that never grew back after radiation to her brain. It looked shredded in wisps. (She actually clipped out pictures from magazines of women with a full head of hair like she used to have.) She never complained about her scarred body from the radical mastectomy. She never complained about her memory loss due to the late effects of radiation to her brain, years after her brain cancer recovery. She never complained about not being able to drive anymore. However, she was bitter at times about the years of medical misdiagnosis. Years later, after her head injury, even in her semi-comatose state, she once said she was happy, during one of the few occasions she spoke in her last five years of life.

She had an extraordinary will to live. She never wanted to give up— not before her brain cancer surgery, during her six-week paralysis after the brain tumor surgery, nor during her five weeks of radiation treatment to the brain when she felt nauseated and could barely walk. At 65, after the brain cancer ordeal, she walked and looked like she was 85, wearing a turban to cover her bare head. Ironically, she had often looked much younger than her years, prior to the brain cancer. After the brain cancer, often people thought she was my grandmother.

In the hospital after her brain tumor surgery, she was paralyzed for six weeks, started losing weight, and lost 25 pounds in the few months that followed, being so nauseated that she couldn't eat. However, after six months of rest, she started to come back slowly.

My mother was a walking rarity after her brain cancer. While statistics differ, a few years after her recovery, the oncologist said that she'd beaten the odds. The odds of her recovery had been one in 100,000. I wondered what the odds were for recovery ten years after her brain tumor.

However, the brain tumor had caused many impairments. Among them, blepharospasm, a condition then affecting one in 5,000 people in the U.S. It involves eye muscle twitching, pain in the eyes as if someone is throwing sand into them, and facial contortions and neck bobbing due to the pain. People who would see my mother often thought she was having an attack of some kind. Bright lights made her eyes worse. It was painful for her to read and watch television, and she was always squinting. An eye specialist said her condition was caused by the brain tumor and was chronic. The brain had learned the blepharospasm mannerisms even after the tumor was removed. For years before her brain tumor surgery, her blepharospasm had been diagnosed as being caused by nervousness, by a number of physicians, ophtamologists, and psychologists. "Go on a vacation cruise for your nervousness," some told her. Her brain tumor also caused some hearing problems, besides the memory problems and dementia. She couldn't live alone. It wasn't a pretty life.

Then, too, years before, she'd been widowed suddenly at age 46. I think that some people get more than their share of problems.

Dealing With Death

People who feel the loss of a parent isn't as bad as the loss of a spouse, don't realize how hard it is to lose an elder that you've cared for as much as you would a child. Grief is grief.

As for grief, after your loved one's death, everyone grieves differently, and there's no time frame. As a caregiver, I was so exhausted after my mother's death, that I just needed to catch up on sleep. Grief has just begun to set in a year later, now that I have time to catch up on my own life. After her death, I was busy handling executor's duties. I didn't experience physical symptoms of grief, such as stomach problems, headaches, muscle weakness, change in eating habits, difficulty breathing, and difficulty sleeping. Nor did I experience emotional symptoms, such as shock, disbelief, anxiety, crying, or fear because my mother had been so sick for such a long time. I went through all those symptoms during her long illnesses. There was, for me, even a feeling of peace. My mother died at home, in the room that was my nursery when I was a baby. She took care of me there when I was helpless, and I, in turn, took care of her there when she was totally dependent on me.

Contrary to what one might think, it's comforting to have a family member die at home. When you walk past her room, it's as if she's still there.

When you start grieving, it does you no good to be around friends and relatives who tell you to snap out of your grief. You can move ahead, but still grieve, not allowing it to incapacitate you. Try to eat well and do purposeful work or activities that occupy your mind.

If your loved one dies in a nursing home, try not to feel regret for having had him die there. We can only do what makes sense to us at the time. But, once again, when your loved one dies, grieve, but also make plans to move ahead with your life. It's certainly time to take care of yourself now. Realize that grief is normal.

If your elder is ill for a long time, perhaps you will feel some relief when he dies. You'll know that when one becomes too sick and isn't going to recover, his time has come.

If in reading this book, you say to yourself that you wouldn't have ever made the decisions that I made for my mother, think again. You never really know how you're going to react to a crisis until you're actually confronted with it. Further, you realize that you made the decision weighing the information you were given at the time. You simply did the best you could, as you try to do with everything in life. Knowing what I know now, I would have taken my mother home from the hospital, never having put her in a nursing home, and taken care of her until my back gave out. If she was still in a coma after a year, maybe I would have let her die naturally, withdrawing the tube feeding. I know that now, but I didn't know it then.

In grieving, you'll find that some of your friends and acquaintances don't like to be around a grieving person. Maybe they don't like to bring up the subject of your loved one dying. Maybe it reminds them of a terrible family death they went through. Some people who are grieving like to talk about death. At least friends and acquaintances should offer condolences, instead of ignoring the death.

I felt a sense of relief when my mother died, that her years of suffering were over, besides feeling a deep sense of loss. I also felt an incredible sense of independence, too. However, I will never get over her death.

We learn to appreciate what we have from watching our elders face illness, and we never take life for granted, after going through their illness with them. We live remembering how precious a family member we cared for was, and still is to us.

Planning For Your Future After Your Elder's Death

After my mother's death, being single, I didn't want to spend the holidays alone at home. However, I didn't want to accept invitations from friends, feeling like a fifth wheel at their family gatherings. Even now, I spend each holiday away from home, on vacation. Just planning for a trip gets me excited about life again. Remember that the most important thing is that your loved one would have wanted you to move on after his death. I'll always have regrets that I didn't take my mother out of the nursing home in the beginning, and I'll take this thought with me to the grave.

However, I always did the best I could.

Once your loved one dies, try to get back on your feet. You probably won't hit the ground running, but two classic books that have helped me are, "How to Stop Worrying & Start Living," by Dale Carnegie, and "You Can Have It All," by Arnold Pantent. My best advice is not to get a job as a caregiver to someone else, even if you think that's all you're qualified to do after years of caregiving. Get out of that mindset.

Thirty years ago, I met a psychologist in the midwestern town I lived in, who worked with people who feared death. She gave lectures on death and asked people to speak openly about their fears. She took people to tour cemeteries. As I now know, perhaps people don't fear death itself, as much as they fear how they will die. Maybe they fear a painful death, for example, with no one to take care of them who is compassionate.

It's a humbling experience to watch a parent die, or to watch anyone die. What appalls me is when I think back on what I once heard a nursing home nurse say, when my mother had just moved into her first nursing home. She was telling another young nurse who was just hired, this: "When you see your first patient die, it's disturbing, but after you've seen four or five die, you're no longer upset by it." This may indicate how quickly a healthcare person can become callous and stop looking at patients as individuals. Even if her 25th patient had died, if she'd known that patient for four months, a year or more at the nursing home, would she still just consider it another death? It sounds as if one is just checking off another death, all in a day's work. What she said, just had a bad ring to it.

There are other things that still haunt me and always will. I remember when we moved our mother into the first nursing home, a few days before Mother's Day. She died five years later a few days before Mother's Day. I brought her clothes to the funeral parlor on that Mother's Day, and looked at her in the Visitation Room there.

I also remember the last Mother's Day she was alive at the nursing home. There was a visit from the oncologist, followed by a visit from hospice, totaling three and one-half hours.

At the nursing homes, I also remember a Christmas when my mother woke up to pneumonia; a New Year's Day in another year when she had pneumonia; and a 4th of July with seizures after my mother was switched from one anti-seizure medication to another that wasn't supposed to sedate her as much.

Illness is particularly bleak in a nursing home. The nursing home environment compounds the insult of illness.

Ultimately, a family member, after the death of a loved one, must move beyond the scenes of illness and death to live the productive life the deceased person would have wanted you to.

Chapter 10

Where Do We Go From Here?

The Nursing Home Dilemma

Today, parents are having children later in life, even well into their 40s. When their children become adults, they may in their 30s, or even in their late 20s, have to make vital and saavy care decisions for their parents.

The American Association of Retired Persons (AARP) recently surveyed more than 2,300 Americans, ages 45 to 55, and found that the majority say they don't expect their children to care for them when they are old. Seventy-two percent of Non-Hispanic Whites and 68 percent of African-Americans 45 to 55, say they don't want their children to feel obligated to care for them in the future. Sixty percent of Hispanics and 49 percent of Asian-Americans feel that way. The survey also found that 42 percent of Asian-Americans care for their parents; 34 percent of Hispanics do; 28 percent of African-Americans do; and 19 percent of Non-Hispanics Whites do.

In an age when prisoners' rights are fought for, it's often disheartening not to see our elders' rights fought for with the same fervor in institutional situations.

As our overall retirement population increases, we, as individuals, cannot afford to pay hundreds of thousands of dollars for care and be antagonized by those in the system when we complain about neglect and abuse of our elders. As I've said before, neglect is abuse, and we need to label it as such. Until we do, we are not a humane society.

Further, this idea of older people needing an advocate in institutions is a sorry admission by society that care isn't adequately being given by institutions to its vulnerable population. An elder needing an advocate simply means that the provider of care isn't monitoring itself and needs to be told what to do.

Remember that as we and our loved ones age, no professional, no matter how brilliant, experienced or revered in his field has the right answers for us about our care and our elders' care. Every person is an individual case, and professionals are often wrong about treatment and prognosis when illness occurs.

Under Hitler's regime, less than "perfect" people, such as the mentally retarded, weren't viewed as being productive members of society. The regime regarded them as unfit to live. We see, at nursing homes, all too often, the attitude that elderly people shouldn't be allowed to live. They are, all too often, purposely neglected to hasten their death. Some nurses, even at religious-affiliated facilities, will openly challenge family members in front of the patient about why their elders are being "kept alive." They diminish quality of life of the elder with their attitude.

We need to stand up as a society and form a grassroots effort that attitudes such as these won't be tolerated. Although the state government can fine a nursing home for shabby care, it can't legislate attitudes. Since nursing home administrators rarely fire personnel, these unprofessional, inhumane attitudes are permitted to fester.

There is something missing in nursing education if people such as these nurses slip through the cracks. After caring for my mother at home for so many years after her brain cancer, and watching her miraculously beat the odds by recovering, it killed me emotionally to see such neglect of her at nursing homes. However, more than that, the common attitude of disgust toward my mother, and I, as her advocate, was particularly distasteful.

Nurses and therapists alike, many of whom spoke callously in front of my mother, while she was fully alert, about their opinions that she would never be able to eat or stand up, don't offer dignity, comfort, or encouragement to the patient and the patient's family. The operative word is "opinion." Medicine isn't science. It remains an art. Didn't they learn that in school?

Their poor attitude filters down to the aides and everyone else who works at the nursing home. A patient is then condemned to neglect. In a nursing home, the staff should ask family members what their goals are for the patient. Even in hospice, nurses ask you what your goals are for a family member who can't communicate. At a nursing home, the goal appears to be to warehouse the patients like vegetables. They tell you that your family member is incapable of doing anything. If staff members attend to each patient, perhaps only 35 minutes each eight-hour shift, how do they truly know what the patient is capable of?

Society often has more compassion for old pets than it does for its elders. I knew a woman who kept giving her 17-year-old dog cancer surgeries, but didn't visit her dying father often. He lived a few blocks away. Many people frown on those who keep treating their frail and ill elders, instead of letting them expire, when, in fact, they have a hard time putting their old, sick pets to sleep.

For the tremendous costs of nursing home care, all family members ask is that in return for payment, their elders receive basic cleanliness, basic safety, and basic respect. The residents and their families are not to be looked upon as a nuisance who do nothing but complain or "nag." My mother's friend who visited her at the nursing home told me she heard one nurse's aide tell a patient to stop nagging. I would even hear nurses complain to nursing supervisors about patients who nagged.

The State's Office of the Long-Term Care Ombudsman puts out a brochure that is called, "Know Your Rights as a Nursing Home Resident." Many of the rules are routinely violated, such as: "You will be free of retaliation. After you or your representative exercises your rights, the facility will not retaliate by increasing charges, decreasing services, rights, or privileges...even suggesting that you leave the facility." I reported that a nursing supervisor and a social worker at two different facilities suggested that I find a different facility for my mother after I complained of repeated care lapses. Each time, I spoke with the ombudsmen, they admitted that the personnel shouldn't have said that. However, they did nothing.

The brochure also says: "The facility staff shall listen to and act promptly upon grievances and recommendations received from residents and families." This is also routinely violated.

While in principle, you have rights, the rights are so commonly abused by staff, that at best, a fine can be levied by the state. State officials feel they can't shut down all facilities for violations, and that if you shut down one, you must shut down all. Yes, poor personal hygiene, cold food, inappropriate billing, inadequate staffing, poor sanitation, and abuse are all violations. However, if the Ombudsman's Office were to crack down on all the violations, it would have to shut down all nursing homes. Even if ombudsmen receive repeated complaints from different families, they often tend to do nothing except talk to staff, or a fine is levied at best.

Nursing home staff members seem to think that they do a better job than what a family member could do at home. If every family knew as much as I did about how little is done, they would conclude that even if they took care of their family member at home and did very little, it would be more than what a nursing home does. At least one's home would be a clean environment, and there wouldn't be germs that aides transfer from one patient to another. If you as a caregiver got sick with a cold, your loved one would still be under better care with you, as you would wear a mask, unlike when staff members in institutions go to work sick and don't even have the decency to wear one.

I found that in moving my mother home for what turned out to be the last eight months of her life, and caring for her on my own, things were so much better. She didn't catch pneumonia that winter—which was routine at the nursing home— and I didn't have to hassle over care issues. Further, in not being in a depressing institution, full of sick people and unhappy staff, this improved my mother's spirits and mine. Everything including the staff's attitude at a nursing home spells death. This is kind of funny, in a macabre sort of way, but at every nursing home I've been in, there appears to be a calendar in each patient's room. The calendar is courtesy of a local funeral home. Why is it that staff is so disrespectful toward patients and family? Yes, we know our elders are going to die, but funeral home calendars don't do anything to lift our moods or spirits, nor do they contribute to quality of life for the patient. The point is, you live each day as best you can, without focusing on death, but rather life. If you focus on quality of life, this improves life.

The idea that one can live adequately in a nursing home is a wishful one, no matter how much the family member advocates or is directly involved in the actual care. It would make sense to take an elder home and even spend $10,000 a month getting some private R.N. care and aide care if your elder isn't eligible for hospice or some other significant healthcare assistance. Say, for example, your elder is bedridden and you spent $168,000 over a two-year period in a nursing home at $7,000 a month, the money would have been better spent over nearly a 17-month period at home, getting some R.N. and aide care, supplemented by some family help. If your elder didn't improve in 17 months and wanted to die, if she got an infection you wouldn't have to treat it with an antibiotic, and she could die a natural death. Although there is often discomfort in not treating an infection, it is certainly no worse than putting someone in a nursing home where infections and pneumonia are routinely ignored and the patient dies.

Unless you know a nurse, you probably wouldn't be able to find private registered nurse help unless you went through an agency that may charge you $70 an hour or more. If you were lucky to know a retired nurse, you could pay her $25 to $30 an hour. However, keep in mind that rarely would an elder need more than one hour of R.N. care a day, if that. A family member can be trained to give virtually any care such as oxygen and bandage sores. Assistance is needed to change or irrigate catheters perhaps every few months at most. As far as nurse's aides, if you go through an agency, you could pay $21 an hour for someone who typically would do little. On your own, you could find an aide for $12 to $14 an hour, and some would be happy, considering that nursing homes pay a little above minimum wage.

At some point, your elder may be eligible for hospice care as discussed in Chapter 5, "Alternatives to Nursing Homes." Hospice is wonderful, not only for the free care, but for the private care.

It's counterproductive to place an elder in a nursing home and try to squeeze some care out of the staff.

I'm sure that in taking a patient out of a nursing home, he will often show more signs of alertness at home. My friend's aunt regained color in her face after being taken out of a nursing home that she'd been in for six months, as did my mother. My friend took care of his aunt at home with supplemental private aide help. When my mother left the nursing home after nearly four and one-half years of institutionalization, she had advanced cancer. However, despite having advanced in age, (she was 80), and having gone through debilitating bouts of pneumonia and infections at nursing homes, she was more alert at home. She was eating more by mouth, having food available to her at all times, and lifting her legs sometimes on command. Being in a clean, non-smelly environment, and not being subjected to abuse, she was revitalized psychologically and emotionally.

The bottom line is, if the patient leaves the hospital comatose, she usually won't improve at a nursing home. The germs, the infections, not begin transferred to a wheelchair, not being kept elevated in bed, room windows left open, aides not following feeding tube precautions, and not being able to eat by mouth—all lead to a further deterioration in health and pneumonia.

We thought we'd give our mother a chance at recovery by placing her at a nursing home with a nurse on duty 24 hours a day. However, a nurse sees a patient only a few minutes on each of the three shifts. No one is in a patient's room to spot emergencies. Therefore, a family member at home can give better care and get emergency help to an elder before a nursing home staff member even discovers there's a problem with the patient.

Over the course of her nursing home years, it became painfully obvious to us that no one except us really cared whether our mother lived or died, whether she ever ate by mouth again, whether her arms and legs became contracted from little range of motion, or whether she died or was harmed by an error made by staff. My brother and I were left to pick up the shattered pieces. It was the most pathetic experience of our lives. We felt we were shoveling sand against the tide in our efforts to get what our mother, as a human being deserved. We will never forget this experience.

It's now estimated that about 40 percent of Americans will end up in a nursing home at some point during their lives for at least a limited time.

Although we can't expect nursing homes to offer one-on-one care despite the staggeringly high cost, you need determination to get the basics for your elder in an institution. Further, you need to advocate for conditions to improve for when it comes your time to be there. Advocacy involves these issues:

- Being kept clean
- Being kept safe
- A clean facility
- Being fed adequately
- Having access to all therapies without excuses being made
- Prompt attention by nurses and nurse's aides
- Responsive social workers and directors of nursing who listen to concerns and problems—without getting defensive and blaming you.
- Group activities and events

One very valuable lesson I learned is that if you have an elder on life support, a nursing home is no place for her. Respirator patients need monitoring on a regular basis, and even nursing homes that accept them can't adequately care for them. If one has a feeding tube, such as my mother did, a nursing home is no place for a tube feeder. The staff is careless with tube feeders. Some staff members don't follow feeding tube precautions. Further, staff and speech therapists are leery to give the okay for even the family member to feed the elder by mouth. Perhaps researchers can figure out a way to make feeding tubes aspiration-free so even if careless nursing home aides don't turn off a feeding tube and lay the patient flat, she won't aspirate.

As far as right-to-life issues and feeding tubes, if a patient is alert, but can't communicate, she will know she is starving to death if she's having trouble swallowing. (This was my mother's case when we opted for a feeding tube in the hospital.) Therefore, a feeding tube is often the natural path to take in these circumstances, unless a patient has an advance directive and has refused it. If a patient is already in a nursing home and stops swallowing, then you should consider if life should be prolonged in a nursing home with a feeding tube implanted, if the patient isn't able to communicate her wishes. If she is already in a nursing home, perhaps she has no quality of life anyway. I knew patients who were in their 80s, even their late 80s, who had feeding tube surgery when they were already nursing home residents. There is no right or wrong answer, despite what staff or onlookers may say. It's something a family member should think hard about on his loved one's behalf, if his loved one hasn't made his wishes known.

The arrogant attitude that staff members know best what is good for the patient is flawed. They only spend a few minutes a day with a patient and don't often see the progress that family members do. They look at the patient as a statistic rather than an individual with potential. I certainly knew my mother's potential more than any doctor or nurse she ever had. In fact, I logged so many hours at the nursing home that one of the housekeepers thought I was a nurse. One nurse thought I was a social worker. Family members who didn't know me, but who saw me around, often thought I worked there.

You can follow medical advice that may or may not be sound. However, healthcare professionals never seem to consider the triumph of the human spirit in recovery, and that one-on-one care by a family member can make the difference in whether one recovers or not.

Attitudes must change. As a society, and particularly among healthcare personnel, we must stop judging what other people's "quality of life" is. Healthy people often look at the frail elderly and memory- impaired as if they are not valuable people. Quality of life is an individual thing.

On a brighter note, after my mother died, I talked to her hospice nurse and gave him my heartfelt thanks for letting my mother die naturally without hurrying her along. He said she deserved the care. If only everyone in nursing homes and in healthcare institutions, in general, realized that patients deserve care.

Nursing attitudes must change. How many times did I hear nurses talk about patients like objects with afflictions? They would say, "He's a hip fracture," for example. Do nursing schools teach this kind of communication? If they do, do they realize that it encourages nurses to focus on the affliction, rather than the fact that there is a human being who suffers from it? It's as if a teacher were to speak of a student by saying, "He's a learning disability." In the latter case, everyone would be shocked.

Nursing homes and hospitals must realize that patients need full care and that family members are there to visit, not to supplement or do most of the care. Even at children's hospitals, I've seen family members do tube feedings. Families are often forced to give care, otherwise their loved ones go without, or the care isn't delivered on a timely basis so it interferes with other scheduled care. Or, the care is executed in a poor manner and causes the patient harm. When care issues aren't resolved, the family member must bite the bullet and pick up the slack. As long as there are nurses who are willing to work at short-staffed facilities, staffing levels won't improve. Worse, these nurses parrot the institution's jargon about how they give excellent care.

Oftentimes, family members pay extraordinary amounts of money to nursing homes, not for the care, but because they need help lifting a patient, as I did.

There is a shortage of aides at nursing homes, in particular. Nursing home aides who could perhaps earn more money if they worked at a restaurant, rather than doing nursing home drudgery, are in short supply. If aides leave nursing homes for home health agencies, the agencies often don't offer aides steady work because sometimes patients aren't with them for a long time. I knew aides who worked for two or three agencies, so they would have the chance of working regularly. The aides I knew who worked privately, if they were good, always seemed to have enough work.

Nursing homes and hospitals need ongoing review sessions for their aides who tend to forget the simplest of care issues, (i.e. leaving windows open in a patient's room.) They need to be monitored by a supervisor to ensure they are performing the required care in a cleanly manner.

However, most of all, cameras are needed in patients' rooms because the frail elderly are among the most vulnerable people in our society.

Employees who do their jobs well at nursing homes are truly special people. They don't let themselves get dragged down by their negative peers, and they go to work each day doing a job that few people would choose to do. Some of these special people remain my friends today, even after my mother's death.

Yes, many nurses at nursing homes and hospitals are conscientious, but they sometimes quit the field because they aren't allowed to give the type of care they feel they should give to each patient.

In a nursing home where your elder is living, you try your absolute best to compliment staff, nurses and nurse's aides alike, especially with kind words. You give them gifts and birthday cards. You sometimes socialize with them outside the nursing home. They must be appreciated and rewarded for their work.

What makes it hard to improve nursing homes is that nurses and aides are willing to work there, no matter how bad the conditions and the pay are. Sometimes they feel they can't do any better and couldn't function at larger institutions such as hospitals. You often see aides who don't understand English well. How will they understand the patients' needs? Feeding tube precautions? They won't. Patients can aspirate on feeding tubes because aides lay them flat. We will see more non-skilled, non-English speaking people work at nursing homes. A nurse-friend of mine at a nursing home told me that at a hospital you have the right to refuse a certain nurse and that you can even fill out a complaint form about the nurse. However, at a nursing home, there is only one nurse per unit out on the floor at a certain time. There is no replacement for her. You would have to have your loved one transferred to a different unit and take your chances there with poor care.

It should be noted, however, that complaints against healthcare personnel at nursing homes and hospitals usually backfire. Other personnel, then, often take a dislike to you, fearing you might complain about them. Or, perhaps the person you complained about was a friend of theirs. It's like a sorority or fraternity. Again, it goes back to a need for a change in attitudes and nursing instruction.

Nursing home staffers often don't care if a patient dies due to errors. I suggested to the director of nursing at one facility that only experienced aides on each shift who knew about feeding tube precautions be allowed to work with my mother. I felt that if they were so afraid of my mother aspirating by taking food by mouth, that they should take equal precautions that she not aspirate because of mistakes made by their aides. Once again, we noted the double standard. It was what was easiest for them, and not what would keep the patient safe. The director of nursing said this couldn't be done. They know that it's hard to prove that a patient died from aspirating on feeding tube formula, because of their mistakes. In this case, they could just say that she died of something unknown, or some saliva she swallowed went down to her lungs, and she caught pneumonia from that.

Ombudsmen may or may not be the answer for you in seeking adequate care at nursing homes. I remember when I complained to one ombudsman about uncleanliness and the aides not wearing latex gloves, she got totally off the subject and said, "You won't get one-on-one care in nursing homes." She said what a good nursing home it was, in compared to the rest. Another ombudsman, who took her place six months later, didn't address himself to cleanliness issues, either. He got off the subject and said, "You won't believe what goes on at other nursing homes."

It's not uncommon for conflicts of interest to exist at nursing homes and hospitals. At the hospital where my mother was receiving bad care and mysteriously lapsed into a coma, the ombudsman had an office at the hospital, and wasn't the least bit interested in hearing our complaints about poor care at the hospital. Since her office was at the hospital, we figured she'd perhaps gotten to know staff and had even made friends with them. Therefore, instead of advocating for the patient, perhaps she was inclined to defend hospital care. I'm sure there are conscientious hospital ombudsmen, but I'm sure there are some who aren't.

The "Reinvention" of Nursing Homes

Despite inadequate care, nursing homes are trying to reinvent themselves by making themselves seem more homey with wallpapering and plants. I've read of nursing homes that operate on-site day care for children, so the elders can share in the joy of children. I've read of nursing homes striving to give less medication. Maybe if they kept patients busy with activities, they wouldn't be so restless. I read of a nursing home that allowed patients to grow cabbage and flowers, and where they were allowed to have birds in cages in their rooms. This is all well and good, and even makes for raising the morale of staff and attracting new staff. However, rather than spend money on some extras, spending dollars on adequate staffing and staff training must be done first, so that care is uppermost on the list of offerings.

If nursing homes truly care about their patients, they must ensure that they aren't being neglected or abused.

Money should be spent on cameras to be placed in every room. It should be noted that in some states, surveillance cameras in nursing homes are prohibited. This law should be abolished. Citizens should lobby for its abolishment. Safety should always prevail over the "privacy" issue. Camera viewing by staff can be discreetly done in medicine rooms next to the nurse's station or in a spot behind the nurse's station. If the aides are doing their jobs adequately, they shouldn't object to the cameras. A director of nursing admitted to me that she doesn't know if CNAs are doing their job unless a family member complains. How many family members even show up on a daily basis? Nursing homes charge by the day for care. They don't want us complaining, but they admit they don't know what's going on. Are we supposed to pay them, be on hand to notify them of care lapses, and then get ignored or even verbally abused when we do ask for the promised care?

Traditionally, patients have literally been paying for rooms and some food, with little care executed poorly, or no care at all for the bedridden who can't speak. That's why it makes more sense to be at home, if possible, or in foster care, where you don't pay for a facility 'round the clock that perhaps only delivers an hour and 45 minutes of care a day, on the average.

It's interesting how nursing home staff, when you talk about taking your elder out, tell you that you won't make it at home on your own. I, and my friends, who had family members at nursing homes, were told this. I made it at home. And, for example, my friend, a single, middle-aged father of two teenage girls, took his father out of a nursing home, too. He was told he'd never make it at home with his dad who was totally blind. He took care of him for two years, besides holding down a job eight hours a day. His blind father would often stay alone during the day.

If nursing homes leave their patients sitting in bed all day or just sitting in a wheelchair with no attention, how can a family member do worse at home? Sitting in a wheel-chair unattended, whether at home or in a nursing home, is the same. The janitor at one nursing home my mother was at, the "absolute best one in town," told me that he found a patient on the floor in his room, bleeding from his head. Apparently, he hadn't been checked on for three hours. He'd fallen down.

My friend's father was blind, but had his mental faculties. When he left the nursing home, he occupied himself while his son was working and his teenage granddaughters were in school.

If there's one thing I regret the most—and being human means having regret—is that I wasn't independent- thinking enough at the nursing home, as I had been after my mother's successful bout with brain cancer. Although I routinely considered taking her out of each nursing home she was in, I should have done so long before I did. I shouldn't have tried to squeeze care out of the management, when many nursing home personnel look at people in my mother's condition as not having a right to good care, nor even a right to be alive. After she'd been in a nursing home for two years, I told the social worker there that I'd like to take my mother home, rather than keep complaining about care issues that apparently couldn't be permanently resolved. I told her I didn't know how long my mother had to live, but that I'd like to take her home to die. The social worker, who had no training as a social worker and who was in her 20s, replied, "When you get old, it's not all that important to die at home." I knew at that time, as I do now, that the lack of common sense in institutional settings is mind-boggling.

Many people end up taking a loved one out of a nursing home when the care is so bad that what little is done is being executed so poorly as to cause the patient infections. Some people who de-institutionalize their elder, do so when they realize they are doing practically all the care, and that care issues aren't being resolved. Some family members get fed up when their complaints are not listened to, and the staff gets belligerent and starts blaming the family for its care problems.

Some nursing home staff try to resolve care issues in good faith, but care usually breaks down again weeks later when there's a turnover of staff or workers get lax again.

If you believe your loved one can benefit from physical and speech therapy, but the nursing home disagrees, take her home. You could perhaps get her doctor to authorize home therapy visits.

In general, nursing home administrators never fire anyone and don't care if you bad-mouth their operation to your elder's doctor and others. There's a shortage of facilities since hospitals dump patients onto them. However, if you take your loved one out, and haven't complained to the state prior to that, you should complain afterwards.

Besides complaining to the state about nursing home care, copy your loved one's doctor and her health insurance with letters documenting poor care, so hopefully word will get out and patients won't be referred to that facility. At the second nursing home my mother was at, her health insurance company got so many complaints about it, that they dropped their contract with the facility.

People who enter nursing homes today are often more ill than those who entered, say, 15 years ago. Back then, people who weren't very ill didn't have as many alternatives open to them as there are today with many assisted-living facilities and more foster homes. It's unacceptable and unfathomable that with the increased acuity in the condition of patients entering nursing homes today, that conditions haven't improved. One nursing home nurse told me that when she began working at nursing homes 20 years ago, she had the same number of patients, but that they were in much better condition, mentally and physically.

If nursing homes are reinventing themselves, as some claim they are, they should focus on "customer" issues to make them not only a friendlier environment, but one that truly is concerned about delivering basic care. Family Councils should be set up at all nursing homes with a nursing home staff member present to answer common concerns and complaints. Nursing homes should provide detailed written materials for each family on care services provided on a daily basis for the daily fees charged.

To not only improve care, but increase staff morale, the nursing home should not only invest in inservice training of all employees, but in giving language training to employees with deficient English skills. We will see more and more foreign-born employees at nursing homes in years to come.

Most of all, nursing homes need to focus on quality of life, and changing their policies that don't allow it. In the case of feeding tube patients, for example, nursing home administrators should allow family members to use their best judgment and decide for themselves if they should feed their elder.

The Flawed Healthcare System In General

The squeaky wheel gets the grease. When you or your family member is in the hospital and isn't receiving what you feel is adequate care, speak up. Ask for the nursing supervisor of that floor. If necessary, keep going higher and higher until the problem is resolved. We are healthcare consumers, and as customers we deserve the right to complain.

Inadequate staffing results in medication errors or other errors at institutions. As many nurses tell me, "Don't get sick, because none of us want to be cared for these days in the healthcare system." Institutions wanting to cut costs, skimp on personnel.

You should ask questions about medication. A nurse-friend told me something that reinforces statistics on medication errors in the hospital. Our friend, who was hospitalized, said that one day, the attending nurse brought medication to her of a different color than what she'd previously gotten. The nurse assured her that it was the right medication, but our friend kept questioning her. Oops, it was the wrong medication meant for the patient next-door. Fortunately, our friend caught the error before the pill was given to her. The nurse actually came back laughing and joking about how our friend was right. What if our friend had been groggy or what if she hadn't been a nurse herself and hadn't thought to question it?

An interesting study on medication errors was done by the Institute of Medicine. After reviewing 6,224 reports of medication errors made in 1999, that 56 hospitals voluntarily reported to the Institute, the Institute's survey found that in 32 percent of the reported cases, the personnel who made the error weren't told a mistake had been made.

If nurses unwittingly make errors, they are often not told about it, if the error is even caught. A nurse-friend who worked at a hospital told me that she was instructed to report errors made by other nurses to her supervisor. However, she said that supervisors routinely never approached the nurse at fault with the error. How can care be improved? At nursing homes, it's worse, because the supervisor doesn't want to embarrass the nurse who makes an error, fearing that the employee might leave, and a replacement can't be found.

If your loved one is hospitalized or institutionalized and you suspect a medication error because he develops a new problem, ask the doctor for a blood test, and specifically ask him if there could have been a medication error. Often, a doctor can't tell, however.

As for reducing nurse's and doctor's medication errors, apparently with computerized doctor-order entry systems for medications in hospitals, many errors can be avoided. Hospitals are now automating their systems for ordering, dispensing, and monitoring medications. Doctors enter medication orders by computer, which avoids errors through handwriting. The goal is to deliver the right drug in the right dose, to the right patient the first time. The system warns the physician if patients are allergic to certain drugs.

Some hospitals have started to use bar code technology for medications. The bar codes contain a drug identification number that indicates strength and dosage. The patient has a bar-coded ID bracelet. When administering a dose to a patient, a nurse can scan in the patient's bar code as well as the bar code on the drug coming from the hospital pharmacy. Providing the codes match, the dose would be administered. However, it will be years before all hospitals will enact this procedure that is quite costly.

Hospitals are dirty places, too. A private R.N. I'd hired to help me with my mother told me she once was a patient in a hospital room with a roommate who was a drug abuser. She had overheard her conversation with the attending nurse. The nurse I'd hired wondered why they'd given her a roommate who could contaminate her. After all, they shared a bathroom and toilet, and the toilet seat would be contaminated.

More food for thought: If, as the Institute of Medicine reports, that 100,000 patients are killed each year in hospitals from "preventable" medical errors, then there's probably thousands more patients who die where the errors aren't caught or acknowledged. Further, what are we to believe about nursing home deaths, where a death is just dismissed as old age-related, and nothing is questioned or investigated. One can readily assume that most likely a high proportion of nursing home patients die due to neglectful care and errors.

The Centers for Disease Control and Prevention found that 90,000 deaths in the year 2000 were caused by hospital infections alone.

Hospital care must also improve, besides nursing home care. In many states, hospitals aren't required to report infections to the state. Lawyers say it's hard to prove that infections occurred due to unclean practices or negligence unless a doctor or nurse is willing to testify.

Legislation should be enacted so that any staff member at hospitals and nursing homes who has knowledge of errors, injuries, or abuse to patients should be required to report them or lose his license, whether or not he had anything to do with it. If he suspects an error, management would be required to follow-up and investigate or lose its license to operate.

Another problem with healthcare is that doctors are becoming less and less influential in the system. Doctors in hospitals are often powerless with nurses who don't carry out their orders that have to do with custodial maintenance of a patient. Nurses often say that nursing policy doesn't allow such and such. (Nursing homes can ignore doctor's orders. The doctor isn't there doing her rounds to check up on things as in a hospital, so a nurse sometimes doesn't follow through.) I remember after my mother mysteriously lapsed into a coma at the hospital, two weeks after her cerebrovascular accident surgery, she was having small seizures consisting of eye twitching—not grand mal seizures. The nurses refused to carry out doctor's orders and transfer her to a wheelchair so she could exercise her lungs and not fall prey to pneumonia. If they'd been afraid of a greater seizure where she'd have fallen out of her chair, they could have fastened a seat belt around her. They knew I was there watching her. A nurse at a another hospital that I later met told me this. (My mother's hospital nurses merely said it was against nursing policy to carry out the internist's and the neurologist's orders in this situation. My mother's doctors told me they couldn't dispute this.) Perhaps the concept of teamwork has been slow to hit the healthcare field.

Nurses need better training. A registered nurse needs only a two-year community college degree. A Licenced

Practical Nurse (LPN), who does virtually everything an R.N. does— except initial assessment of the patients' condition when he is admitted to the institution—has only about one and one-half years of education. These days, it's rare to hear of anyone doing anything professional with so few years of education.

I've heard even young nurses, fresh out of nursing school, both in hospitals and nursing homes, talk about the patients as if they were a nuisance. Many seem to talk about enjoying a turnover of patients when, "You don't have the patients for too long." Are they being taught adequately in nursing school? Certainly, there are wonderful nurses, and I know they must be ashamed of some of their colleagues.

After my mother's metastatic breast cancer, that spread to her brain, was treated, the nurse told my mother that she would need a guardian after she left the hospital. This upset my mother, as she'd felt that at the age of 65, she could function with assistance, and didn't need a guardian. I'd asked her doctor if he or anyone else had written this in her chart. He said nothing of the kind had been written in her chart by anyone. I feel that nurses should refrain from making comments such as these to a patient. If it's true, it's better left said by a doctor.

Another nurse in a doctor's clinic, months after my mother's brain tumor surgery, upset my mother by telling her that her leg pain might signal "something serious." When my mother got upset and started asking questions that the nurse thought were unintelligent, the nurse told me, "Your mother understands very little." I said, "What a thing to say." After that, at least she realized her error, she backed down, and started speaking politely to us.

Some nurse's attitudes can be damaging to a patient. Bad attitudes of nurses are more common than expected. Certainly, there are bad apples in every profession.

When an elder is ill, you can probably improve her situation through caregiving at home, rather than run the risk of your elder being cared for by some institutional nurses who might not want to do their job to the best of their ability. Even if the doctor gives a bad prognosis for recovery, it should be kept in mind that no one can accurately predict recovery. However, some nurse feel compelled to talk about the patient's negative prognosis, rather than just deliver the care as required.

If nurses study ethics in nursing school, and I'm told they do, perhaps more of these courses need to be included in the curriculum. We don't want nursing students to regard elderly patients as vegetables. We don't want them to become nurses who will give them less care than they might give to a younger patient, thereby causing further decline in their health. I hope we are not getting to the point in healthcare where nurses and doctors are picking and choosing who they want to treat and who they don't want to treat.

As far as improving care at nursing homes and hospitals, perhaps nursing schools could give extra credit to nursing students who work as CNAs in their spare time at facilities. Nursing students hopefully have better cleanliness skills than the average CNA, so patients might get better CNA care. The pay at nursing homes and hospitals for CNAs may not be enough to attract nursing students, but perhaps the extra credit would.

Baby Boomers must unite. They are 76 million strong. That's a tremendous number. By the year 2020, it's projected that hospitals will be short 515,000 nurses, exactly the time when most Baby Boomers will be pushing 70 and flooding the system. It's not just a question of being short of nurses, but being short of qualified nurses who'll want to take care of the elderly. A nursing student in my neighborhood recently told me she had no desire to take care of elderly patients, as she said she didn't like the elderly. I wondered if her nursing education taught her that a patient was a patient, regardless of his age.

Staff at nursing homes and hospitals must realize that their job is not only to treat patients with respect, but also their family members with respect. I hope that nursing schools—particularly those with the two-year programs—don't get into quickly cranking out "technicians" to meet the increasing shortage of nurses, but that they turn out graduates who actually become real professionals. When I was a teacher at high school level, I respected both my students and their parents. Professional demeanor, besides actual job skills, is very important.

Doctors need to raise their level of professionalism, too. I remember one internist came to visit my mother in the hospital after her head injury. She seemed to be recovering at this time. Later, she lapsed into a coma. The doctor discussed with me, right in front of my mother, whether she should be resuscitated if she had a heart attack. Later on, the neurologist had no answers as to why my mother mysteriously lapsed into a coma. When I called him at his office with some questions, two days in a row, he told me I was "always bothering" him. Further, the oncologist who came to visit her at a nursing home, a year later, looked at her breast tumor, and right in front of her, said she had cancer. My mother was semi-alert at the time. Could nurses have picked up the bad habits of doctors?

Years before, after my mother's brain cancer surgery, she was having pains in her leg. Earlier that year she had had surgery to repair torn cartilage in her lower leg. I was talking to her orthopedic surgeon, and he said the pains in her leg might signal bone cancer. In reality, she didn't have bone cancer. However, I later found that this was to be typical of doctors' attitudes toward my mother for ten years after her brain cancer. Each time she had a persistent pain somewhere, it must be lung cancer, stomach cancer, or bone cancer, according to the doctors. It turned out to be just a pain, and the doctors were jumping to conclusions. This doesn't help the patient or the family member, both of whom are constantly kept off balance with doctors' alarmist attitudes, before they've checked out anything.

Often, in the medical profession, professionals never seem to get at the heart of the matter. When my mother's third cancer appeared at the nursing home, a lesion on the surface of her breast, her internist and her oncologist, said that despite her bedridden, mentally lethargic state, she should have surgery to remove her tumor. They said that surface tumors eventually ulcerate and smell foul like human waste. They said no caregivers would want to come to take care of her. Well, she died four years later, not of cancer, and her tumor never ulcerated. She died from a recurring bladder infection. Of course, in her weakened state, it's only common sense that had she had cancer surgery, she wouldn't have survived the surgery for more than a week after it. What would have been the point of cutting her up? Just to let her die?

We could have let our mother die four years sooner than she did, by not giving her medication to treat her third cancer. However, we felt there was a lot left of our mother, despite her weakened condition. We felt that you treat what you can treat with a drug—not with surgery or radiation—if you're bedridden.

Doctor-wise, if I had the chance to do things differently, I would have taken my mother, after her brain cancer recovery, to a different internist. I figured out that doctors at medical schools are usually more on top of things than your average doctor in private practice. The alternative is to get a referrel for a good doctor from someone you know who's had bad health problems, or chronic problems that the doctor has successfully taken care of. These bad health problems should be in the same area your loved one has had problems with. For example, I would have taken my mother to an internist who'd treated many patients with neurological problems. Perhaps, I should have even taken her to a geriatrician.

Currently, there are over 50,000 pediatricians in this country, but only about 8,000 geriatricians. As Baby Boomers age, we'll need more geriatricians.

How Society Regards Elders

According to the National Alliance for Caregiving, about 23 million households have at least someone caring for an elderly relative or friend, and about two and one-half million of these caregivers are themselves elderly. Studies have shown that long-term stress on elderly caregivers often causes problems with their immune system. (I was only 33 years old when I became a caregiver and it ended 16 years later.) Elderly caregivers are more prone to heart disease and cancers.

In China, able-bodied elders volunteer to help the frail elderly in their homes. In turn, the government keeps track of their time spent and ensures that they themselves will be taken care of by other volunteers when their time comes.

We need a more humane society, especially for elders. Historically, in this country, as a culture, we haven't revered our elders. You often hear elders speak disparagingly of themselves as "has-beens." Further, we need to hold healthcare people to the same standards we hold our teachers to and other professionals. Neglect shouldn't be tolerated.

When you see Americans spending so much money on their pets and having such an endearing attitude towards their aging pets, you wonder about how you rarely see family members on a regular basis visiting their elders in facilities. I knew a woman who never spent a day as a caregiver for her dying mother who had mutiple sclerosis. Her mother could no longer walk, and was bedridden from it. However, the woman I knew stayed home from work for a few days to care for her dying dog who was paralyzed and needed to be carried outside to urinate. He was a very heavy dog.

Communities in the U.S. can help elders. It would be easy for churches to send volunteer parishioners to homes or nursing homes to sit, read, and chat with individuals, rather than to groups of patients.

Just as a state's Long -Term Care Office sends out ombudsmen to nursing homes, perhaps it could also organize volunteers to go out to nursing homes to read to individual patients and entertain them.

As for hospitals, if your elder is being thrown out prematurely, you have the right to contact the Peer Review Organization in your state to appeal a discharge. You can appeal any loss of Medicare benefits, while your elder is in the hospital. You can find the PRO contact information in the publication, "Your Medicare Handbook," available at your local Social Security Administration Office. Or, to get the toll-free PRO phone number for your state, call the toll-free social security number as listed in your local phonebook.

As we see our elders fail, some of us distance ourselves from them, not just because we don't have the time to deal with them, but we fear aging and becoming like them. However, if we don't advocate for them, we will soon be faced with the same shabby care that was available for them. Some of us Baby Boomers have only 20 years left before we become infirm ourselves. Yesterday, after spending some time working on this book, I saw a person I grew up with that I hadn't seen in 30 years. She was a blond and now has completely gray hair. Although I still have my dark hair, in looking at her, I pondered the measure of my aging in my old friend's face. It was daunting.

Preparing For Our Care

People of the Baby Boomer Generation, are often those who like to micro-manage their lives. We've seen prenuptual agreements, for example. I guess Baby Boomers often attempt to control every aspect of life. Sometimes, one can control how one dies. Oftentimes, not. What if, for example, you had Alzheimer's, and were totally "spaced out," but you could still eat when you were fed? Many people end up in nursing homes like this, and the only way you can avoid it is if you kill yourself before your Alzheimer's becomes advanced. How many people are capable of doing this? When you start to fail, how do you know how long it's going to take you to fail completely, to where you can't function without help? Will you hook yourself up to the exhaust pipe of the car? At what point? The majority of us aren't capable of doing ourselves in, nor should we have to. In an intelligent, advanced society, there should be intelligent options available to us all.

I believe that everyone should have an Advance Directive, whether or not it ends up being useful to them.

Once again, consider an Advance Directive for yourself, especially if you have no children who will care for you or make decisions for you, as is my case. An advance directive document is more than a Living Will. A Living Will expresses your wishes for life-saving treatment. It comes into play only if you have a terminal illness or are in a state of permanent unconsciousness. An Advance Directive guides your healthcare at any time you are unable to communicate even temporarily.

In a crisis, a directive can reduce stress on a loved one. If your directive authorizes one person as the decision-maker, you may avoid family disagreements. One nurse told me: "I have an Advance Directive, so if I'm totally out of it, in a coma, my family won't get cold feet, and not feel that they can't make a decision to terminate my life."

An Advance Directive has different parts. You choose a representative or "health care power of attorney." The person you appoint should be included when creating your directive so he knows your wishes. Since I am presently single, my attorney is my representative.

In filling out the directive, first consider if there are types of disabilities you don't think you could live with. If you needed a respirator, would you want one? If you feel you want to continue eating no matter what, then you don't want a feeding tube if you are unable to eat. In this case, you'd obviously die naturally. However, consider if you'd want a feeding tube if the doctor thought your condition was temporary. Would you want a feeding tube if you had a progressive illness and were in a debilitating state? Consider what your spiritual values are. Unfortunately, you must consider the cost of care. As you can see, there are shades of gray, and you need to consider all sides of the argument.

A good idea is to do what I've done. That is, give your doctor a copy of your Advance Directive, besides giving one to your representative and to a family member.

You can revise this document at any time, but be sure to destroy the old copies. A sample of an Advance Directive is available on the American Medical Association website at www.ama-assn.org.

By 2020, seven million people will be 85 or older, according to the National Institute on Aging.

With Baby Boomers having had fewer children than their parents, and many Baby Boomers having gotten divorced and some subsequently estranged from their children, who will care for you? There are many Baby Boomers who don't have children. Hopefully, Baby Boomers like me will not be a silent generation, but will start a grassroots effort to improve care now, so that when we need it, it will be available.

Many children of Baby Boomers will probably be raising young children and caring for elderly parents at the same time. When you are old and feeble, you may be unaware of your deficits. You may be unappreciative of your adult children caring for you. You may be roaming the house at 3 a.m. because you're confusing nighttime and daytime. Would you want your adult child caring for you under these circumstances? Most of us wouldn't. At the very least, as a society, we need more adult day care services available, so that it's feasible for family caregivers to keep elders at home, if they wish.

None of us want to be dependent on anyone else. We also recognize that facilities and foster homes, and other outside living options are businesses first, even if they classify themselves as being in the healthcare or senior services field. However, as businesses, they must deliver service. We must expect that of them, just as we expect our healthcare insurance to kick in. I go back to my mother's situation in that she was originally told that substantial private R.N. care wasn't available to her in her home. Later, she was told that her health insurance wouldn't cover an occupational therapist to order equipment such as wrist splints. We later found out that this wasn't true in speaking to more healthcare professionals and in harping on the doctor for referrels. For example, splints that were first denied, may be later okayed, if you can prove that by not having them, a physical or medical problem may result. The case of my mother's wrist splints was an example. She wasn't able to move her hands to pick up things, so she wasn't a rehab candidate whereby splints would be useful to keep her wrists from contracting more. However, in reality, she was eligible for splints only because the doctor stated that her fingernails would dig into her palms without the wrist splints, and may, therefore, cause infections.

Just like some things in life, you never get everything you ask for in healthcare the first time you ask. You must persevere. As a society, we must not accept old age and infirmity as a time to just roll over and die, without getting back what we've put into the system all during our lives. We must train ourselves to be wise consumers in healthcare and start demanding care from the system now.

Appendices

This section includes selected organizations and websites offering information about care options for the elderly, and general information and help for families and caregivers.

It also includes a glossary of helpful general healthcare/legal terminology, and abbreviations used by nurses in their charts.

Finally, it includes some recommended books for families with elders.

Appendix A

Selected Organizations/Websites
Offering Information About Care Options

Alzheimer's Association; (www.alz.org); (312) 335-8700; 225 N. Michigan Ave., Ste. 1700, Chicago, IL 60601.
Offers support groups, local chapters, and educational materials on this progressive, degenerative brain disease.

American Association of Retired Persons; (www.aarp.org); 1-888-OUR-AARP; 601 "E" St., NW, Washington, DC 20049.
For persons 50 years of age and older, seeks to improve every aspect of living including health. Especially helpful for its publications. Includes a bi-monthly magazine, a news bulletin published 11 times a year, and all kinds of special resource materials on a range of issues including health, caregiving, and finances for older Americans. Its website also has basic information about grief and loss and online discussion boards.

American Bar Association Commission on Legal Problems of the Elderly; (www.abanet.org); (202) 662-8690; 740 15th St., NW, Washington, DC 20005.
This commission, created in 1979, can give you information about the legal aspects of planning for incapacity.

American Health Care Association; (www.ahca.org); (202) 842-4444; 1201 "L" St., NW, Washington, DC 20005.

Federation of state associations of long-term healthcare facilities. Promotes standards for professionals in long-term healthcare delivery and quality care for patients in a safe environment.

American Society on Aging; (www.asaging.org); 1-800-537-9728; 833 Market St., Ste. 511; San Francisco, CA 94103.
Largest organization of professionals in the field of aging. Serves to enhance the skills and knowledge of those working with elder adults.

Area Agencies on Aging. Phone numbers can usually be found in the local telephone directories under county government listings.

Assisted Living Federation of America; (www.alfa.org.); (703) 691-8100; 11200 Waples Mill Rd., Ste. 150, Fairfax, VA 22030.
For providers of assisted living, state associations of providers, and others interested in the industry. Offers information, for example, on how to query an assisted living facility about its care.

caregiverzone.com; (510) 229-1104.
Referrel services for eldercare. Also offers information on wellness programs, and "work/family balance" for caregivers.

careguide.com—A website that is a good resource for finding out about home health agencies.

carescout.com—A website that provides vacancy information and quality ratings for nursing homes and other facilities. (As with other resources, quality ratings are sometimes misleading for a number of reasons, including the fact that facilities change management often.)

Centers for Disease Control and Prevention; (www.cdc.gov); (404)-639-3311; 1600 Clifton Rd., NE, Atlanta, GA 30333.
Run by the federal government, it offers guidelines for hospitals to follow regarding infection prevention.

Eldercare Locator; (www.aoa.dhhs.gov); 1-800-677-1116.
Financed by the Federal Administration on Aging, it provides information about services for the elderly in your area. Will refer you to appropriate local agencies, helping you find programs for home-delivered meals, transportation, adult day care, senior centers, nursing homes, etc.

elderweb.com—A website that offers links to useful websites.

extendedcare.com—A website that allows users to "talk" with a geriatrician.

Family Caregiver Alliance; (www.caregiver.org); 1-800-445-8106; 180 Montgomery St., Ste. 1100, San Francisco, CA 94104. A non-profit information clearinghouse for caregivers of those with chronic and disabling illnesses. Also offers links to other websites.

Gerontological Society of America; (www.geron.org); (202) 842-1275; 1030 15th St., NW, Ste. 250, Washington, DC 20005.
Comprised of educators, researchers, and practitioners of gerontology who wish to improve the quality of life as one ages.

Hospice Association of America; (www.nahc.org/HAA); (202) 546-4759; 228 Seventh St., SE, Washington, DC 20003.
Home care and hospice services. Works to heighten the

public's visibility of hospice services. Provides a voice for hospice providers. Sponsors and promotes research related to hospice services.

Medicaid; (www.hcfa.gov). Federal government healthcare information for needy elders. For your local office, check your phonebook.

Medicare; (medicare.gov). Federal government healthcare information for senior citizens. Contact your local Social Security Administration Office as listed in your phonebook.

National Academy of Elder Law Attorneys; (www.naela.org); (520) 881-4005; 1604 N. Country Club Rd., Tucson, AZ 85716. Will refer you to an elder law attorney who can help you address legal matters and related healthcare and financial issues. (You can also contact your state's bar association.)

National Adult Day Services Association; (www.nadsa.org); 1-800-558-5301; 722 Grant St., Herndon, VA 20170.
Provides names and locations of adult day care centers in your area. You can even inquire through this association about lobbying legislators and state officials to increase programs in your area.

National Association of Professional Geriatric Care Managers; (www.caremanager.org); (520) 881-8008; 1604 N. Country Club Rd., Tucson, AZ 85716.
Promotes quality services and care for the elderly. Provides referrel service. This association could be helpful, in particular, to family members who live far from their elders for referrals to care managers throughout the country.

National Citizens' Coalition for Nursing Home Reform; (www.nccnhr.org); (202) 332-2275; 1424 16th St., NW, Ste.

202, Washington, DC 20036.
Advocates to raise care standards for people in nursing homes.

National Council on the Aging; (www.ncoa.org); 1-800-424-9046; 300 "D" St., SW, #801, Washington, DC 20024.
National network of organizations improving the health and independence of older persons. Its members include senior centers, adult day care centers, area agencies on aging; senior housing facilities, etc. Its website will also give you information on subsidy options for caring for your elders.

National Family Caregivers Association; (www.nfcacares.org); 1-800-896-3650; 10400 Connecticut Ave., Ste. 500, Kensington, MD 20895.
Founded in 1993, this organization works to meet the needs of family caregivers and improve the caregivers' quality of life. Offers caregiving tips, information, education, and community outreach programs. Advocates for respite assistance for caregivers. This association has published a resource guide on caregivers' associations.

National Institute on Aging; (www.nih.gov/nia); (301) 496-1752; Building 31, Room 5C 27, 31 Center Dr., MSC 2292, Bethesda, MD 20892.
Sponsored by the federal government, the Institute conducts biomedical, social, and behavioral research to increase knowledge of the aging process.

National Patient Safety Foundation; (www.npsf.org); (312) 464-4848; 515 N. State St., Chicago, IL 60610.
Offers brochures and fact sheets for patients that provide guidance on how they and their families can check safety procedures in hospitals. This information is also useful for showing people how to ask questions that might seem rude

or challenging to medical staff. Among them: asking staff members if they've washed their hands to prevent infections or asking nurses if they've double-checked the medication. This foundation believes hospitals have an ethical duty to disclose errors.

People's Medical Society; (www.peoplesmed.org); 1-800-624-8773; PO Box 868, Allentown, PA 18105.
Promotes citizen involvement in the cost, quality, and management of the American healthcare system. Seeks to train and encourage individuals to study local healthcare systems, practitioners, and institutions. Assists individuals in maintaining their personal health.

United Way—Check your phonebook for your local office that can provide you with information about programs for elders in your area.

U.S. Department of Health and Human Services; (www.hhs.gov.); (202) 619-0257; 200 Independence Ave., SW, Washington, DC 20201.
The Department oversees the Health Care Financing Administration, and it provides information on choosing a nursing home. It has pushed to improve staffing at nursing homes and training for aides.

USSearch.com—A website that can check the criminal background of a person. Good for checking out caregivers.

Visiting Nurse Associations of America; (www.vnaa.org); 1-800-426-2547; 99 Summer St., Ste. 1700, Boston, MA 02110. Non-profit home health care agencies.

Volunteers of America; (www.voa.org); 1-800-899-0089; 1660 Duke St., Alexandria, VA, 22314. Provides local human services programs, including day care for elders.

Appendix B

General Healthcare/Legal Terminology

A

advance directive—A document that guides one's healthcare at any time one is unable to communicate, even temporarily.

aspiration—When liquids go down into the lungs, often manifested by breathing difficulties. "Silent aspiration" refers to when someone shows no sign of having aspirated—no coughing, choking, nor difficulty breathing, etc.

assisted living facility—For elders who don't need nursing care, but who need assistance with dressing, bathing, and other daily living skills.

B

bed bath—Comprehensive sponge bath from head to toe.

bedsore—With immobile people, a sore caused by laying down too long in the same position. It is also caused by not being cleaned up regularly after urinating and defecating.

behavior modification—Language used at nursing homes that usually means sedating an elder who is hard to control.

blue pad—Disposable cotton pad that absorbs overflow of urine if diaper leaks.

BM—Bowel movement.

C

catheter— A rubber tube inserted into the body to remove urine from the bladder.

CMA—Certified Medication Aide who is a Certified Nurse's Aide. A CMA is certified to dispense medications at some nursing homes.

CNA—Certified Nurse's Aide or often called a Certified Nursing Assistant.

contractures—A permanent shortening of a muscle, such as an arm bent at the elbow.

D

DNR—A patient who is labeled "Do Not Resuscitate."

DNS—Director of Nursing Services.

drain sponge—Not a sponge, but an absorbent gauze that fits around a tube, such as a feeding tube entryway. The gauze is intended to soak up residue, such as feeding tube formula.

drawsheet— A small sheet or pad used by a caregiver to pull up an immobile patient in bed.

E

edema—Bloating, swelling of skin.

elder law attorney—One who specializes in legal issues for elders and who can answer related healthcare and financial issues. He can also refer one to a geriatric care manager or social worker who can be privately hired to find caregivers.

evening shift—Swing shift at a healthcare facility.

F

feeding tube—A tube that a patient receives through surgery that can deliver liquid sustenance and medication directly to the stomach. This surgery is available to people who have trouble swallowing.

G

geriatric care manager—Someone who helps an elder arrange for care services. He can also help arrange for legal and financial services.

geriatrician—A physician who specializes in caring for geriatrics, that is, elderly patients.

gerontologist—Someone who studies old age.

gravity pole—For a feeding tube patient, the pole is used to hold a feeding tube bag that hangs from it. You can raise the pole higher so the feeding tube formula will drip faster, or lower it, so the formula will drip slower.

H

hoyer lift—A machine that can be pumped manually to lift and transfer an immobile person from her bed to a wheelchair.

I

incontinence—The inability to control natural evacuations.

intermediate care—Nursing home care after a patient leaves the skilled nursing unit of the facility. Intermediate care is self-pay, unlike skilled care that is covered by Medicare and private insurance.

L

living will—A document that details the circumstances under which medical care is to be terminated. Adult children should know if these documents have been prepared and where they are kept.

long-term care insurance—Insurance that covers all long-term care, not just nursing home care.

LPN—A Licensed Practical Nurse. He/she is a nurse who can do everything a registered nurse can do, except an assessment when a patient is admitted to a nursing home.

lubricating jelly—Gel used to insert a suppository.

M

mechanical soft food—Food that can be mashed with a fork, unlike solid food.

moon boots—Cloth booties for a bedridden person that help prevent sores to ankles and feet.

N

nebulizer—A plug-in vaporizing device that makes it easier for a patient with plugged up nasal passages to breathe.

night shift—Graveyard shift at a healthcare facility.

O

occupational therapist—One who treats patients having physical or mental disabilities through specific exercises. Works with a patient on everyday skills such as getting dressed. Also fits a patient for wrist/hand or arm splints.

ombudsman—Volunteer with the government, assigned to a healthcare facility to field complaints of patients and their families. She acts as a liaison with staff to attempt to resolve problems.

orthotist—One who fits a patient for leg splints.

P

palliative care—Comfort care and pain control for a dying patient.

peg tube—A feeding tube that is sutured in and cannot be replaced unless the patient has another surgery.

phlegm—The thick discharge from the nose and throat that accompanies a cold.

physiatrist—A physician specializing in physical medicine, that is, physical therapy.

power of attorney—A document that enables a designated person to act on behalf of someone else in specific transactions. The designated person will have authority to manage the person's finances and make everyday life's decisions for him when he no longer can. It can be limited when it is drawn up and terminated at any time. Regular power of attorney is automatically revoked when the person dies. (Durable medical power of attorney is a document that allows a person to choose someone to make medical decisions on his behalf if he becomes incapacitated.)

pressure sore—See "bedsore."

R

recreational feeding—Feeding a patient with swallowing difficulties on a limited basis, not for nutrition, but for enjoyment.

resident care manager—In a nursing home unit, an R.N. who does paperwork and develops a care plan for each patient.

residential care facility—A facility with limited residents who need custodial care.

restorative aid—Range of motion exercises.

restorative aide—A certified nurse's aide who performs range of motion exercises.

S

skilled nursing unit— Hospital or nursing home care, covered by Medicare and Medicaid benefits.

speech therapist—One who specializes in either evaluating and rehabilitating patients with communication problems or swallowing difficulties.

splints—Braces that help retard contractures in arms, wrists, fingers, and legs, and help retard foot drop and twisting of the ankles.

sponge bath—In lieu of using a bathtub, the patient is cleaned with damp soapy washcloths while in bed, then rinsed with damp washcloths, and dried with a hand towel.

stoma—The tissue around the entry passage for the feeding tube. The tissue can become enlarged and bleed if it is irritated by carelessly pulling on the tube.

suctioning—Performed by using a suction pump to draw mucous upward from the throat.

T

thickened juices—For patients with swallowing difficulties, these can be purchased at a medical supply store in a large plastic bottle or in individual snack size cartons. They have corn starch consistency. One can also buy thickening powder at the medical supply store to thicken juices and even other foods.

toothette—A miniature sponge on a stick that can be used instead of a toothbrush to swab the mouth. Used by patients who have trouble swallowing.

transfer belt—An elastic wasteband placed around a weak patient. It is used to help lift and balance him, when transferring him from his bed to his wheelchair, or when helping him ambulate.

tray table—Used in a hospital or nursing home, a table on wheels that slides over the bed to hold a tray of food or a plastic tub for a sponge bath.

V

ventilator—Respirator.

Common Abbreviations Used By Nurses

The following are helpful to know if you read your elder's chart, and you should, from time to time:

abd—abdomen
a.c.—before meals
ADL—activities of daily living
ad lib—as desired
Adm—admitted or admission
amb—ambulatory
amt—amount
approx—approximately

b.i.d.— twice a day
BP—blood pressure
BRP—bathroom privileges

C-centigrade
Ca—cancer
Cath—catheter
CBR—complete bedrest
c/o—complains of (refers to patient stating health problems)
CPR—cardiopulmonary resuscitation
CVA—cerebrovascular accident (stroke)

dc or d/c—discontinue
drsg—dressing
Dx—diagnosis

F—Fahrenheit
fld—fluid

GI—gastrointestinal

H2O-water
H.S. or h.s.—hour of sleep
ht-height

in—inch
IV—intravenous

L-liter
liq—liquid
lt—left

meds—medications
mid noc—midnight
min—minute

neg—negative
nil—none
no—number
noc—night
NPO—nothing by mouth

O2—oxygen
OT—occupational therapy

p.c.—after meals
per—by, through
p.o.—by mouth
prep—preparation
p.r.n.—when necessary
Pt—patient
PT—physical therapy

q—every
q.d.—every day
q.h.—every hour
q2h, q3h, etc.—every 2 hours, every 3 hours, etc.

q.h.s.—every night at bedtime
q.i.d.—four times a day
q.o.d.—every other day

R—rectal temperature
ROM—range of motion

stat—immediately
Surg—surgery

t.i.d.—three times a day
TPR—temperature, pulse, and respiration

VS—vital signs (temperature, pulse, blood pressure)

w/c— wheelchair
wt—weight

Appendix C

Recommended Reading

Brain Repair, by Donald G. Stein, Oxford University Press, New York: 1995.
A comprehensive book on brain injury. It also illustrates that the beliefs and attitudes of caregivers and medical staff influence whether or not the patient makes a recovery of any kind.

How To Get Out of The Hospital Alive: A Guide to Patient Power, by Sheldon P. Blau and Elaine Fantle Shimberg, MacMillan, New York: 1997.
Discloses the most common medical errors and how to avoid them, and provides practical measures on how to become an informed participant in one's treatment. (Note: This gives families ideas that they can apply to nursing homes, besides intermittent hospital stays of their elders.)

My Turn to Care, by Marlene Bagnull, Thomas Nelson Publishers, Nashville, TN: 1994.
Offers comfort to caregivers. Shares the struggles and joys of more than 100 individuals who care for their aging parents.

Recalled to Life: The Story of a Coma, by Esther Goshen-Gottstein, Yale University Press, New Haven, CT: 1990.
Clinical psychologist Goshen-Gottstein's husband fell into a coma and wasn't expected to recover. Almost four months

later, he emerged and eventually made an almost complete recovery. The rights and ethics of coma patients are
included in this account of her husband's struggles.

Index

Order Form

Please send me ____ copy(ies) of **Everything You Need to Know About Nursing Homes:** The Family's Comprehensive Guide to Either Working With The Institution Or Finding Care Alternatives.($19.95 each, softcover).

Shipping & Handling by USPS Book Rate for one book is $3. (First Class is $5 per book). Please inquire about multiple orders and foreign orders.

Name:
Address:
City/State/ZIP:
Phone: (   ) _____

My check, payable to Civetta Press, in the amount of $____ is enclosed.

Please mail to: Civetta Press, PO Box 1043, Portland, OR 97207-1043, USA.
Our phone is: (503) 228-6649.

Your satisfaction is guaranteed.

Among other bestselling titles we have in stock, are:
You Can Be A Columnist
Beginners' Guide to Writing & Selling Quality Features
The Analogy Book of Related Words
Your Original Personal Ad
Big Ideas for Small Service Businesses

Ask for our catalogue! These books are also available at special quantity discounts for bulk purchases. For details, contact Alice Andresen, Special Sales Dept., Civetta Press.

SAN: 200-3171